Family Health Care

Debra P. Hymovich

Associate Professor
School of Nursing
University of Rochester

Martha Underwood Barnard

Assistant Professor
University of Kansas Medical Center

McGraw-Hill Book Company

A Blakiston Publication

New York   St. Louis   San Francisco   Düsseldorf   Johannesburg
Kuala Lumpur   London   Mexico   Montreal   New Delhi
Panama   Rio de Janeiro   Singapore   Sydney   Toronto

Family Health Care

567890KPKP798765

This book was set in Times Roman by Rocappi, Inc. The editors were Cathy Dilworth and Sally Mobley; and the production supervisor was Sally Ellyson. The drawings were done by Eric G. Hieber. The printer and binder was Kingsport Press, Inc.

The family symbol on the cover of this book has been adopted by the Society of Teachers of Family Medicine and several graduate training programs in family medicine. It was designed by Mrs. Alexander Styne of Miami in 1965.

Library of Congress Cataloging in Publication Data

Hymovich, Debra P
    Family health care.

    Includes bibliographies.
    1. Nurses and nursing.   2. Family medicine.
    I. Barnard, Martha Underwood, joint author.
II. Title. [DNLM: 1. Family.   2. Public health
    nursing. WY 108 H996f 1973]
RT61.H93   362.1'4   72-12743
                           ISBN 0-07-031656-2

To our families

Contents

List of Contributors

Martha Underwood Barnard, R.N., B.S.N., M.N.
Assistant Professor
Departments of Human Ecology and Nursing Education
University of Kansas Medical Center
Kansas City, Kansas

Beverly Henry Bowns, R.N., Dr. P.H.
Associate Professor and Chairman
Community Health Nursing
Department of Community Health
Vanderbilt University School of Nursing
Nashville, Tennessee

Carolyn Brose, R.N., B.S.N., M.S.
Assistant Professor
Department of Nursing
University of Kansas Medical Center
Kansas City, Kansas

Maxine Cadena
Director
Associate Degree Nursing
El Paso Community College
El Paso, Texas

Lynn P. Carmichael, M.D.
Director
Division of Family Medicine
University of Miami School of Medicine
Miami, Florida

Mary Reardon Castles, Ph.D.
Assistant Professor
School of Nursing and Allied Health Professions
Department of Nursing
St. Louis University
St. Louis, Missouri

Edward R. Christophersen, B.A., M.A., Ph.D.
Assistant Professor
Department of Human Development
University of Kansas
Lawrence, Kansas

Barbara J. Clancy, R.N., B.S.N., M.S.N.
Assistant Professor
Department of Nursing Education
University of Kansas Medical Center
Kansas City, Kansas

Rene Clark Davis, R.N., B.S.N., M.N.
Director of Health Occupation Education
Lincoln Center for the Human and Mechanical Arts
Gainesville, Florida

Loretta C. Ford
Dean and Director of Nursing
School of Nursing
University of Rochester
Rochester, New York

Lucille D. Gress
Assistant Professor
Department of Nursing Education
University of Kansas Medical Center
Kansas City, Kansas

Katherine Gustin, M.S.W.
Chief Social Worker
Department of Pediatrics
University of Kansas Medical Center
Kansas City, Kansas

Jo-Eileen Gyulay, R.N., B.S.N., M.S.
Pediatric Clinician
Department of Nursing Service
University of Kansas Medical Center
Kansas City, Kansas

Gerald Handel, Ph.D.
Department of Sociology
The City College
City University of New York
New York, New York

Debra P. Hymovich, R.N., Ph.D.
Associate Professor of Nursing
School of Nursing
University of Rochester
Rochester, New York

Rosemary Kilker, R.N., B.S.N., M.S.
Associate Professor
Department of Nursing Education
University of Kansas Medical Center
Kansas City, Kansas

Joan T. Large, Ed.D.
Associate Professor in Nursing
Health Science Center
College of Allied Health Professions
Temple University Department of Nursing
Philadelphia, Pennsylvania

Susan Nelson McCabe, R.N., B.S.N., M.N.
Lecturer
Georgetown University
Washington, D.C.

Jed B. Maebius, Jr., L.L.B., L.L.M.
Attorney
Maebius and Duncan, Attorneys at Law
San Antonio, Texas

Nancy K. Maebius, R.N., B.S.N., M.S.N.
Doctoral Student
University of Texas
Austin, Texas

Miriam T. Manisoff
Director
Professional Education
Planned Parenthood—World Population
New York, New York

Margaret Shandor Miles
Assistant Professor
Department of Nursing Education
University of Kansas Medical Center
Kansas City, Kansas

Martha L. Mitchell, R.N., M.S.N.
Assistant Professor
School of Nursing
University of Wisconsin
Madison, Wisconsin

Ora Rios Prattes
Nurse Clinician
Bexar County Hospital
San Antonio, Texas

Jean L. Sparber, M.S., A.C.S.W. (deceased)
Medical Social Worker
Children's Hospital
Morristown, New Jersey

Ruth F. Stewart, R.N., M.S.
Associate Professor
The University of Texas
School of Nursing at San Antonio
San Antonio, Texas

Marvin B. Sussman, Ph.D.
Chairman
Department of Sociology
Case Western Reserve University
Cleveland, Ohio

Carol Taylor
Professor
Department of Anthropology
University of Florida
Gainesville, Florida

Mary J. Tudor, R.N., B.S.N.
Candidate for Master's Degree in Nursing
School of Nursing
University of Washington
Seattle, Washington

Michael A. Viren
Candidate for Ph.D. in Economics
University of California, Santa Barbara
Instructor
Department of Human Ecology
University of Kansas Medical Center
Kansas City, Kansas

Betty L. Wilkerson, R.N., B.S.N., M.A.
Assistant Professor
Department of Nursing Education
University of Kansas Medical Center
Kansas City, Kansas

Lorraine Wolf, B.S.N., M.A.
Assistant Professor
Department of Nursing Education
University of Kansas Medical Center
Kansas City, Kansas

Jean A. Yokes, R.N., M.S.N.
Associate Director of Nursing
Bistate Regional Medical Program
St. Louis, Missouri

Raeone S. Zelle, R.N., B.S., M.N.
Nursing Consultant
Alta California Regional Center
Sacramento, California

Preface

Professional personnel concerned with today's health delivery systems are seeking improved methods of providing health care to the masses while attempting to keep this care personal and individualized. Nursing plays a key role in delivering this individualized health care. Nurses have an advantage in developing and utilizing unique methods of delivering health care because they are with individuals and their families the great majority of time in all health care settings. One unique method being developed for improved health services is the emphasis on the entire family unit rather than on just one individual member.

We believe, as nurses, educators, and citizens, that this trend to emphasize the entire family unit is a realistic and reasonable one. It is one which emphasizes the dignity and personality of the family as well as the dignity and personality of the individual. It is a realistic approach to helping people to help themselves because they can avail themselves of the strengths of their nuclear, extended, or communal family. Therefore, it seems only fitting that a book should be compiled to bring together in a single volume selected multidisciplinary references which are applicable to the nursing of members of family units.

Part One of this book presents a variety of considerations which can be applied in planning the delivery of health care. We believe it is important for all members of the health team to be aware of other theories and experiences when working with families. This awareness can make it possible to use knowledge from specific disciplines where it is most appropriate in order to deliver optimum health care.

Part Two discusses the expanding and contracting family. It is time for all health team members to be aware of the normal needs of families at different stages of their development. Only when the normal is known and understood can delivery of care be directed toward health maintenance and health promotion.

Part Three illustrates a variety of crisis events that families may encounter during their life span. This is not to say that these are the only critical situations families experience. Rather they represent a variety of critical events from which commonalities can be identified and applied in other family crisis situations.

It is imperative that nurses become informed, and inform others, of how nursing can be practiced by considering the family unit. We have, therefore, compiled original contributions from nurses working with family units, and from individuals in professions from which nurses must obtain basic knowledge related to families.

We do not pretend to give you all the concepts and theories related to working with the family. We want you, whether students or practicing health team members, to use this material as a basis for application in your individual health care situations and as a stimulus for ideas related to new and effective roles for delivering health care to families.

Debra P. Hymovich
Martha Underwood Barnard

Acknowledgments

The development of a book such as this can occur only with the cooperation and encouragement of family, friends, and colleagues. We would like to acknowledge the support and assistance of those who made this book possible.

The authors are especially grateful to both of their faculties, who made many important suggestions. Special thanks go to Dr. Margretta Styles, Dean of The University of Texas School of Nursing at San Antonio, and to Dr. Martha Pitel, former chairman of the University of Kansas Department of Nursing Education. They gave us the freedom in our professional environments that allowed the creation of ideas for this book. Thanks also go to those nurses, physicians, and members of other disciplines who contributed so much of their time and effort to writing the necessary chapters for this manuscript.

We would also like to acknowledge those members of the health team who advised us during the preparation of this publication. Special thanks go to: Edward Defoe, M.D., Chairman of the Department of Human Ecology,

University of Kansas School of Medicine; Margery Duffey, Ed.D., Chairman of the Graduate School, Department of Nursing Education, University of Kansas School of Medicine; Loretta Ford, Ph.D., Chairman of the Department of Community Health Nursing, University of Colorado; Kermit Krantz, M.D., Chairman of the Department of Obstetrics and Gynecology, University of Kansas School of Medicine; Jerome Lysaught, Ed.D., Program Director of the National Commission for the Study of Nursing and Nursing Education, Rochester, New York; Susan N. McCabe, R.N., M.N., lecturer, Department of Nursing, Georgetown University; Shirley Martin, Ph.D., Dean of the School of Nursing, Florida State University; Herbert Miller, M.D., Chairman of the Department of Pediatrics, University of Kansas School of Medicine; Juanita Murphy, Ph.D., Dean of the School of Nursing, Arizona State University; and Patricia Jane Phillips, R.N., M.N., Clinician, School of Nursing, Vanderbilt University.

We would also like to express our appreciation to the students who offered their suggestions for this book. This type of cooperation between faculty and students narrows the communication gap and serves to make the content more relevant.

We would like to thank the many authors and publishers who have given permission to use their data and publications. It is this type of cooperation that will make it possible to unite the efforts of a variety of individuals to share their knowledge in order to strive for quality care for many families.

We are especially grateful to Jan Brown, Anne Hammons, Heather Taylor, Wanda Smith, Beverly Warren, Mary Kovac, and Arlien Mann for their secretarial assistance. They helped us meet our deadlines.

We would also like to thank the McGraw-Hill Book Company for making this book possible, and especially Joseph Brehm and Cathy Dilworth for their cooperation.

Our warmest and sincerest appreciation goes to Howard Barnard for his kindness and patience during the development of this book.

Debra P. Hymovich
Martha Underwood Barnard

Part One

The Family: General Considerations

This section presents a variety of considerations which can be applied in planning the delivery of health care to families. It is important for all members of the health team to be aware of other theories and experiences when working with families, and this awareness can make it possible to use knowledge from specific disciplines where it is most appropriate in order to deliver optimum health care.

Part One discusses the development and meaning of family nursing and the role of the family nurse clinician. The sociological, legal, and economic aspects of family life as they relate to health care are examined. Because of the wide range of cultural backgrounds and life-styles that the nurse will likely encounter in her professional role, the last three chapters in Part One are devoted to an examination of the nurse's response to cultural differences. The Mexican-American family and the low-income family were selected, as examples, to illustrate the way that these cultural differences may become barriers to the delivery of effective health care.

1

Chapter 1

The Development of Family Nursing

Loretta C. Ford

Tracing the development of family nursing in the emergence of professional nursing preparation and practice is a frustrating endeavor. Factors and forces within the profession, in related disciplines, and in the context of social evolution make the identification and analysis complex and multidimensional. Time and relationships of movements and events overlap, lack sequential evolvement, and, for all intents and purposes, appear unplanned. In one sense, family nursing has grown in response to the zephyrs and hurricanes of change within nursing as well as in external forces.

In another sense, the elusive quality of "becoming" rather than "being" characterizes the state of the art and science of family nursing today. To capture a composite picture of this growth, four major dimensions are explored: advances in nursing and nursing education; contributions of professional organizations; theory development in nursing and related disciplines; and changes in needs, demands, and aspirations of society. A preliminary review of the history of nursing education and practice serves as a point of departure.

3

The concept of family nursing has always been with us in nursing. Some arenas of practice, notably public health nursing, have claimed more interest, expertise, opportunities, and responsibilities for family care than others in nursing practice. Delivering service in the patient's home fostered the nurse's insights about the family as a resource in the maintenance or disruption of health and also afforded opportunities to view holistically the problems and progress of patients and families.

Public health nursing in its initial stages began by providing care to the sick poor; it later emerged as a force in augmenting preventive health services and family care. As society grew and specialized by grouping people in schools, industries, and communities, specialized nursing practice evolved. Public health nurses struggled with the problems of specialization and finally laid claim to a practice known as *generalized nursing services*, or *family nursing*. Essentially it meant nursing care of the sick and health counseling and teaching for all members of the family under the sponsorship of governmental or voluntary health agencies. Some agency programs, of course, while directing their efforts toward specific disease eradication or other specialized goals, used family service as their basic philosophical orientation. Notable among these was the tuberculosis control program sponsored by the federal government in the forties.

Early in the growth of public health nursing practice, nurses recognized that their preparation in hospital schools was inadequate to serve families. Demands for advanced preparation in institutions of higher education were met first in 1910 by Columbia University. The movement of nursing education programs into collegiate settings began. Braving the resistance to change, many courageous nursing leaders introduced concepts of family care in the basic nursing curricula (Committee on Education, 1919; Committee on Grading, 1934; Report of the Committee, 1923).

Admittedly, the theoretical orientations often were lacking; however, the operational aspects which gave recognition to the family as a unit of service and study were identified as principles. No effort will be made to recount this very early history verbatim. It exists and is well documented in the literature of the field (Gardner, 1936; National Association for Public Health Nursing, 1939).

It suffices to say that the history of public health nursing practice is replete with undulating curves of crises and plateaus reflecting the changes and stresses in society. Unfortunately, despite these early advantages to promote family nursing care, often agency policies and procedures controlled nursing practice, unconsciously undermining the basic stated philosophy of family care. Referral policies, established daytime hours of duty, health insurance coverage limitations, reimbursement policies from government sources, mechanized recording, and the demands for certain types of disease-identification statistics all required operationalizing the nursing service given by public health nurses to an individually oriented care system. As Freeman points out, some record systems organized for the collation, storage, and retrieval of data were devised for care of an individual, not a family unit (1967).

Other factors mitigated against delivering family nursing care. Nurses themselves played a large part in giving lip service to family care concepts and in actuality practiced nursing as they had basically learned it in hospital settings. Nursing care plans frequently revealed that service was rendered to individual patients, rather than to the family. Though the National Organization for Public Health Nursing enunciated a cardinal principle in 1932 that identified the family as the basic unit of service, as Freeman points out, "practice does not always follow precept" (1970, p. 109). Influxes into the public health nursing field of ill-prepared nurses at certain times in history, such as in pre- and post-World Wars I and II, undoubtedly accounted for the widening gap between promise and performance in the delivery of family care.

Following World War II, changes in undergraduate and graduate collegiate nursing education influenced positively the development of family nursing. Content from the social sciences was explored and selected for its applicability to nursing curricula. Introductory courses in sociology and advanced courses on the study of the family as a basic social group and an institution in society were included in many programs. In special certificate programs, public health nursing courses offered extended study of the family and the community.

As the scope and nature of nursing came under scrutiny by nursing educators, an intensive examination of educational processes was begun. Collegiate schools introduced a new field teaching pattern which made public health nursing faculty members primarily responsible for the student's education during clinical experiences in the community. When the National League for Nursing Accrediting Service required that public health nursing courses be integrated into all generic baccalaureate educational programs by 1963, emphasis on the family in patient care became an integral component of every professional nurse's education. All faculties were required to have basic public health nursing preparation. Nursing itself was fast being professionalized. As nurses began to formulate basic conceptualizations about nursing, there was movement away from the medical model, disease-oriented, largely technical programs. Many nursing school faculties engaged in all-out efforts to create curricula based on a philosophy and goals commensurate with nursing's commitment to care for people. Debates about nursing's goals and identification of the client were heard in national and local arenas. The search for the body of nursing knowledge began.

The emphasis on research, the recognition of the care concept as a philosophical commitment, the efforts to redirect nursing potential to clinical rather than managerial responsibilities in the health care system, the desire for autonomy in clinical practice, and the demands for rigorous scientific and theoretical bases for changing and developing nursing practice all contributed to the growth of an increasingly sophisticated knowledgeable group of professionals.

Conceptual frameworks were created. Nursing was introduced as an integrated subject matter; clinical resources were expanded; and the student's clinical study was balanced with general education courses. Some programs quickly launched into extensive use of ambulatory care settings for learning experiences. Preventive and promotional aspects of nursing and health care were emphasized. As new basic curricula evolved, advanced preparation for leaders in nursing received increasing attention. Certainly, psychiatric nursing with its early financial support from the federal Mental Health Act led the field in the expansion of graduate programs and in the preparation of clinicians (Peplau, 1959). The patterns of operation for the distribution of those original grant funds, the mid-fifties National Institutes of Health study on families of schizophrenics, the increasing interest and research in family therapy in psychiatry, the federal government's later commitment to community mental health programs influenced greatly the contributions that psychiatric nurses have made and are making to the growth of family nursing as a field of study (Joint Commission on Mental Illness and Health, 1961).

Psychiatric nurses entered the community from a relatively stagnant position in hospital care to find the dynamic, exciting world of families and the community ready and willing for their specialized psychotherapeutic skills. Early hospital discharge of the mentally ill forced public health nurses to examine their abilities to cope with family problems in this relocation effort and seek consultation from psychiatric nurse clinicians and others in the mental health field. Emphasis on health counseling of the family group, team delivery of mental health care, and the reduction of the mystique of psychiatric diagnosis to behaviorally describable terms all added appreciably to the development of understanding among nurses and helped immeasurably toward working constructively with families.

Other nursing specialists, notably those in maternal and child care, have demonstrated extended interest in family care, focusing initially on the mother-child dyad and later on parenting. Historically, midwifery used a family-centered approach, particularly in home delivery services when family resources were explored and activated in preparation for care of the mother and newborn in the home setting. Leading the way for parents' classes, nurses in such well-known agencies as the Maternity Center Association of New York and the Child Study Association in association with the Children's Bureau also promoted the development, over time, of nursing care of the family (Auerbach and Taylor, 1960; Corbin, 1960).

Philosophically, the uniqueness of this approach in group education was to meet expressed needs and concerns of parents through the nurse's group leadership role, and not through a preplanned course of instruction.

Probably the decision to prepare nurse clinicians at the graduate level was a major step in redirecting the educational endeavors of the profession. Certainly, professional organizations played a major part in this, and their influence in the development of family nursing can be traced throughout history.

Early, the National Organization for Public Health Nursing championed the cause of family nursing practice; later the National League for Nursing assumed leadership through its community commitments and its influence in nursing education. Only a few specific details can be mentioned here. The NLN's Committee on Perspectives began agitating for expanding nursing's role and serving families and communities through improved patterns of health care delivery (National League for Nursing, 1967). Changes in the National League for Nursing accreditation criteria also played a part in emphasizing care of the family and the community. Efforts of the 1967 Records Committee NLN-PHS committee are also worthy of mention (National League for Nursing, 1970). The product of their labors, the family record system, focused on assessment and intervention using the locus of the family. The American Nurses' Association also gave direction for nursing practice and nursing education. The *Position Paper* (1965) was followed by a *Statement on Graduate Education in Nursing* by the ANA's Commission on Nursing Education (1969). The latter helped identify as the major purpose of graduate programs the preparation of clinical specialists for leadership responsibilities. The commission's charge to the profession was to advance the science of nursing through research. The ANA organizational restructuring which provided for Divisions on Practice, a Congress for Nursing Practice, and an Academy of Nursing called national attention to a core value in nursing—the direct care of people. Statements on the standards of practice will be forthcoming from the Congress for Nursing Practice as charged by the ANA board of directors.

In 1967, the following definition was approved by the Division on Community Health Nursing Practice:

Community Health Nursing Practice is a field of nursing practice for which there exists a body of knowledge and related skills which is applied in meeting the health needs of communities and of individuals and families in their normal environment such as the home, the school, and the place of work. It is an area of practice which lies primarily outside the therapeutic institution (ANA, 1967).

Other divisions struggled with definitions, some of which included family concern. Attempts to prevent duplication and overlapping now are in progress with the eventual goal of establishing standards of nursing care. In addition to the American Nurses' Association's and the National League for Nursing's activities, the Western Council for Higher Education for Nursing's actions deserve recognition. In 1958 the graduate seminar of the Western Council on Higher Education for Nursing (WCHEN) of the Western Interstate Commission on Higher Education published *Guidelines for Developing Master's Degree Programs in the West* (1958). These guidelines publicly announced the belief of Western deans and some graduate faculty that clinical nursing should be an integral part of graduate education in nursing. Further the graduate seminar sought action. It applied for and was granted project funds from the United States Public Health Service for graduate faculty in Western schools to clarify and delineate clinical content appropriate to the four major nursing areas: maternal and child nursing; psychiatric nursing; medical-surgical nursing; and public health nursing, later called community health nursing. Reports on this project were published in 1967 (*Defining Clinical Content*, 1967). The impact of these reports on the total nursing community has never been researched. However, Western faculty members involved in the years of collaborative effort attest to the great insights they gained from this rare learning experience. The Public Health Nursing Section of the American Public Health Association, initially through a special joint ad hoc committee, with the American Nurses' Association formulated a statement on the nursing specialist in public health nursing (Public Health Nursing Specialist, 1967). This statement emphasized expertise in family and community nursing practice.

Probably no force has been so potent or recent as that provided by theorists and researchers in the social and behavioral sciences. In describing the development of the family as a field of study, Christensen identifies four time spans and phases: (1) preresearch—activities until the midnineteenth century; (2) social Darwinism—from end of preresearch period to the twentieth century's beginning; (3) emerging science—the first fifty years of the twentieth century; and (4) systematic theory building—from 1950 to the present and into the future (1964). Obvious strides in theory building were made in the sixties. Efforts to theorize and conduct research about families as a social phenomenon brought together many disciplines, and, to a great extent, encouraged cooperation and collaboration in the study of this complex social entity—the family. These multidisciplinary contributions derived from collaborative studies of the family have greatly motivated many teachers and scholars of nursing to seek advanced preparation and conduct research about families.

Identification and categorization of conceptual frameworks by Hill and Hansen (1960) afforded the field of family study a tremendous growth spurt. They also served to attract community health nurses whose long-standing interest in the family served as a primary motivator. Christensen's 1964 *Handbook of Marriage and the Family* provided a comprehensive overview of the field of family study and brought together many eminent authors and researchers. In a compilation of conceptual frameworks for family analysis, Nye and Berardo presented eleven frameworks in an effort to advance theory building by introducing "orderliness into research processes and findings" (1966, p. 6). Many nursing teachers in graduate programs, particularly in community health nursing, found these published works on family helpful resources for the newly organized clinical nursing courses. Some students used the conceptual frameworks for the development of assessment tools and for testing nursing intervention techniques. Clinical studies in nursing evolved from the theories and research of these behavioral scientists—particularly in the sixties.

Recently, as the decade ended, historical perspectives and future projections were in order. The *Journal of Marriage and the Family* gave public recognition of this point in history by publishing decade reviews in three parts. In one of these reviews, a comprehensive and astutely analytical article by Broderick traces a decade of development of family theory (1971).

Essentially the development of family theory in the sixties advanced the field of family nursing appreciably from a relatively static, philosophical concept to a dynamic, operational testing ground. Social scientists' contributions to systematic theory building have had a great influence in altering circumstances, identifying conceptual frameworks for testing and analysis, and providing direction and substance to the field. Emphasis on scientific approaches through research about family life has encouraged scholars in nursing to view these aspects of family nursing. Though few erudite studies have been published to date, current explorations offer much potential.

Perhaps most significantly, nursing is joining with other disciplines from related fields whose basic interests and competencies in the family may someday ensure team approaches in family care, in multidisciplinary educational programs, and in research. In projecting future directions, Broderick (1971, p. 153) suggests three new strategies for future research: (1) systematic theory building which would in Hill's suggestion provide an organized research effort in "systematically abstracting general principles from empirical generalizations"; (2) multiple perspective strategies which promote the integration of specific social processes related to family life using the established conceptual frameworks; and (3) modern systems analysis which uses complex, simulated computer programming for cognitive mapping and information networks.

This latter strategy requires extended periods of time for data collection and skilled analysis. The continuity of care responsibilities and the new emerging community and statewide health information systems which Glasser (1971) describes in a recent article may make modern systems analysis particularly fruitful for research in family nursing.

Efforts in theory construction in nursing are recorded by King in her publication, *Toward a Theory for Nursing* (1971). The contributions of Rogers, Quint, Brown, Gunther, Orlando, Abdellah, McCain, and others, while not specifically directed toward family nursing, deserve recognition for lending force and direction to the total field of nursing (King, 1971). Within their focus on nursing practice, one finds concepts and constructs particularly applicable to family nursing.

But the growth of family nursing as a field of study and practice in large measure is dependent upon powerful, dynamic, societal forces. The expanding knowledge base about man and technology, the evolving philosophies of equality and humanism, the changing value system, the concern for population growth and the environment all have their impact. One of the most remarkable influences today is the demand to activate the long-enunciated democratic philosophical concept of equality for all—including health care. The implications of this are not only for the development of quality health services but also for health care to be comprehensive and primarily oriented toward the promotion of health and the prevention of disease. Many health service organizations today are restating their goals in terms of high-level wellness, which Dunn (1961, p. 3) defines as:

> An integrated method of functioning which is oriented toward maximizing the potential of which the individual is capable within the environment where he is functioning.

Dunn applies his concept to individuals, families, and communities in an ecological framework. Though the terms *health, wellness,* and *illness* are difficult to define, often highly subjective and culturally determined, and impossible to measure precisely, society is beginning to recognize positive health as a value, a goal, and a right. Society's demands, needs, and aspirations are making rapid changes in all health arenas—including nursing practice and educational programs. Tired of fragmentation in service, high costs, barriers, and the inertia and unresponsiveness of the health care system consumers are taking action.

With this powerful movement in society, health professionals find themselves in the center of a revolution in the health care system. One such outcome of consumer input affecting family care is the emerging neighborhood health center phenomenon, encouraged and supported by the Economic Opportunity Act of 1964 (Curry, 1971).

Efforts to make health care accessible, adequate, available, and acceptable to deprived populations required ecological and creative approaches. It meant serving families in their neighborhoods, using patterns of health care delivery which were not conducive to the highly specialized, infinitely technical, and controlled professional practice arenas. Health care in these centers tends to be holistic, humanized, and informal. Cutting the red tape rituals of the formalized health care system became necessary if groups of deprived people were to be brought into the mainstream of our society through the health care system. Health then becomes a mechanism for social progress as well as a social goal and a right. Individual rights extend to family and community rights—giving the consumer of health care decision-making power. Consumers of health services assume major responsibility in planning, developing, and managing their own health centers. Health professionals become learners and followers in certain aspects of the neighborhood health programs.

From the consumer groups, the indigenous family health worker came into existence. Functioning as case finder, interpreter, and liaison personnel between the consumers and providers of care, the family health worker introduced a new element in health care delivery patterns. Articulating roles for the team delivery of care became a necessity—and the transition was not always smooth and efficient. Nor is the concept of neighborhood health centers totally new. Rosen's historical review documents the rise and fall of early neighborhood health centers (1971). The need for a national health policy is glaringly apparent throughout history.

Only recently, a national health policy directed toward developing a comprehensive health strategy for health maintenance was announced. This strategy employs health maintenance organizations and area health education centers (U.S. Department of Health, Education, and Welfare, 1971). The mechanism of family health insurance plans using the public and private sectors is proposed to provide competitive, capitalistic, and pluralistic components of the nation's political economy. This is the new health care system look for the 1970s. Will nursing, and more particularly, the family nursing proponents be ready? Perhaps.

In the late sixties, society's needs and demands for primary care fostered the development of new health workers. Now family nurse practitioner programs are becoming increasingly visible ("Editorial," 1971). Their first appearance is recorded at the annual meeting of the American Public Health Association in October 1964 when Dr. Duncan E. Reid of the Harvard Medical School introduced his concept of a family nurse practitioner. Primarily Reid's practitioner would provide the major portion of health care for normal expectant mothers and for newborn care in satellite community health clinics. In discussing Dr. Reid's proposal, Wiedenbach (1965) astutely analyzes some of its shortcomings and adds the professional nursing perspective, promoting comprehensive maternal and child care through advanced preparation for collaborative physician-nurse relationships in practice. Just prior to this, Siegel et al. (1965) had reported successful work in expanding the role of the nurse in well child care in California (Ford and Silver, 1967).

By this time, national concern for the crisis in health care, and more particularly, the horrendous problems of preparation and utilization of the country's health manpower began to be heard in medical circles. Physicians and others realized that doctors were not meeting total health care needs of people; indeed they should not and could not be expected to do this. The dwindling supply of general medical practitioners, the lack of responsiveness of the health care system to meet people's needs, the health manpower crisis, and the insistent demands of society for quality and comprehensive health care all contributed to experimenting with new roles for nurses and other health personnel. Siegel's work was followed by other projects which were designed to tap nursing's potential for expansion. The Pediatric Nurse Practitioner Project at the University of Colorado and the studies at Montefiore, Massachusetts General, and the University of Kansas Medical Center are excellent demonstrations of the time and directions which pioneered nursing's future (Ford and Silver, 1967; Ford et al., 1966; Stoeckle, 1963; Lewis and Resnik, 1967). All these projects developed a clinically oriented, independent nursing role with collaborative, interdependent functioning with physicians in the ambulatory health care systems.

Although some of this effort was made to relieve the physician of his heavy workload, this pressure forced a new look at current, available resources and some cooperative arrangements on the part of health professionals to work together for a common goal—to provide quality health care to people. Further, it encouraged nurses to take a hard look at their role and its articulation with fellow team members.

The advent of the expanded role of the nurse for specific age groups and conditions was a phasing-in of the current interest and direction for the development in the late sixties of a *family nurse practitioner*. There are as many definitions of this term as there are programs, projects, and interested people.

Conant (1970-1971, p. 5) describes one such project and illuminates the model with the following framework:

> The family nurse practitioner is a practitioner who is prepared to make independent judgments and to assume principal responsibility for primary health care of individuals and families in organized services. She assumes major professional responsibility for decision making in relation to health needs. She works collaboratively with physicians and other members of the health team in the delivery of

health services to individuals and families. Her practice is community oriented, related to needs, concerns, and priorities of the consumers.

The family nurse practitioner will have responsibility for the following:

A Wellness
  1 Health maintenance of all age groups—provision of continuing care to assist the patient and/or family to function at their individual optimum level of wellness
  2 Prevention
    a instituting known procedures to prevent illness
    b screening procedures for purposes of early detection, primary prevention, health counseling, and appropriate referral
    c health teaching and counseling of patients and families related to need and interest
    d periodic examination of well infants, children, and adults
B Illness
  1 An initial assessment and evaluation of the health status of the patient with needed diagnostic procedures to enable the family nurse practitioner to make one of three decisions for the care of the patient:
    a immediate intervention with or without medical consultation
    b arrangement for emergency care
    c referral of the patient to the physician
  2 Provision of on-going health maintenance and clinical management of stable chronically ill patients
  3 Identify the impact of the health status on the individual and family in order to:
    a help the patient and/or family cope with the situation
    b plan for continuity of care

The nurses who completed the initial course for family nurse practitioners say that what they learned is the link that has been missing previously in their nursing practice. No longer do they have to stop when someone presents symptoms of illness, instead they can evaluate and make plans in relation to their assessment of the patient's condition.

Some people view the family nurse practitioner as one who not only serves as the primary care specialist for individual members but also is qualified to serve the family as a unit. This nurse relates to the family in an interactional relationship offering continuous coordinated health care to the total family as a group. Few of the programs articulate the more sophisticated definition of family nursing, where the practice of nursing is defined in terms of concepts of family care and sophisticated nursing practice, e.g., working on a contractual basis with the family as the unit of service, making complex multidimensional assessments of the family group's resources and "cope-abilities," applying therapeutic interventions from autonomous interpretations of family interactional patterns, and employing prediction models for future family development. A current major problem is the variety of programs and models, the level of educational preparation of the candidates, and the eventual certification of the nursing practitioner. The words *practitioner* and *clinician* have variant meanings and do not always differentiate types and levels of preparation. In the early models of practitioner programs, the basic preparation was the baccalaureate degree in nursing. Not all later models demanded this educational base. In the minds of nurse educators, the nurse clinician is clearly a product of graduate education.

Concepts of the nurse's role in primary care are now under exploration by nursing leaders. A statement by the Western Council of Higher Education in Nursing boldly directs nurses toward exciting new roles as primary care takers (*Western Interstate Commission on Higher Education,* 1971).

In discussing the past, present, and future development of family specialists without identifying any specific discipline, Mace (1971) lists two criteria for the contemporary family specialist giving direction and substance for the future: (1) The family specialist's primary function is to deal exclusively with the family itself; and (2) he is prepared from a scientific base and with specialized skills.

Nursing has not yet articulated such criteria to give direction for the development of programs in family nursing at the graduate level. Currently the state of the art is understandably fuzzy. Family nurse practitioners and community health nurses, maternal and child nursing specialists, and psychiatric nursing clinicians all promote their own territorial claims. In the meantime, families in the community are seeking comprehensive health care which will assure them the quality of life they have been promised and deserve. Today the horrendous crisis in the health care system is causing nurses to take a new look at their roles and goals. There appears to be a decided shift to search out nursing's professional role in health maintenance as a primary care agent, emphasizing the delivery of family services. Recommendations of the National Commission for the Study of Nursing and Nursing Education include developing the science and art of nursing through research, expanding role articulations in the delivery of health care, creating statewide planning committees for nursing education, and increasing governmental support for education and research (Lysaught, 1970). Pointing toward the current fallacies in the organization of the health care system, which unselectively lumps the well with the sick, Garfield (1971) suggests a four-pronged approach which separates the well from the sick and the worried well from the early sick. Norris (1970) adds her influence with her insightful article about the nurse's role as one of the gatekeepers of the health care system. Ideas such as those presented by the National Commission on Nursing and Nursing Education, Garfield, Norris, and others have evolved from the acute and astute concerns about the inability of the present health care system to meet even minimum standards of quality health care. The continuing misutilization and maldistribution of health manpower resources, the escalating costs of health care, and the potential for society's consumers to erupt into violent action have catapulted health professionals into action—finally. In terms of delivering family care, it may be later than we think, particularly if the assumption is that the family of the future will be the same as it is today or was yesterday. Toffler (1970) proposes that families of the future may be very different in structure, organization, and function. Communes, trial marriages, single-parent families, homosexual unions, foster parents, and grandparent arrangements may replace the contemporary family. Extensive diversity of family life styles, new patterns of childrearing practices, and transient interpersonal encounters can be expected. New theoretical orientation on changing family relationships will be needed to understand the future phenomenon of family life. As technology advances, permitting man's freedom to create and innovate in work and play, new patterns of daily living will evolve, demanding diverse approaches to the humanization of care. New roles for professional health workers are imminent. Families are concerned about the quality of their lives—not only from the materialistic base but also from the aesthetic and ecological points of view. Threats to future generations from environmental pollution, stresses of the pace of change, etc., are becoming the major concerns of many families and groups. How well will nursing be able to cope with the problems of preparing future practitioners for family nursing? Developmentally, family nursing of the type families will need, demand, and desire is in its infancy. It is a time of searching and thoughtful becoming. Now is the time to take advantage of these growing years.

BIBLIOGRAPHY

American Nurses' Association: *Division of Community Health Nursing Practice,* New York, April 1967. (Mimeographed)
———: *A Position Paper: Educational Preparation for Nurse Practitioners and Assistants to Nurses,* New York, 1965.
———: *Statement on Graduate Education in Nursing,* New York, 1969.
Auerbach, A. B., and R. G. Taylor: "An Experiment in Training Nurses for Leadership," *The Bulletin for Maternal and Infant Health, A Symposium: Education for Parenthood,* American Association for Maternal and Infant Health, Inc., 1960.
Broderick, C. B.: "Beyond the Five Conceptual Frameworks: A Decade of Development in Family Theory," *Journal of Marriage and the Family,* 33:139-159, 1971.
Christensen, H. T. (ed.): *Handbook of Marriage and the Family,* Chicago: Rand McNally and Company, 1964.
Committee on Education of the National League for Nursing Education: *Standard Curriculum for Schools of Nursing,* New York: National Nursing Association, 1919.

Committee on the Grading of Nursing Schools: *Nursing Schools Today and Tomorrow,* New York, 1934.

Conant, L. B.: "The Nature of Nursing Tomorrow," *Image: Sigma Theta Tau National Honor Society of Nursing,* 4:2, 1970-1971.

Corbin, H.: "Development of Parent Classes in the United States," *The Bulletin for Maternal and Child Health, A Symposium: Education for Parenthood,* American Association for Maternal and Infant Health, Inc., 1960.

Curry, F. J.: "Neighborhood Health Centers, Planned, Developed, and Managed by Neighborhood Groups, Should Be a Top Priority in Bringing Tomorrow's Medicine Today," *California's Health,* 1971.

Dunn, H. L.: *High Level Wellness,* Arlington, Va.: R. W. Beatty, Ltd., 1961.

"Editorial," *American Journal of Nursing,* 71:489, 1971.

Ford, L. C., and H. K. Silver: "The Expanded Role of the Nurse in Child Care," *Nursing Outlook,* 15:43-45, 1967.

Ford, P. A., M. S. Seacat, and G. A. Silver: "The Relative Roles of the Public Health Nurse and the Physician in Prenatal and Infant Supervision," *American Journal of Public Health,* 56:1097-1103, 1966.

Freeman, R. B.: *Community Health Nursing Practice,* Philadelphia: W. B. Saunders Company, 1970.

————: "The Criterion of Relevance," *American Journal of Public Health,* 57:1522-1531, 1967.

Gardner, M. S.: *Public Health Nursing,* New York: The Macmillan Company, 1936.

Garfield, S. R.: "Prevention of Dissipation of Health Services Resources," *American Journal of Public Health,* 61:1499-1506, 1971.

Glasser, J. H.: "Health Information Systems: A Crisis or Just More of the Usual?" *American Journal of Public Health,* 61:1524-1530, 1971.

Hill, R., and D. A. Hansen: "The Identification of Conceptual Frameworks Utilized in Family Study," *Marriage and Family Living,* 22:299-311, 1960.

Joint Commission on Mental Illness and Health: *Action for Mental Health,* New York: Basic Books Inc., Publishers, 1961.

King, I. M.: *Toward a Theory for Nursing: General Concepts of Human Behavior,* New York: John Wiley & Sons, Inc., 1971, chap. 1, pp. 2-6.

Lewis, C. E., and B. A. Resnik: "Nurse Clinics and Progressive Ambulatory Patient Care," *New England Journal of Medicine,* 277:1236-1241, 1967.

Lysaught, J. P.: *An Abstract for Action,* New York: McGraw-Hill Book Company, 1970.

Mace, D. R.: "The Family Specialist, Past, Present, and Future," *Family Coordinator,* 21:291-294, 1971.

National Association for Public Health Nursing: *Manual of Public Health Nursing,* New York: The Macmillan Company, 1939.

National League for Nursing: *Record System Guide for a Community Health Service,* New York, 1970.

National League for Nursing Committee on Perspectives: *Change, Collaboration and Community Involvement,* New York: National League for Nursing, 1967.

Norris, C. M.: "Direct Access to the Patient," *American Journal of Nursing,* 70:1006-1010, 1970.

Nye, I., and F. Berardo: *Conceptual Frameworks for the Study of the Family,* New York: The Macmillan Company, 1966.

Peplau, H. E.: "Principles of Psychiatric Nursing," in S. Arieti (ed.), *American Handbook of Psychiatry,* vol. II, New York: Basic Books, Inc., Publishers, 1959.

Report of the Committee for the Study of Nursing Education: *Nursing and Nursing Education in the United States,* New York: The Macmillan Company, 1923.

Report of Joint Ad Hoc Committee of A.N.A.-A.P.H.A.: *Public Health Nursing Specialist,* 1967. (Mimeographed)

Rosen, G.: "Public Health: Then and Now—The First Neighborhood Health Center Movement—Its Rise and Fall," *American Journal of Public Health,* **61**:1620-1637, 1971.

Siegel, E., and S. L. Bryson: "Redefinition of the Role of the Public Health Nurse in Child Health Definition," *American Journal of Public Health,* **53**:1015-1024, 1963.

———, R. Dillehay, and C. J. Fitzgerald: "Role Changes within the Child Health Conference: Attitudes and Professional Preparedness of Public Health Nurses and Physicians," *American Journal of Health,* **55**:832-841, 1965.

Stoeckle, J. D., B. Noonan, R. M. Farrisey, and A. Sweatt: "Medical Nursing Clinic for Chronically Ill," *American Journal of Nursing,* **63**:87-89, 1963.

Toffler, A.: *Future Shock,* New York: Bantam Books, Inc., 1970.

U.S. Department of Health, Education, and Welfare: *Toward a Comprehensive Health Policy for the 1970's: A White Paper,* Washington, D.C., 1971.

Western Interstate Commission on Higher Education: *Defining Clinical Content, Graduate Nursing Programs: Community Health Nursing,* Boulder, Colo., 1967.

———: *Defining Clinical Content, Graduate Nursing Programs: Maternal and Child Nursing,* Boulder, Colo., 1967.

———: *Defining Clinical Content, Graduate Nursing Programs: Medical Surgical Nursing,* Boulder, Colo., 1967.

———: *Defining Clinical Content, Graduate Nursing Programs: Psychiatric Nursing,* Boulder, Colo., 1967.

———: *Guidelines for Developing Master's Degree Programs in the West,* Western Council on Higher Education for Nursing, Boulder, Colo., 1958.

———: *Statement on Primary Care in Progress,* Western Council on Higher Education for Nursing, Boulder, Colo., 1971.

Wiedenbach, E.: "Family Nurse Practitioner for Maternal and Child Care," *Nursing Outlook,* **13**:50-52, 1965.

Chapter 2

Family Systems in the 1970's: Analysis, Policies, and Programs*

Marvin B. Sussman

Abstract: This paper contains a brief review of some of the salient discoveries and theoretical formulations which provide the most powerful explanation of the issues and problems faced by different types of families in their dealings with institutional systems and bureaucratic organizations. Specifically covered are variant family forms; structural properties of kin family systems; family/organizational linkages; major tasks and functions of families; the kin network as a mediating-linking system; and changes in the internal role structure of the family. The second section deals with practical applications, needed policies, programs, and strategies for increasing the level of competence of human service systems to meet the expectations, capabilities, interests, and aspirations of members of variant family forms found in pluralistic societies.

When confronted with a suggested subject like "Strengthening the Home

* Reprinted from Marvin B. Sussman, "Family Systems in the 1970's: Analysis, Policies, and Programs," *The Annals of the American Academy*, vol. 396, July 1971. By permission of the publisher.

and Family," one might be tempted to respond with the usual rhetoric of "what ought to be"—the "For God, country, and Yale" gambit, plus motherhood and, to be safe, a quick reference to the women's liberation movement. But this is contrary to my self-concept. I am much more comfortable in analyzing "what is," and my recommendations for action have a decidedly pragmatic, if not existentialist, flavor. My ideological position is that all behavioral science research faces the ultimate test of salience by the power of its explanation and usefulness to the solution of the problems of the human condition.[1] The basic issue is, How can the quality of life be improved for individuals of varying capabilities, motivations, and ambitions who live in pluralistic societies with extensive differentiation and complexity in occupations, organizations, associations, and family forms?

Having stated a capsulated version of my philosophical posture, I will proceed to dissect the social, political, and academic developments which sustain a particular perspective on the social system commonly identified as a family. This analysis, while particularly oriented toward the American scene, is by no means restricted, since similar developments and social movements are to be found in transitional and complex societies.

There are two main sections of this paper. The first covers theoretical formulations and research, which provide a perspective for looking at the family as a group and its linkages with nonfamily organizations and institutions in the 1970's. Included are:

1   variant family forms
2   structural properties of kin family systems
3   major tasks and functions: family-organizational linkages
4   kin network as a mediating-linking system
5   internal role structure: accommodations to exigencies of the 1970's.

The second section deals with practical applications, needed policies, programs, and strategies for increasing the level of competence of human service systems to meet the expectations, capabilities, interests, and aspirations of members of variant family forms found in pluralistic societies.

VARIANT FAMILY FORMS

Ethnic historians and race-relation sociologists and psychologists have long emphasized the pluralistic characteristic of United States society. Over the years there has been quibbling in academic halls over whether a melting pot was cooking an amalgam composed of ethnic and cultural distillates called

---

[1] See Marvin B. Sussman, "The Sociologist as a Tool of Social Action" in *Sociology in Action,* Arthur B. Shostak, ed. (Homewood, Ill.: Dorsey Press, 1966) pp. 3-14, for a statement of this position.

"American," or whether this society was persisting as a salad bowl with its shapes and hues of ethnic, religious, and racial identities. The argument is by no means over, but the salad bowl adherents are winning out in this decade.

Surprisingly, this notion of pluralism, or variability and differentiation of groups, did not take hold among students of the family. This may be a sensitive area which supports the rhetoric of "what ought to be"—an ideal family form according to some preordained, and often religiously sanctioned, set of values. The power and pervasiveness of this belief in the ideal family have resulted in the formulation of research questions which do not capture empirical descriptions of what family systems are actually like in the real world. Forms that vary from the traditional nuclear family of husband, wife, and children living in neolocal residence with the male as breadwinner and female as homemaker have been viewed as deviant. Research in the 1950's and 1960's on the working mother of the single-parent or dual-work family was mainly concerned with the deleterious effects of such gainful employment upon children. The implications were that women should be "in the home where the good Lord intended them to be," and in the case of the single parent, to marry or remarry as soon as possible. Very little attention was accorded to the meaning and significance for women of working, the circumstances under which women took jobs, or the implications for the reallocation of roles within the dual-career family.[2]

This preoccupation with the model nuclear family pattern and efforts to preserve it at all costs prevented sociologists from describing what was becoming most obvious to non-sociological observers of the American scene: a pluralism in family forms existing side by side with members in each of these forms having different problems to solve and issues to face. Moreover, few individuals over a lifetime remain in a single type of family structure, although the majority have some experience in the traditional nuclear family.

TRADITIONAL FAMILY STRUCTURES

The most prominent traditional types of family structures now existing, and variations on these structures, are:[3]

1 Nuclear family—husband, wife, and offspring living in a common household.

---

[2] Rhona Rapoport and Robert N. Rapoport, "The Dual Career Family," *Human Relations*, 20, 1 (February, 1969), pp. 3–30.

[3] An analysis of variant family forms is found in Marvin B. Sussman et al., "Changing Families in a Changing Society," 1970 White House Conference on Children, Forum 14 Report (Washington, D.C.: Government Printing Office, 1971). Margaret P. Brooks, Research Associate, Institute on the Family and the Bureaucratic Society, has suggested a modification of the original typography, which is incorporated in this presentation.

    a Single career
    b Dual career
        1 Wife's career continuous
        2 Wife's career interrupted
2 Nuclear dyad—husband and wife alone: childless, or no children living at home.
    a Single career
    b Dual career
        1 Wife's career continuous
        2 Wife's career interrupted
3 Single-parent family—one head, as a consequence of divorce, abandonment, or separation (with financial aid rarely coming from the second parent), and usually including pre-school and/or schoolage children.
    a Career
    b Non-career
4 Single adult living alone.
5 Three-generation family—may characterize any variant of family forms 1, 2, or 3 living in a common household.
6 Middle-aged or elderly couple—husband as provider, wife at home (children have been "launched" into college, career, or marriage).
7 Kin network—nuclear households or unmarried members living in close geographical proximity and operating within a reciprocal system of exchange of goods and services.
8 "Second-career" family—the wife enters the work force when the children are in school or have left the parental home.

Emerging experimental structures which have an effect on children include:

1 Commune family
    a Household of more than one monogamous couple with children, sharing common facilities, resources, and experiences; socialization of the child is a group activity.
    b Household of adults and offspring—a "group marriage" known as one family—where all individuals are "married" to each other and all are "parents" to the children. Usually develops a status system with leaders believed to have charisma.
2 Unmarried parent and child family—usually mother and child, where marriage is not desired or possible.
3 Unmarried couple and child family—usually a common-law type of marriage with the child their biological issue or informally adopted.

The implications of variant family forms for legislation, policy, and programs to help families are obvious. No single policy, legislative act, or program will be equally supportive of all types of family structures. There will be more discussion on this topic later.

The problem of strengthening variant family forms is complicated by such intervening variables as the stage in the life cycle and the socio-economic status of the family. When a traditional nuclear family becomes a single-parent one, the problems created by this transition and the mechanisms for handling them will vary according to the cause(s) which induced this change: whether the new single parent has small children, yet requires gainful employment (or training), or whether the parent is middle-aged with grown children and requires resocialization into a career or new uses of leisure. Consequently; the age composition, size, and socio-economic status of each family undergoing this structural transition will create issues and problems for the human service systems of the society.

It is becoming increasingly common for individuals over the life cycle to move from one family form to another, either because of design or circumstances. Consider the following case: For the first five years of his life, Craig lived in a three-generation rural household with his siblings, grandparents, and a number of aunts, uncles, and cousins. During this time he had many parent surrogates and adult role models; one in particular was his grandfather. Near his fifth birthday, his parents and two siblings left the farm and migrated to a city about one hundred miles away. His father found a job as an unskilled factory worker. The income was insufficient to support the family, so when Craig entered primary school his mother took a job as saleswoman at a downtown department store. Three years later the father, who could not "make it," deserted. Financially the family was secure, because Craig's mother proved to be a competent businesswoman and was soon promoted to the position of department manager. Two years after the father left, a divorce was granted; a year later, the mother married a widower with two children.

It is unnecessary to continue the family life career of Craig to illustrate that over a period of six or seven years he lived in four variant forms of the traditional nuclear (intact) family: the three-generation household, dual-work, single-parent, and remarried. Each of these forms presented different issues and problems for Craig, his parents, and his siblings. These involved changes in interaction patterns, the role system and socialization patterns within the family, and modifications of the linkage of the family with nonfamily groups and organizations.

Possible explanations of the causes of variant family forms, or at least their greater visibility and increased incidence, are varied and speculative.[4]

1 Traditional institutions have reached the limits of their capabilities to absorb and embrace the adherents of the "new culture." One alternative for

---

[4] Marvin B. Sussman, "The Family" in *Encyclopedia of Social Work* (New York: National Association of Social Workers, 1971), pp. 329-340.

members of the "establishment" who hope to continue societal control is to further recognize pluralism by increasing the options for individuals and families of different forms, especially where these forms are characteristic of certain disenfranchised and deprived minorities.

2   A different and somewhat contrary explanation states that powerful elites feel comfortable about their ability to control large-scale change and at the same time perceive tolerance of non-conformity and deviance to be politically salient. Variant behavior and structures become increasingly overt as the more frequent, minor, negative sanctions are removed.

3   American society is in the beginning of a social revolution. It is at a stage when old-order institutions are being attacked, and experimental family forms like communes represent opposition and confrontation with the old culture's way of life. The thrust of some social revolutionaries is to create new forms of the family based on ideologies and arrangements which accommodate the differential capabilities, aspirations, motivations, and needs of its members.

STRUCTURAL PROPERTIES OF KIN FAMILY SYSTEMS

A plethora of research by family sociologists during the past two decades has established the pervasiveness of a kin family network in urban environments built upon principles of exchange and reciprocity.[5] This network embraces numerous family forms. The delay until the early 1950's in recognizing this network was due, in part, to conceptualizations which emphasized that social mobility was the most characteristic feature of complex bureaucratic societies. According to this view, the nuclear family, consisting of a married couple and their minor children, appeared to be the unit best suited to meet the normative demands of the economic system—to move where there was the best opportunity for higher income with parallel improvements in social status, prestige, and power.[6] The functionality of the nuclear family is still maintained by a large number of investigators. For them, the unit is treated as coterminus with the entire institution of the family today in the American milieu. Talcott Parsons considers it to be a completely integrated unit which has survived by virtue of its superior adaptability. It can bend and reshape its structure according to the needs and demands of more powerful bureaucracies. This view is reinforced by law, policies, and programs which label the

[5] For a review of research supporting this view and presentation of empirical data, see Marvin B. Sussman and Lee G. Burchinal, "Kin Family Network: Unheralded Structure in Current Conceptualizations of Family Functioning," *Marriage and Family Living,* 24 (August, 1962), pp. 231-240; idem, "The Urban Kin Network in the Formulation of Family Theory," in *Families in East and West,* Reuben Hill and René König, eds. (Paris: Mouton, 1970), pp. 481-503; and idem, "Adaptive, Directive and Integrative Behavior," *Family Process,* 7 (September, 1968), pp. 244-249.

[6] A theoretical formulation which goes contrary to the theme of dominance of the economic system over the family is found in Marvin B. Sussman and Betty E. Cogswell, "Family Influences on Job Movement," *Human Relations* 24 (December, 1971), pp. 477-487.

nuclear family as the unit which has corporate responsibility for its affiliated members.

At the same time, however, social scientists have been aware that all possible social interactions are not exhausted by contractual arrangements between bureaucratic organizations and discrete units such as the nuclear family. In urban as well as rural settings, nuclear families living in separate households are functionally related so as to form kin family networks. These extensions of the family remain viable through a system of unequal exchanges of services and financial aid which, in goals, norms, and values, vie with other primary and bureaucratic systems for the loyalty of those who are participants. Trust, expected reciprocity, and being able to "count on" the kin member are the most salient characteristics of this system.

Studies of middle-class and working-class urban families reveal visitation among members with financial aid, advice, and child care as primary modalities. These studies reveal extensive intrafamily and interfamily relationships in a continuous state of change and with differential influence on the behavior of the actors. Linkages are forged or rendered inoperative on the basis of intra-network values. Network relationships are by no means stable; conflict as well as coöperation exists. There is an ongoing struggle among family units in each network for the achievement of in-group goals, as they attempt to meet their own needs and to achieve desired rewards. When shared goals cannot be identified among component units, disintegration of the kin network may result.

A study of family units at differing generational levels revealed cultural factors to be highly influential in assuring family continuity.[7] Notable among these were differences in the socio-economic cultural background of marriage mates; the types of courtship and wedding ceremony that preceded the formation of a family unit; differences in child-rearing philosophy and practice; and the extent to which a help pattern was developed between parents and their married children. Proximity of residence was found to be another factor in determining the influence of those mentioned above, as it was utilized by the family to forge closer links or, alternatively, to lessen tensions.

MAJOR TASKS AND FUNCTIONS: FAMILY-ORGANIZATIONAL LINKAGES

In the 1970's, as in the past, all types of families function with varied degrees of proficiency as facilitating, mediating, and confronting systems for their members, who have differing aspirations, capabilities, and potentials. Fam-

---

[7] Reuben Hill, *Family Development over Three Generations* (Cambridge, Mass.: Harvard University Press, 1971), and Marvin B. Sussman, "Relationships of Adult Children with Their Parents in the United States," in *Family, Intergenerational Relationships, and Social Structure,* Ethel Shanas and Gordon Streib, eds. (Englewood Cliffs, N.J.: Prentice-Hall, 1965), pp. 62–92.

ilies adapt and influence behavior of their members and outsiders simultaneously. They adjust to complex urban life and at the same time modify the development, structure, and activities of contemporary social institutions and organizations. Because of variations in form, families differ in their adaptation and in their efforts to mitigate the demands of nonfamily groups and to influence the behavior of outside organizations such as the school, welfare agency, or factory. Consequently, the main tasks of families are: (1) to develop their capacities to socialize children, (2) to enhance the competence of their members to cope with the demands of the organizations in which they must function, (3) to utilize these organizations, (4) to provide an environment for the development of identities and affectional response, and (5) to create satisfactions and a mentally healthy environment intrinsic to the well-being of a family.[8]

In complex societies, there exist many alternative patterns for meeting contingencies. In the urban setting, a great variety of jobs, schools, residences, and facilities are available to family members, with the largest number of options available to the higher social classes and elites.[9] For some families, especially those of the middle and upper classes, the problem is sometimes too many choices, or "option glut."[10] For ethnic and racial groups, such as Mexican Americans, blacks, Puerto Ricans, Appalachian whites, there is option scarcity often coupled with pressure to limit or take away existing alternatives. As children acquire additional skills through informal and formal training systems, the potential range of options increases. "Enlightened" elites as well as social reformers recognize the differences in option availability when they work to expand the available options for more and more people in such life sectors as education, leisure, welfare, and work.[11]

Although the number of options available to an individual varies according to his class, and ethnic and racial status, some families of every background seem able to enhance the capacity of their members to choose from available options and to perform competently in new roles and within a variety of organizations. Other families seem less able to do so, producing instead various manifestations of individual and familial malfunctioning. We know that the way in which community, social, welfare, and educational systems support or constrain the child and his family has some impact upon

[8] Op. cit., M. B. Sussman et al. These notions are the bases of the White House Conference on Children, Report 14, "Changing Families in a Changing Society." Marvin B. Sussman was chairman of this committee and drafted the report.

[9] See working papers of the Cross-National Family Studies Project, Marvin B. Sussman, principal investigator, Case Western Reserve University, and "Policy, Family and Constraints," paper presented at Groves Conference on Marriage and the Family, April, 1970.

[10] This is the reverse of too few options and was suggested by Robert Rapoport of the Human Resources Centre, Tavistock Institute of Human Relations, London.

[11] See Marvin B. Sussman, "Competence and Options: A Theoretical Essay, Implications for Nutritional Research," in David Kallen, ed., *Proceedings of NICHD-PAHO Conference on Assessment of Tests of Behavior from Studies of Nutrition in the Western Hemisphere* (forthcoming).

the development of competence in the use of options. Moreover, in modern societies the growing needs and demands for social, educational, and welfare services, as well as preventive and therapeutic health care, are extending beyond the capacities of even potential professional and paraprofessional manpower. As a result, the family—as a social unit with caretaking, therapeutic, socializing, expediting, and handling activities—is a vital and sometimes unrecognized partner of bureaucratic service organizations having health, welfare, and rehabilitative objectives. [12] Thus, the competency of the family unit in managing these societal relationships is an increasingly important issue.

In summary, the salient prerequisites for individual and family survival are competence in using bureaucratic organizations, the family's success in developing these management capabilities, and the family members' uses of options within a framework of satisfaction for self and concern over the welfare of others. Families which "make it" are those which have become aware of and use options and develop successful linkages with nonfamily organizations. The family, being a relatively small group of individuals usually intimately related to one another, forms a closed system. As a rule it does not join with other, non-kin families to develop an organization similar to existing institutional bureaucracies that are most resistant to outside influences and change. As a consequence, it and its larger kin network play their most significant societal role as a mediator between its members and bureaucratic organizations, as it provides socialization and competence in coping with the normative demands of bureaucratic systems. Mediation, if it is perceived as successful, has to involve action which results in compromise without an undue loss of position, integrity, or power by participants. It involves a reciprocal process of being able to influence as well as being influenced.

A party to any transaction which is shorn of its strength and power to act on behalf of its members cannot maintain its integrity. It becomes subordinate. Any unit—family, group, or organization—must provide sufficient support and success in transactions so that its members believe it is worthwhile to maintain over time.

THE KIN NETWORK INFLUENCE

The kin network and its member families may assist in individual adaptation to the larger society and in some instances influence organizational policy and practices. Education, for example, implies learning new roles as well as new knowledge. Much of the socialization in the student role is actually achieved

[12] For a fuller explanation of this notion, see Marvin B. Sussman, "Family, Kinship, and Bureaucracy," in Angus Campbell and Philip Converse, ed., *Social Change and Human Change* (New York City: Russell Sage Foundation, 1972), pp. 127-158.

in the family setting; although the latter takes place in the school, the family often exercises considerable influence over its performance. The educational program of the school takes cognizance of the social class of the families it serves, their patterns of socialization, and home environmental conditions. It must cater to these as well as to the needs and demands expressed by its pupils. [13]

All families are not equally prepared to perform this mediating function. Research has revealed that the extent to which they are able to perform it depends upon their location and activity in the kin network, life-cycle stage, and experience with organizations. The community status of a family is affected by its kin connections. The position and attitudes of member units of the kin group also affect such matters as family planning, family size, and sponsorship in achieving educational and occupational objectives. This network can be an opportunity structure insofar as it accepts the priorities of the bureaucratic society and has the socio-economic resources to deal with it. Middle-class and upper-class families tend to have the most advantageous linkages through kin for purposes of mobility, and the greatest competency in using the network to achieve individual and family goals. Lower-class families, however, may consider that the intrinsic advantages of familism take precedence over those of increased mobility. The unskilled enjoy little security in the larger social sphere, a condition which encourages dependency upon kin for services which support economic as well as emotional ends. Thus, family cohesiveness, persistence, and continuity are not necessarily coincident with the effectiveness of the family unit in coping with the larger society.

It is apparent that the resources of some families leave them at a disadvantage in those transactions which take place outside of primary groups. In the mediation process, the bureaucracy may rely on the professional expert as its representative. He has been formally socialized for this role and is permitted, through his mandate for public service, to go beyond organizational goals and to concern himself in part with public or primary group needs. [14] Nevertheless, primarily he supports the more extensive concerns of the bureaucratic institutions with which he is associated. He is likely to possess more resources to be used in the bargaining transaction than are available to the representative of the primary groups, and he is under constraints to mediate in the best interests of his employing organization.

[13] Marie Haug and Marvin B. Sussman, "Professional Autonomy and the Revolt of the Client," *Social Problems,* 17 (Fall, 1969), pp. 153-161.

[14] Eugene Litwak and Henry J. Meyer, "Administrative Styles and Community Linkages of Public Schools," A. J. Reiss, ed., *Schools in a Changing Society* (New York: Free Press, 1965), pp. 45-97; idem, "The School and the Family: Linking Organizations and External Primary Groups," Paul Lazarsfeld, W. Sewell, and H. Wilensky, eds., *The Uses of Sociology* (New York: Basic Books, 1967), pp. 522-543; "A Balance Theory of Coördination Between Bureaucratic Organizations and Community Primary Groups," *Administrative Science Quarterly,* 11 (June, 1966), pp. 31-58.

Functionaries of bureaucratic organizations often co-opt primary group members in the mediation process. Even when families or their representatives are given a "piece of the action" through mediation, the degree of shift in their superordinate/subordinate power relationship is determined by the linkers from the bureaucratic organization. The experiences of black families with programs sponsored by Aid to Families with Dependent Children and the Office of Economic Opportunity provide examples.

If primary groups are going to influence the mediation process and are to have any effect on the policies and programs of organizations and, more importantly, maintain the integrity of their own internal structure, then they must socialize their members into the means for coping with mediating relationships of this character. The goals and functions of both the primary group and bureaucratic organization must be understood, and a competence developed in dealing with the complexities of their interaction.

The kin network may be a veritable gold mine for linkers with mediating skills and connections in different life sectors. Initial findings from a pilot study of a barrio in Puerto Rico indicate that members of the kin network and *compadre* system take on "specialist linker roles." If a family member needs a loan, is in trouble with the police, requires a social security number, wants a job, needs to obtain a driver's license, or wants to make a trip to the mainland, he goes to an "expert" kin or *compadre* family member, if such is not present in his household. This individual links the family with the bureaucratic organization and frequently may educate the help-seeker into the use of options as well as socialize him into mediating and handling skills and new roles required by the bureaucratic structure. [15]

INTERNAL ROLE STRUCTURE: ACCOMMODATIONS TO EXIGENCIES OF THE 1970's

A detailed analysis of changes in the internal system of the family in the 1970's would fill a monograph-length manuscript. Our objectives here are simply to illustrate modifications in role relationships and task allocations within families, and to raise some questions of issues and problems of these families without providing definitive answers. The dual-career family will be used to demonstrate the kinds of changes occurring in the interaction system.

Accurate statistics on the incidence and prevalence of this family form are not available. However, analysis of census data since 1948 on mothers who were or are currently employed gives some measure of prevalence and incidence rates. From 1948 to 1969 the percentage of mothers in the labor force with children less than six years old increased from 13 to 30, and mothers with children aged six to seventeen increased from 31 to 51. Non-

[15] Cross-National Family Research Project, Caguas, Puerto Rico, working document. Institute on the Family and Bureaucratic Society, Case Western Reserve University, Cleveland, Ohio.

white groups had a disproportionate number of mothers who were sixteen years or over and were gainfully employed during this same period. In March, 1969, of the 9.8 million mothers in the work force, 1.2 million were nonwhite; 64 percent of the nonwhites compared to 47 percent of the whites had children six to seventeen years of age; 44 percent compared to 27 percent had children under age six; 52 percent compared to 33 percent had no children under age 3. These figures suggest the necessity for a large proportion of nonwhite mothers with small children to enter the labor market. [16]

As married women continued to enter and re-enter the labor force during the 1960's, the dual-career family became more accepted in contemporary American life. In March, 1969, the proportion of families in which the husband and someone else worked was almost 52 percent. That "someone else" was far more likely to be the wife than a son or daughter. [17] The proportion of multiworker families among nonwhites was 11 percent higher than among whites.

The amount of the husband's income is directly related to the decision of many women to go into gainful employment. In families with both parents present, mothers with children over six years but under seventeen are more likely to enter the labor market with each increasing year of age of the youngest child. It appears that mothers with younger children are not markedly influenced to go into gainful employment in proportion to the husband's income. [18]

In addition to the need or desire for income, there are other reasons why women enter the labor force; for example, aspirations for a career, boredom at home, and a labor shortage in certain occupations. Regardless of the reasons for women increasingly entering gainful employment, the adults of such families do have responsibilities for the socialization of their children and for providing the youngsters with love, attention, and affection.

Earning money is one source of power, and a woman's working usually means re-allocation of roles and tasks within the family. If, as in better educated groups, the woman is pursuing a highly skilled or professional career line, the family has more problems regarding mobility and child management than other family types. How does one handle problems arising from differential success of the husband or wife? If a decision is made to move, what adjustment is required in the career change of the marital partner? [19]

[16] SOURCE: U. S. Department of Labor, Bureau of Labor Statistics. Table titled, "Labor Force Participation Rates of Mothers (Husband Present), by Race and Age of Children, March 1969." From statistics to be included in *Profiles of Children,* chartbook of the White House Conference on Children and Youth, 1970.

[17] Ibid. Table titled, "Employment Status of Family Head and Labor Force Status of Wife and Other Family Members, by Color, March, 1969."

[18] Table titled, "Labor Force Participation Rates and Percent Distribution of Mothers (Husband Present), by Income of Husband in 1968 and Age of Children, March 1969."

[19] The nonmonetary factors affecting job mobility are discussed in Sussman and Cogswell, op. cit.

What are the special problems of having children? Do dual-employment parents have more guilt feelings than traditional parents about neglect of their children? Does working provide new options, with consequences such as a reduction in fertility? What do such families require in the form of educational, counseling, social and other supportive services and conveniences, which will enable them to pursue their careers successfully and meet their emotional, physical, and social needs and those of their children? What new uses of social and physical space are now required to enhance the functioning of this newly established major family form? What "built-in environments" can be created which will provide the uses of living space most conducive for the self-fulfillment of individual aspirations and needs? [20]

For each of the variant family forms, a similar set of questions can be raised—with answers to be found within a framework which recognizes multiple problems and suggests solutions, policies, and programs tailored to fit the life style of that form. Such an approach demands an acceptance of pluralism in structure, belief, and action.

RECOMMENDATIONS FOR SUPPORT OF MARRIAGE AND FAMILIES

In the 1960's, the increased variability in family forms has become more visible. Diversity is based on the right of individual Americans to live in any family form they feel will increase their options for self-fulfillment and help them achieve a desired quality of life. This may be a measure of this society's modernity. An enduringly pluralistic society must recognize that individuals of different capabilities and motivations may find self-fulfillment in any one of the family forms currently in existence in American society.

The type of family structure will affect socialization processes and outcomes. It is assumed that a society is interested in supporting those family structures which foster healthy physiological, emotional, and social growth of children. We are generally aware of the desirable conditions for character and personality development in the traditional nuclear family, but we have little knowledge of the positive qualities inherent in the environmental conditions of variant and experimental family forms.

It cannot be overemphasized that members of each family type have needs, problems, capabilities, and aspirations; some they share with members of other family types and some are limited to their own family form. The major task is to use our advanced technology and scientific discoveries to

---

[20] A fuller analysis of this concept will be found in Marvin B. Sussman, "A Prospectus: Construction of Built-In Environments—Housing and Services," 1970. Institute on the Family and Bureaucratic Society, Case Western Reserve University.

support all family forms by harnessing and re-allocating the resources on nonfamily groups and organizations to improve conditions for children, parents, and other related kin. To accomplish this we must build policies, structures, and environments around people rather than fit people into mass-produced formal systems and unimaginatively created physical, social, and interactional space.

Government agencies such as Housing and Urban Development, Office of Economic Opportunity, and Statistical Reporting Service can institute this approach by examining their on-going programs and exploring the possibilities of rearranging their policies and activities in order to meet the needs and aspirations of variant as well as traditional family forms. The essential approach of a unified agency program would be a "client-centered" one, in which conditions and environments (communities) are designed around families, rather than trying to fit families and their members into social and physical space on the economic principle of least cost and on narrowly conceived professional expertise.

The need is to abandon the traditional model of superordinate/subordinate interaction in providing services for families. In the 1970's, there are increasingly notable exceptions to traditional types of programming, where members of the family have been viewed as subordinate and in need of being "acted upon" by more knowledgeable and powerful professionals who have organized themselves into intellectual elites. One such international program is within the Home Economics Service of the Nutrition Division of the Food and Agricultural Organization of the United Nations. The "Planning for Better Family Living" program (PBFL) is a family-focused population program developed within FAO to reach rural families. Under this descriptive title is subsumed a multi-faceted educational program operating within theoretical constructs and tested methods used in field programs of FAO, where the objective is to provide families with an increasing number of options suited to members of different aspirations, capabilities, and motivations. Within the context of this varied program there will be extensive population-planning education, together with other services geared to needs of the varying recipient populations.[21]

"LAYERED MODEL" ABANDONED

One salient feature of this program is that the traditional "layered model" of research and action, where the researcher and programmer are dominant and manipulative, is being abandoned. On the premises that action without research into needs is folly and that research into human problems without

---

[21] The author is under contract with FAO to assist in the research activities of this project.

action is stupidity, the developers of this program are involving the families themselves from the very beginning. Commencing in countries in East Africa and then in other nations which request this program, the focus is on learning by doing, and changing behavior and values by reciprocal socialization. Student and teacher, novice and agent, will operate within a situation which fosters reciprocity in decision-making and mutuality in exchange of knowledge and the giving of self. Family members will be encouraged to become full participants in the research and teaching processes, and will be considered as integral members of the team in achieving the objectives of PBFL.

Although it may be true that the majority of children find optimal conditions for effective socialization and character development in the traditional nuclear household, it is also necessary in a pluralistic society that governmental agencies supplying supportive services to families remove restrictions that prohibit services to children and their families simply because the style of their lives in labeled deviant. This is equally true whether the life style is forced by conditions beyond their control or in an attempt to devise new forms of family living, new patterns of socialization, and new ways of earning a living.

On the scientific level, further active assistance may be offered through research grants, demonstration programs, economic maintenance, or long-term loans for projects designed to investigate living and working processes in varied family forms, focusing on the implications of these structural systems for all aspects of the development of children. Such research and demonstrations must be thoroughly reviewed and evaluated, and mechanisms must be created for the communication and exchange of ideas among participants.

Forum 14 of the 1970 White House Conference on Children issued a strong recommendation to:

> Establish a people-oriented, national institute for the family for action, advocacy, implementation, legislation, and research.

> Recognizing that the family is the dominant socializing agent and the primary interface between the individual and society, its central position must be considered by the White House Conference on Children in making recommendations for improving the well-being of our nation's children.

> It is vital that children living in all types of family structures, including single-parent, traditional, dual-work, and commune, have equally available options for self-fulfillment.

> Present human service systems tend to fragment and undermine the family. All such delivery systems should be redirected to provide services and support through and to the family as a unit with recognition of the different needs, strengths and weaknesses of varying family forms. Therefore, we recommend

that an Institute for the Family be established by the Congress as a quasi-public organization. The process for its operation should be assured by establishing a trust fund through a per capita assessment drawn from federal taxes.

This Institute should have a broadly representative Board of Directors and be adequately staffed for carrying out its functions. These functions are [to]:

1 Serve as an advocate for families and children.

2 Provide the mechanisms for assuring follow-up and implementation of the White House Conference recommendations at all levels.

3 Develop and support demonstration, action, research, and evaluation programs which focus on building new environments for families and children; reorder existing services and programs to fit around desires and aspirations of families, and to involve families in their development and implementation.

4 Examine existing legislation for its effects on variant family forms.

5 Take action against legislation, regulations, and practices which are punitive to children because of their discriminatory policies against the integrity of families or variant forms of parenting.

6 Provide technical assistance to state and local programs for families and children.[22]

This institute is much needed and the proposed program of services for families and children is long overdue. Finally, all recommendations for improving the quality of life for families are strictly academic, unless there is a re-allocation of societal resources buttressed by government policies and programs which will provide an adequate guaranteed annual income for all families. With such an economic base, the way would be paved for the complementary activities of supplying more adequate education, food, housing, and the material amenities of living. In order to provide a greater number of real or meaningful options for an increasing proportion of all families, basic survival resources are essential. Only then can programs of family life education, including elements of family planning, home management, nutrition, maternal and child care, growth and development, interpersonal competence, and socialization make any sense.

QUESTIONS AND ANSWERS

Q: I am concerned with urban renewal, which was fleetingly referred to when HUD was mentioned. I was afraid Dr. Sussman would come to the end of his speech without making any reference to a guaranteed family income or to something like a negative income situation. Since he did refer to it briefly at the very end, I would like to ask him if he would comment more fully on the guaranteed family income and family income tax?

[22] "Changing Families in a Changing Society," pp. 232-233.

A: I support guaranteed family income. I think all the other programs of uplift don't take on much significance unless there is the economic means of life. I just got back from abroad, meeting with people from what we call the "developing countries" of the world, and saw the programs of providing nutrients, and improving interaction within the family—all far removed from reality because of the basically deprived economic conditions.

When I served years ago on a number of grant-giving agencies, we got in an application for a grant which was going to provide a population a very small sample of what I call the "dancing girl treatment services." It was to provide them ten different kinds of services, "nails on wheels," psychiatric care, home visitation, television, all sorts of support services. (I think support services are important within their context.) The research project was going to demonstrate that if you provided all these services you could increase the longevity of the relatively aged population. One of my colleagues who was more quantitatively oriented than I—he runs a big center at the University of Michigan—figured out that this research project was going to cost fifteen thousand dollars per year for each person that was going to be helped and studied.

He said, "What would my Congressman say if he saw this application?" I in my devilish way made the crass suggestion, "Why don't we give them each six thousand dollars and save the government nine thousand dollars per head, and then study the consequences of this?"

I think that if you were to begin to shift around the economic resources, reallocate them, you would begin to see confidence develop in many ways— that often the program does not require the heavy hand of the professional.

Q: If I understand one of your main points correctly, it seems to me that it is quite revolutionary, so I want to make sure I understand it correctly. If two homosexuals adopt a child or two lesbians adopt a child, or if a hippie commune raises children, are you saying that these families are to be treated in a kind of value-free way by the government, and that they are to be dealt with simply as families?

Are you saying that the general attitude toward such families is to be ignored by the governmental agencies? If you are saying this, how do you expect this to happen, as long as society has the attitudes it has toward these activities and this type of family?

A: That is a great question to ask. I won't hedge on it. I think a pluralistic society like ours—and I think it is a great one—has to survive on its tolerance, on allowing people to make their own decisions as to what is best for them.

I happened to look a little bit into the communes. It has become very fashionable to study them; I am not studying communes, but I did take what seems to be a high-powered forum committee out to New Mexico. I decided not to meet in Washington or Philadelphia—too much tradition there—but to take them out to the West, where these communes were. I think even the monsignor on our committee was quite impressed by the honest efforts of the young people to find themselves in a new form of family life, if you will.

I guess I'll have to say that I would go for this kind of toleration. This doesn't necessarily mean that I would choose to live in one of these groups; I am too old, anyway, and I need not tell you what my preferences are. But I think I would stick by their right to do this, and I would fight for the prevention of hoeing them down, of eliminating them. I don't know what the consequences to children are. I think we ought to find out. We certainly have not done so great a job with our children in the traditional manner.

Q: I'd like to ask Mr. Sussman how planning for an improved family through the use of our technological and economic capacity will avoid the problems of social unrest? As Mr. Cutler illustrated in his discussion of the "J" curve, when one is shown something better, his satisfaction with his present state will diminish rapidly and his unrest will be increased.

A: I don't know whether my own work would enable me to handle the global issue you raised. I mentioned using science and technology because I am working with a group which is trying to create new kinds of environment, in terms of physical and social space which you can actually build—what I call a built-in environment—that would meet different problems which now exist. Let me give you a very commonplace example.

There are some family forms that need the kind of housing in which there is a large space, you might call it community space. You can, using the technology we have, at the same cost as you build the very conventional, unimaginative, what we call "plantation estates"—public housing—begin to work it out. We have computer systems that we can feed data into and give you exactly what it would cost to develop an imaginative environment for a family—a large family, if you will.

Or, if you have a family that doesn't want this, or wants the option of not eating in the sterile kitchen we built for them, but of perhaps eating as a group, you could find out what the cost would be, in housing projects for those of middle income or working-class income, to provide the different options of living. When I talk about built-in environments, I am thinking that some of the fundamental unhappiness, the alienation and frustration, comes about from being unmotivated in the usual sterile environments. I would begin there.

I am not sure I can answer your question. I could handle the big problems of unrest, but I have a feeling that the unrest begins in the monotony, the being constrained, the being forced, the being pushed, and not having much to say about what is happening to you. How many people who develop new institutions, or new communities, really pay attention to the people whom they are going to help?

Q: I am with the Philadelphia Bar Association. I was very intrigued with the answer that you gave a moment ago and I was thinking about it. Let me share my thoughts with you.

How is it possible, in a society with a system of private ownership, of private property, as our society is, with laws relating to adultery, fornication, sodomy, and the like on the one hand, and laws relating to the devolution of property upon death and such things as wills acts and intestate acts on the other—how is it possible, with these things on the books as they are, and with the Supreme Court holding, as it did just a few days ago, that an illegitimate child cannot succeed to the property rights of a deceased parent—how is it possible to work it all out? With these things built so strongly into the superstructure of this society, would it not be impossible, without changing the concept of property and the meaning of property and the way property is distributed, to have these forms that you just have spoken about become viable entities within a pluralistic society?

A: This is an excellent observation and question. I think some of the existing legislation structures are being put to the test; they are constantly being put to the test. I just finished a study of inheritance in the family and what it does or doesn't do to the family. I am hoping that as a consequence of this study, with a whole set of recommendations, there may be some reform in the probate process itself and in some of the legislation governing inheritance of property.

I raised these very questions with the people living in the communes. These matters ought to be studied so we can see what the impacts are. I am not convinced as you are that changes cannot be brought about. I see vast changes in divorce laws in this country. I see vast changes in abortion laws in this country. I suspect that it takes the legal system several hundred years to catch up with the world, but it finally does.

Q: I would like to ask a practical question about the low-income individuals living in public housing. How can you expect these people to live on an income of $138 a month and pay a rent of $74? What good are your ideas if people don't have enough to eat?

A: You are perfectly right. I am with you, and I think this is where the basic income, the guaranteed income, is necessary—modifying the social security system. Some efforts are being made to do this. It is one of the essential problems for a minority of people. There are many people who live with relatives, but I am not saying this is a substitute for having an adequate income. I think anything that the professional suggests or recommends, any of these human service systems of providing a better life, has to have the economic base.

I would almost say that each of the forums in the White House Conference came up with the central theme of a reallocation of resources to provide these minimum levels of life for the underprivileged, the aged, and all the groups that we have labeled as deviant. I think that anything else is a sort of trimming on the cake.

Q: As a parent, I am concerned about family disruption in the urban environment. I have children in the Philadelphia public school system and I am in the Home and School Association and I have observed the problems in the urban area up close. It is my observation that much of the disruptive behavior of young people in the urban environment can be linked to families that for a variety of reasons have given up on the management of their children.

You referred to the concept of child management, which I thought was fundamental. The children as a result of this abandonment are relying on their own devices. This results in a great deal of anti-social behavior on the part of groups sometimes characterized as gangs, and in a great many other problems produced by the present urban environment.

A: Maybe we have to work on the resocialization of parents. I don't think much has been done here. We have tended, in much of the effort to "socialize" children, to get the reciprocation of socialization. I think that perhaps even the way we look at it is part of the problem. It is not simply parents shaping and forming children to conform with a growth process involving both. A lot of it has to do with the in-puts the child gets from his parent group, and in school. We find in studying very poor ghetto families that children are much more effective as socialization agents for their parents, because of the exposure to new experiences, new knowledge, and the like.

I wanted, too, to be a sort of devil's advocate in answering the question about disruption. I always felt that a little disruption is very good, that it preconditions for change—makes you begin to think. Many of us have been "shook up" in the last few years by disruptions and we have begun to examine our own cherished hypotheses as a consequence of this.

So, I don't know whether you are talking about blood-thirsty eating or the kind of disruption that one has to learn how to live with in a complex society, which may be part of the training of the child in handling confrontation—I should say (which I did not stress in this paper), in becoming fairly proficient at confrontation. As a matter of fact, I think families might be able to get a better "handle" on the society by helping their children learn skills, and also by confronting injustice rather than accepting it.

You are asking a very direct question because you are bothered by disruption and you are saying, How can we get these parents to do something about it? I am simplifying a very complex question, but I shall ask you to think with me: Who are these parents? What are some of the other hang-ups they have? What other problems are they having—in their marriages? in making a living? What do they know about population control? Maybe they have too many children to pay much attention to any one of them.

There are a lot of things like that about which I can't say, "I'll go in there and preach to them, and I'll get them to do this or that." You just can't do it.

Chapter 3

The Family Nurse Clinician*

Beverly Henry Bowns

Ours is an era of social reorganization which had little to do with careful and effective planning. Much of the change was the result of powerful and uncontrolled social forces. A discernible change has occurred in the health care system, and the *family nurse clinician* is one product of this change. Like an unveiling, the facade has been removed, and the games health professionals have been playing are recognized for what they are—needless manipulative maneuvers. The relationships are becoming more honest, and, more often, actions are in consort. The nurse is no longer to be excluded from the rewards of job satisfaction so important to the professional. As a professional he will have the authority to use his competencies openly and freely and so be recognized for those accomplishments. Anderson (1968) addresses this serious issue of ambiguity in nursing, and Lysaught (1970) indicates the destructiveness of role deprivation. It will be some time before we are able to measure

* This article describes a graduate program for the family nurse practitioner developed by Dr. Beverly Bowns while at Vanderbilt University School of Nursing, Nashville, Tennessee.

the impact of this one change on the delivery of health care since we are not clear about who does what for whom, and in what way, that seems to make a positive difference. Quality care for every recipient is a common goal, but what is to be minimal acceptable quality care and how it is to be monitored are yet undetermined.

EVOLUTIONARY CHANGE

Changes in nursing have been evolutionary ones and not so much a matter of expanding the role. Updating knowledge and skills is a responsible educational pursuit. The report by DeBakey on heart disease, cancer, and stroke (1967) identified the serious lag between application of scientific knowledge to the benefit of the consumer and the initial discovery of the knowledge. When the situation became acute enough and the consumer disgruntled enough, like a convulsion, a multifarious display of effort was initiated, and each new plan was expected to improve the health care of mankind. So it happened that the family nurse clinician was not the only product; the health care market was flooded with new health care workers.

Like a "social patent" each new health worker is labeled, and the label is expected to miraculously communicate to others all the things this person can do under that label. Actually consumer and provider alike are now confused. Unfortunately the image of a nurse may have become even more "diffused"; we were already struggling with the misnomer of "registered nurse" which had three interpretations for the citizen and taxpayer. This social issue has been a singularly costly one, as support of nursing and nursing education has lost out at times when the congressman could not determine what the dollar was going to buy for him in nursing care or nursing education.

Education and Titles

Pediatric assistant, pediatric nurse practitioner, pediatric nurse associate, physician assistant, ambulatory care assistant, physician associate, medex, primex, and family nurse clinician are only some of the titles being used. The January 1972 issue of *Nursing Outlook* discusses extensively the views of some nurses about these "new" roles.

The 500 or more programs across the country fall into three main categories. The product of each category bears the title of the program: (1) physician's assistant or associate, (2) nurse practitioner, and (3) nurse clinician. The *physician's assistant* is trained by a physician to be his subordinate and carry out those technical skills which will free the physician for those tasks more appropriate to his level of training; the education occurs in a physician's office on an apprenticeship basis, in hospital clinics, in agency clinics, in continuing education programs, or in medical schools; the length of the program may vary from 6 weeks to 2 years plus a 1-year internship; the student may receive no credentials at all, a certificate, or a degree; eligibility for entry to the training experience may be determined by physician selection and personal training in his office, referral of nurse by physician, military corpsman experience, or a high school diploma with or without 2 years of college. The title of *associate* was to have identified the specially trained person who works as an extensor of the physician and requires more training, as in Silver's Program at the University of Colorado School of Medicine (American Academy of Pediatrics, 1971). Two difficulties have arisen through the use of this term: (1) some physicians prefer the term be reserved for physician-physician relationships, and (2) nurses resent the term as another "facade mechanism" to make the role of physician's assistant more acceptable to them.

The title *nurse practitioner* is considerably more confusing since the nurses are more often than not physician's assistants and must function in a subordinate position to the physician; the training may be within or outside an institution of higher learning; it may be for as short as 6 weeks or as long as 2 years; the training may be under the direction of a single physician or by nurse-physician collaboration or by physician-nurse teaching teams; the program may be housed in one or the other of the two professional schools, or in an agency; requirements for entry may range from a physician's referral and accompanied agreement to act as preceptor to his student to meeting the admission requirements of a graduate program in an institution of higher learning. At successful completion of the program the student may receive no credentials, a certificate, or a bachelor's or a master's degree. The term *nurse practitioner* generally refers to a nurse with a baccalaureate degree or a nurse who has taken postbaccalaureate work leading to a certificate to be a pediatric nurse practitioner. The term is a misleading one unless one is generalizing about members of the profession of nursing practice. A practitioner can be anyone who is engaged in the practice of his profession or occupation; more simply it refers to anyone who practices something specific. In the culinary arts, it could refer to a practitioner of the art of gourmet cooking.

Medex and Primex are two educational programs which are under study and have received considerable governmental support. *Medex* is a 15-month program developed by a physician and is tailor-made for corpsmen to certify them as physician assistants.

Another program of this kind has been developed at Duke University under the direction of Howard (1971) and admits corpsmen, others with medical experience, and most recently, *nurses.* Similar to many collegiate nursing programs, this is also a 2-year college program for students who have completed 2 years of college. University schools of nursing with undergraduate programs are competing for student brainpower. On campus the competition has been more in terms of other professional school choices, and off campus it has been in terms of associate degree and diploma programs. Even so, baccalaureate programs have continued to increase their enrollment year after year. Medex programs introduce a new demand on the pool of prospective student nurses and an attractive one to some. Nurses and nurses-to-be desire to become more involved in patient care; and the "expanded role" of these programs, on the surface, seems to many to provide that opportunity. Like the layman, nurses are becoming confused by the increased variation of programs and the job careers to which they lead. The baccalaureate programs will have to meet this new competition for student brainpower.

Primex is a continuing education program to prepare family nurse practitioners and accepts all R.N.'s to the program (diploma, A.D., or B.S.) (Walker, 1972). It is a valuable program in that it prepares the nurse who is already on the job, who requires this training to fulfill her job functions, and who does not choose to work toward a degree. As schools of nursing begin to include more and more of this content in their undergraduate programs, Primex and pediatric practitioner programs will become less necessary. The baccalaureate graduate will have those very same competencies and more.

A *nurse clinician* is a master clinician. This is a person who has a master's degree in nursing or a nurse with a master's in an allied field; the candidate has met the admission requirements of the university of her choice; the program may range from 1 year of intensive graduate study to 2 years that includes an "internship"; at successful completion of the work, the student receives a master of science degree. In the future and until the matter of legalities in practice are resolved, the master clinician may also receive a certificate, i.e., midwifery. The term *clinician* connotes a high level of expertise and professional stature as an independent agent who can be depended upon to carry out her own decisions and assume her own responsibility for those decisions. She is equally competent as an interdependent team member who can work in consort with other professionals as a colleague. Although the legal aspects receive considerable attention, they are not irresolvable. The political-economic issues may be of much greater magnitude and are more likely to place undesirable controls on nurses' functions in the planned advancement of health care services, as health in this nation has become "big business."

HEALTH CARE PROVIDER

How can the health care system be changed to provide care that is acceptable, available, and accessible to the consumer? What aspects of the changes need to be made collaboratively by nursing and medicine to alter the present role relationship, thus reducing the territorial factor while increasing the flexibility of the system to make it more responsive to consumer needs?

Identified Need for Change

It is generally recognized that a state of crisis exists in health care and health care systems in this nation (U.S. Congress, 1970). The dilemma is commonly attributed to the manpower shortage among the health professions and to the lack of an adequate system for delivery of health services. These two factors are so interrelated that any action to correct the malfunctioning of one may be expected to have an effect in bringing about change in the other. This chapter addresses the problem from the standpoint of the educational preparation of existing manpower—the professional nurse, namely, the community health nurse family clinician. The titles *community health nurse family clinician* and *family nurse clinician* are used interchangeably.

The assumption is that there is a chain effect in the system whereby a nurse on the health care team who is trained to function at a high level of competency can be depended upon, by her professional colleagues, to make accurate, independent judgments in the area of primary care; can be relied upon to perform the interdependent role of health care in consort; will more adequately meet consumer health demands and needs; will experience greater satisfaction from the expert application of her knowledge and skills; and will attain the professional status that produces greater career commitment. This will attract more young people to nursing plus retain more nurses in active practice. Adequately prepared and appropriately utilized manpower provides a built-in human force to facilitate and create positive change over time. In this way, by avoiding obsolescence, we can hope to prevent the necessity for the expensive remedial, stopgap measures mentioned earlier which are presently required to patch this system's deficiencies.

The evidence indicated that physicians and nurses cluster in large centralized medical centers (American Nurses' Association, 1969). Nurses with expertise in episodic care specialties are needed in these centralized areas if we are to achieve the regional planning recommended in the report by De-Bakey (1967). However, the trend of the vanishing general practitioner is real and one that requires a concurrent readjustment in our health care delivery system. Preventive and promotive health care management must become as much a part of health management as episodic care is, if we are to have quality care and it is to be randomly distributed and not assigned to specified groups by age, location, race, or social class.

The change required is one that avoids preparing only nurses specialized in the care of episodic illness or the reinforcement of the traditional hierarchial management of care. The objective is to free capable people to function as nurses with independent clinical expertise, in the diversified way most needed for ambulatory care, which is *majority care* (U.S. Department of Health, Education, and Welfare, 1970).

The need for primary care personnel becomes clear when one considers that in 1 year over 100 million visits are made to out-patient services in contrast to the 25 million admissions to the general hospital short-term care facilities (Ribicoff, 1970, pp. 18–20). Knowing that at least one-half of those receiving short-term care in hospitals would benefit from follow-up care when they return to their homes and that people who are in early stages of illness require care gives some indication of the size of this aspect of the problem. In a nation as advanced as ours, preventive and promotive services that would reduce the numbers of people becoming ill in the first place become a vital factor of the equation.

Inappropriate use, as well as inappropriate distribution, of personnel confounds the manpower shortage. For example, pediatricians spend over 60 percent of their time attending minor illnesses and examining well children (Bergman, 1966). Physicians in internal medicine state that 90 to 95 percent of the disease entities they encounter are easy to diagnose and treat, and only 5 to 10 percent of the diseases will be difficult to diagnose (Beaudry, 1970).

Consumers in core city and isolated rural areas are confronted daily by the need for services that are not available to them. Much of the service could be provided by the nurse, but she lacks the preparation for competent action. These nurses have had first-hand experience with programs like Medicaid which are compounded by social upheaval and increased consumer demands.

The large number of community health nurses who have requested or are requesting to enter programs which prepare them to meet these needs is evidence that they recognize the need for additional skills. Interviews with these nurses would indicate that the existing programs do not prepare them adequately for services they are expected to deliver or that they believe to be best for their patients.

The educational system is responsible for preparation of these practitioners and sets the standards for the practice of that service; that is the position taken by this author. *A diversified health care worker is a nurse* capable of functioning appropriately in some of the same ways as a physician while retaining an ability to give quality nursing care to families needing (1) care of common illnesses, (2) care of chronic long-term illness, (3) preventive services, (4) family health counseling, and (5) health education. All are functions that make it possible to bring about change in the quality and in the delivery of health care. This more completely prepared professional would be vital to the health maintenance and disease prevention aspects of the health system (Lysaught, 1970).

In principle, it has been shown that the generalist is a useful resource and is available, accessible, and acceptable to the recipients of care. Much of the evidence indicates that it is the community health nurse who continues to provide the bulk of health services in the rural and ghetto areas. In some instances, she is the only immediate resource for health care. Because of the increased responsibility placed on nurses working in these areas, they could benefit greatly by having the knowledge and skill of a nurse clinician, either by entering the program themselves or by accepting graduates from the program in these areas of greatest need.

The situation is an amenable one, and preparing a nurse clinician to enter the health care system for the purpose of delivering better health care to more of the population is a positive action. The diversification of proficiencies the family nurse clinician will have acquired from an educational program of study meeting these goals will have a fulcrum effect of coordination that seems to be lacking in the health care delivery we experience today.

Nurses and physicians involved in the education of nurses at the level defined above are convinced that the education must be more advanced than that for physician assistant or nurse practitioner. More than having some time saved, the physician and every other team member must have the peace of mind that high-level decisions can be made reliably and the assurance that the person making the decision will accept responsibility for the actions. A team unit is no more effective than the individual strengths of its members.

The training of a family nurse clinician requires 1 to 2 years of postgraduate education. The basic education must be of equally high quality. Students entering the master's degree program at Vanderbilt University, for example, must have a baccalaureate degree from a National League for Nursing accredited collegiate school of nursing, have a grade point average of 2 point on a 3-point scale, and have acceptable scores on both the Graduate Record Exam and the Miller Analogies Test.

The baccalaureate program curricula requirements are the sound, scientific base upon which a family nurse clinician program must rely. Most would agree that well-rounded baccalaureate programs appeal to the brighter students and enhance the scope of the intellectual thinking that contributes to creativity. These programs attract people with the desired potential. A scientific base for nursing is essential; and general chemistry, general organic chemistry, botany, physics, general zoology, anatomy and physiology, bacteriology, sometimes microbiology and epidemiology, pathophysiology, and advanced organic chemistry are included. In the applied sciences sociology, anthropology, political science, general psychology, and psychosociological courses are prerequisite for nursing majors. In some schools introduction to research methods, statistics, advanced mathematics, and calculus are included.

The nursing courses are generally focused on producing what is referred to as the "thinking nurse," and old, traditional curricula have given way to those labeled as "integrated." Problem solving and the cognitive process, psychosocial aspects of nursing, physiopsychosocial nursing care, interview and observation techniques, advanced physiology and illness, advanced physiology and wellness, ecology of community health, family health, long-term illness, and the aging process are examples of the content in undergraduate programs. These generic programs are intended to prepare the first-level generalist. An analogy in medicine is the general practitioner.

Some changes have appeared fairly recently, and we now hear about the baccalaureate program which will produce a generalist with certification as a midwife in addition to a bachelor's degree. Other schools plan curricula where a core of basic general nursing knowledge is obtained, and then the nurse may choose acute episodic care nursing or community primary care nursing at the undergraduate level of her education. Still others provide pediatric practitioners (certified) within the degree program. The B.S. degree, plus a certificate, is usually designed to give the nurse a sound generalist background, while in her senior year she is given the opportunity to complete work in a primary interest area and become certified in that semispecialty.

The graduate program is to produce the highly specialized, skilled clinicians as exemplified by the family nurse clinician program. By basing the advanced education on undergraduate work, the educator makes use of skills the student already has, such as identifying nursing needs through skillful interviews, observation and communication skills which are well-developed, and the ability to make a nursing diagnosis and determine a plan of care. As capable as the bachelor degree graduates may be in these skills, much more is required of the nurse in the community of our time. A marriage of nursing theory and skills with primary care knowledge and skills combines the required proficiencies in a single person who is where the patient is when the care is needed and can effectively and efficiently give that care. Much can be said for having such a person available to patients.

The program goals are fourfold: (1) to provide the nurse with content and experiences essential to *preventive* and *promotive* health care maintenance; (2) to provide training in the *curative, restorative,* and *preventive* components of illnesses; (3) to provide interdisciplinary learning situations for learning teammanship in ambulatory health care; and (4) to do research on the effectiveness of the family nurse clinician in relation to consumer satisfaction, clinician job satisfaction, and employer satisfaction.

The program design provides learning situations in the community: evaluation of health status of families and communities, improvement of family problem solving and coping skills in adapting to change, understanding of political implications in community action groups, and direct guidance to families. These are the *preventive* and *promotive* functions inherent in health maintenance.

Adjunct to the first goal is to prepare the nurse to give primary care to ambulatory patients at their point of entry into the health care system. More simply he is where the consumers are, and so he is available and must be prepared to care for them. The theoretical content and clinical experiences needed are those inherent in the care of emergencies, diagnosis of common illnesses, management of stabilized chronic disease, rehabilitation and long-term care of the aging, comprehensive screening skills, all in order to give safe, accurate, quality care and to make appropriate expedient referrals. These are the *curative, restorative,* and *preventive* components of nursing care of the ill.

Unquestionably the "team concept" of health care is not a reality nor an effective functioning unit of today's health services delivery system. Cardinal to this position is the fact that we are not certain who the "team" is, who we want it to be, or even what we mean by health team care. In the author's interpretation one thing is a certainty—the consumer is a team member in all instances. Critical to the problem is the prototype for educating professionals in "parallel tracks" rather than in "collaborative work situations." It is no wonder we are unsuccessful in formulating collaborative health care teams in professional practice. So, rather than settle for course work together, the team in consort must have clinical learning experiences together while they are students.

A fourth goal is the evaluation and research that are needed to gain a better understanding about clinician-patient transactions, i.e., what the clinician does, when it is done, who else is giving care, and what circumstances seem to be of greatest help to the consumer. Our nation has the potential for scientific education and effective implementation of skills, and the measurement of the success is the educated talent available for health service.

Role Description

Unlike primary care, prevention of illness sometimes requires unsolicited entry into the lives of individuals and families. It is in this setting that health problems are hidden or denied. One way to cope with this situation is to have teams of health workers cooperatively managing population units which are identified by geographical boundaries or by clinical catchment areas. The family nurse working in this fashion will be in a better position to assess community actions needed to meet family and community health needs. The community approach to health is a reasonable one where the combined resources can be brought to bear on a health problem. By incorporating the functions of primary care and preventive care in a single health profession, more effective management of the health care of individuals, families, and communities can be accomplished. The family nurse clinician will be able to bring competency to the problem by using his skills in other organizational arrangements such as a member of group practice with physicians; outpatient staffs; agency staffs such as the Frontier Nursing Service; or core city neighborhood centers, satellite clinics, public health centers, visiting nursing service, and mental health centers (see Figure 3-1).

In the area of primary care, the family nurse clinician will be capable of assessing, diagnosing, and treating common illnesses of ambulatory patients at the point of entry into the health care system. Through a careful history-taking process, the interpretation of laboratory findings, and a physical examination, the nurse will determine the health status of individuals and families. The nurse is responsible and accountable for four broad areas of decision making:

1 If the data collected and assessed indicate that the family obtained medical assistance when it was appropriate and demonstrated an ability to carry out prescribed recommendations accurately and effectively, then the family would be considered capable of managing its own health care in terms of illnesses. In these situations the clinician would rely on other team members, professional (school participants, social workers) and nonprofessional (babysitting services, neighborhood workers), to help meet the family's health needs of primary prevention and promotion of health. Under the clinician's guidance, health programs may be "tailor-made" for each family's health potential.

2 If the individual and family health assessment presents a specified set of short-term primary care treatments with predictable outcomes, and if the expected results are not realized within a reasonable time, the clinician will initiate another course of action.

3 When the prescribed treatment of a common illness does not produce the expected response, the clinician will collaborate with the appropriate specialist, the pediatrician, the psychiatric social worker, pediatric nurse clinician, and similar professional persons. Alternate actions will arise which may or may not be the clinician's responsibility, and the referral will be completed. It is expected that the case will be referred back when the highly specialized care is accomplished, and mechanisms for maintaining continuity will be an integral part of the clinician's actions.

4 The evidence obtained from the assessment process presents a complexity of alternatives that does not identify a specific disease entity but clearly denotes the need for follow-up by a specialist, the case would be referred and the screening data forwarded to the specialist for diagnosis and care. Interceding for the patient in this manner will expedite the delivery of care by getting the consumer to the proper resource with less stress and time

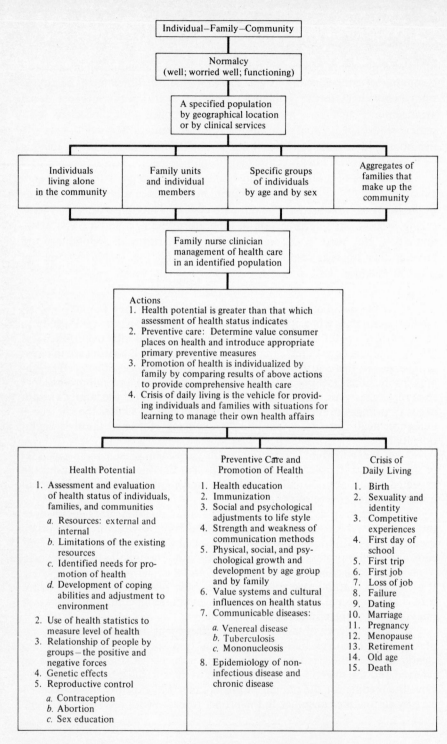

Figure 3-1 Health maintenance and disease preventive components in the management of health care of individual families and communities.

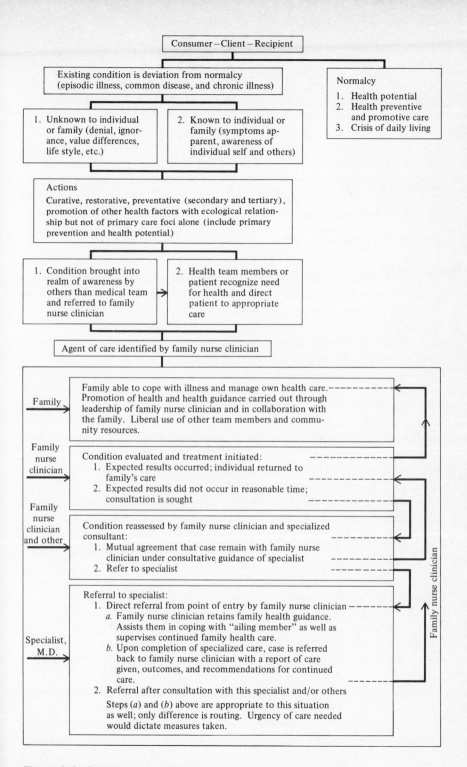

Figure 3-2 Primary care component of management of health care of families and individuals.

loss. The specialist is saved the routine "work-up" on the patient. The family nurse clinician would continue her services to the family, coordinating her efforts with those of other team members.

As described, the family nurse clinician is a member of the health care team who can be depended on to take independent actions as well as those interdependent ones associated with team practice (see Figure 3-2).

EDUCATIONAL PURSUIT

Program of Study

Prerequisite to the successful training of a family nurse clinician is a program of study and experiences imperative to providing the best possible clinical expert to meet the prescribed standards. The curriculum design presented in this section is not a static one, and content and experiences change when faculty and student evaluations identify a better means of meeting the defined goals. Other evaluation results are systematically collected and analyzed to be used in redesigning courses for the following year.

The program this author is most familiar with is completed within 1 calendar year, over three 16-week semesters and does not conform to the school's calendar of two 16-week semesters and a 10-week summer session. It is a rigorous, intensive, action-learning program of study that has broken with the traditional educational patterns of the school in which it is housed. The program was developed collaboratively between a school of nursing and a school of medicine. The teaching is accomplished by nurse-physician teaching teams in all clinical courses and in two of the more didactic courses.

In the first semester, in addition to statistics, advanced physiology, and pharmacology, there is an intensive lecture-laboratory series in physical examination and history taking which is liberally distributed across the 4 months of the first semester and sets the common framework for future course study and experiences on the clinical rotations.

A three-semester family nurse clinician seminar in community health nurse clinical practice runs concurrently with the other studies.

In the first semester of this series of seminars, the focus is on the student's current experiences in the role socialization process. This is achieved through group team sessions and through extensive reading and discussion sessions about the numerous other programs that prepare other kinds of health care workers.

The last two semesters of the seminar the nurses are assigned families in the community. In these sessions the concepts and principles of psychosocial health care which are to be integrated in all the clinical interactions with recipients of care are introduced. The family nurse seminar is also the arena for synthesis of concepts and principles learned in the other courses and clinical activities, thus helping to promote the integration of primary care with nursing care functions. This dual process of comprehensive care continues throughout the two semesters with special emphasis on family nursing care functions.

Upon completion of the seminar, there are four 2-month rotations: (1) adult physical illness, common and chronic; (2) child health care, both well children and those with common illnesses; (3) gynecology and obstetrics which includes delivery, planned parenthood, and care of patients in menopause; and (4) community health clinical experience in a rural and an urban community. Research methodology and an epidemiologic study of the area assigned for the summer rotation complete the course requirements.

The first year of employment after graduation is considered a residency experience. The salary the family nurse clinician will receive in residency is equivalent to that of a master's degree nurse. At the end of the first year, the salary will be negotiable and should fall somewhere between that of a master's degree nurse and that of a physician.

As the program matures, much of the physical examination and history-taking content will be moved to the undergraduate level; this is the prevailing pattern in other nursing schools in the country. Pathophysiology may necessarily need to receive special emphasis in the undergraduate years as this seems to be one of the weaker areas of the nurse's prior education. Learning the normal and moving toward the abnormal would be the desirable sequence.

Introduction to research and statistics certainly is undergraduate work and can only strengthen the scientific productiveness of nursing students as would the early introduction of epidemiology and community health organization.

Political science would be most useful. This does not preclude that more advanced course work in some of these same areas is not to continue. The strengthening of the undergraduate work simply provides a sounder base for any graduate nursing program, including the family nurse clinician program.

It is evident that flexibility in curriculum design must be possible and tolerable to the school's administrative leaders. Flexibility is necessary, and freedom to break with tradition within reasonable limits is essential.

For example, students would not be required to repeat work they have already had or already know. A midwife entering this program would be evaluated by a nurse-physician team of the faculty experts in obstetrics and gynecology. If the student was found to meet the school's required standards, then the student would omit that portion of her studies. If she met most of the requirements, she would be permitted to take only that content required to bring her knowledge up to the expectations of the program faculty.

Program Strands

A most valued and dominant educational concern of the nurse-faculty teaching team member is that of *relating all learning experiences to the family developmental unit* in a community setting which may or may not be conducive to healthy living. This ecosystem approach provides the framework for the integration of psychosocial, economic, political, and cultural community organization theoretical concepts to nursing care practice. The *role socialization process* is so completely a part of the learning experience and the success of the role function that it, too, is a dominant strand in the program.

Contributing strands to the theoretical framework of the teaching-learning process are: (1) therapeutic communication, (2) health education through problem solving (a teaching-learning process), (3) man's adaptation to environmental forces, (4) diagnosis and the decision-making process, (5) family group dynamics (6) continuity and coordination of nursing care to patients and their families, (7) application of research in clinical practice and use of epidemiologic methods and vital statistics in identifying researchable problems having implications for nursing.

Through the team-teaching method, application of nursing theory to the clinical experiences will be enhanced. This is to say, conceptual content recognized as being theory common to both disciplines will enable nurse-faculty teams to blend primary care with all other nursing care actions in the student learning situation. In these ways the curriculum will provide for the achievement of the objectives.

Objectives

The major objective of the curriculum is to prepare the graduate community health nurse to function as a family nurse clinician in the ambulatory setting in the delivery of comprehensive health care to the family unit through involving the family in its own health education process and through the purposeful use of techniques and strategies of care that help families to cope with the crisis of daily living.

Some of the contributing objectives are as follows:

1 To demonstrate an ability to analyze health problems, across all age groups, in a systematic, scientific manner which utilizes a sound theoretical framework for nursing actions

2 To be able to demonstrate the competent application of knowledge and use of skills following an accurate assessment of the physical, psychological, and social health status of family units and of individuals

3 To be able to evaluate the appropriateness of the implementation and the results of planned health care actions in relation to mutual nurse-consumer goals

4 To be able to assess the forces which are directly and indirectly affecting the community's health and to plan for facilitating change through consumer-health profession collaborative efforts

5 To continue to define and evaluate the role of the family nurse clinician in order to initiate changes in the health care system

6 To work collaboratively with other health workers (professionals and nonprofessionals) in the continued reorganization of the health care system's method of delivery by initiation of those changes essential to improve the quality of care the consumer receives

7 To participate with nurse clinicians and other researchers in the formulation of nursing theory that embraces the ecological approach to health care

8 To function as a family nurse clinician role model, as an independent entrepreneur in giving direct care, as an interdependent member of a health care team, and as an educator in clinical practice

Socialization Process Strand

Although the socialization process has been mentioned as a concern, it requires more detailed discussion. Other program directors, in earlier programs, discovered that supplying the student with greater knowledge did not ensure that he would achieve fulfillment in the working world of the health care system. Both nurses and physicians had difficulty accepting the fact that these new practitioners could function differently and with a greater range of competencies.

The socialization process of the family nurse clinician into a new role cannot be left to chance and to idiosyncratic talents of the nurses graduating from this program. The role deprivation phenomenon previously experienced by nurse midwifery in this country, before the sixties, is to be avoided. The clinical experience will provide the real situation where the students will be left to depend on their own coping abilities in order to function. A seminar for discussion and sharpening of problem-solving skills will accompany the clinical experiences. As discussed earlier, the graduates of the program are to be placed in positions where the employer or colleague (1) desires the family nurse clinician, (2) is willing to participate in the evaluation involved, and/or (3) has some clearly communicated perceptions that denote an understanding of how this new health worker can work independently as well as interdependently using all the knowledge and skills with which he is prepared. To assure that purposeful efforts are made to accomplish the role socialization, a specialist in human behavior was added to the program to teach this content area.

The socialization phase of the program, as developed by Dr. Edwin Bartee, professor of management, will consist of an experience-based process of education in which the graduate nursing student will be exposed to four different phases of learning.

1 *Personalization phase* This phase will give emphasis to the individual student as a learner in a small-group context. Matters related to giving and receiving feedback, helper and receiver roles, individual roles in task groups, independent learning, and self-actualization will be dealt with. Role playing and game exercises will be used to facilitate the learning process.

2 *Collaboration phase* Issues related to group dynamics, leadership, tolerance for conflict, group norms, and evaluation will be given emphasis in this phase. The student will be placed in circumstances that will emphasize his role as a group member contributing to common objectives.

3 *Institutionalization phase* In this phase the student will be exposed to learning experiences that give emphasis to the relationship between informal and formal relationships. Particular issues related to organizational structure, institutional norms, tolerance for ambiguity, and role performance will be dealt with in an experience-based mode of learning.

4 *Socialization phase* This final phase will facilitate the student's self-awareness as a social being. Problems related to communication, empathy, and cooperation with other professionals and with client personnel will be given particular emphasis. Developing a greater tolerance for individual differences will be a main thrust of this final phase.

Experimentally, Bartee has conducted sessions to help professionals learn to work collaboratively and to learn more about each other. A student family nurse clinician participates in these sessions. It is planned that faculty and students of both professions will form groups of this kind to determine how they can work with each other (and with others) in the clinical setting for the benefit of the patient.

CONCLUSION

The professional health worker has been oriented primarily toward the family as individuals rather than as a unit. This has had an adverse effect on the consumer as it feeds into the pattern of illness. As Satir (1967, p. 2) has stated, family members can and do interfere with an individual's recovery by overprotectiveness and by perpetuating the person's illness; family members use illness of one of the members as a defense to excuse themselves for any number of malfunctioning behaviors. It is a reasonable and realistic consideration that we prepare a nurse clinician for family care at a high level of professional competency. This requires a diversified worker who is prepared to function across all age groups with families within a specified segment of the population, use his own competencies to their limit, and enlist the talents of others when that is the logical means of meeting the consumer's needs and demands. The family nurse clinician may conduct morning clinics in chronic disease, common illness of children, well child clinics, family clinics, maternity clinics, family-planning clinics—a different clinic each day of the week. In the afternoons he may make home visits to specific families with complex problems where family counseling is needed on a continuous but short-term basis. He may work with a group of consumers and a team of professionals to initiate new health facilities or to find new ways of modifying the health care delivery system to make it a more satisfactory one. He may provide inservice education to other nurses and develop teams of workers to assist in clinics, community agencies, out-patient departments, or physicians' offices. He may act as consultant to laymen, legislators, community leaders, other professionals, etc. Specialization among the professions is required; but the diversified family nurse clinician is needed equally as much, if not more, since his concerns are with majority care, that is, ambulatory care of the well, worried well, and the borderline "nearly well." He can work wherever he happens to be: in a sophisticated group practice of physician specialists or in an outpost in Alaska.

BIBLIOGRAPHY

American Academy of Pediatrics: *An Accumulative Listing Reference List of Paramedical Training Programs in Pediatrics,* 1971.

American Nurses Association: *Facts about Nursing,* New York: American Nurses Association Publication, 1969.

Anderson, O. W.: *Toward an Unambiguous Profession? A Review of Nursing,* Center for Health Administration Studies, Graduate School of Business, Chicago: University of Chicago, 1968.

Beaudry, C., et al.: "Decision-making and Diagnosis," *Diagnostica,* 17:22, 1970.

Bergman, A. B., S. W. Dassel, and R. Wedgwood: "Time-Motion Study of Practicing Pediatricians," *Pediatrics,* 38:245–263, 1966.

DeBakey, Michael E.: *Report to the President (A National Program to Conquer Heart Disease, Cancer and Stroke),* Washington, D.C.: U.S. Government Printing Office, I, 1967.

Grupenhoff, J. T.: *Ad Hoc Committee on the Nation's Health Crisis,* H. R. Bill 18515.

Howard, R. D.: "Physician's Assistant Program," paper given at Tennessee Conference on Roles, Law, and Practice, sponsored by TNA, guests TMA and THA, 1971.

Lysaught, J. P.: *An Abstract for Action: National Commission for the Study of Nursing and Nursing Education,* New York: McGraw-Hill Book Company, 1970.

Ribicoff, A.: "The Healthiest Nation Myth," *Saturday Review,* 53:18–20, 1970.

Satir, V.: *Conjoint Family Therapy,* Palo Alto, Calif.: Science and Behavior Books, Inc., 1967.

U.S. Congress, Senate: *National Health Insurance and Health Security,* 91st Cong., 2d Sess., S. doc. 4297, 1970.

U.S. Department of Health, Education, and Welfare: *A Conceptual Model of Organized Primary Care and Comprehensive Community Health Service,* 1970.

Walker, E.: "Primex: The Family Nurse Practitioner Program," *Nursing Outlook,* **12**:28-31, 1972.

Chapter 4

Family Medicine

Lynn P. Carmichael

The traditional concepts and established methods of medical practice in the United States are currently being challenged at many levels by a dissatisfied public. The emergence of family medicine as an academic discipline represents a distinct departure from these established patterns by providing a new kind of medical care. Without relinquishing medicine's traditional concern and responsibility for the maintenance of life, family medicine places equal emphasis on the maintenance of health and the quality of life. By accepting as its area of responsibility and expertise the continuing health maintenance of the family, family medicine offers a more meaningful and affirmative approach to meeting the health needs of contemporary society.

DEVELOPMENTAL BACKGROUND

At the beginning of the twentieth century in the United States, physicians were preoccupied with becoming recognized as members of a legitimate profession based on scientific knowledge and methods. Throughout the previous century, a scarcity of licensing regulations had permitted virtually anyone who called himself a doctor to treat patients as a medical practitioner. Numerous healing cults had engendered a plethora of mystical "healers" and magical "cures." A proliferation of proprietary schools of medicine with few regulatory or educational standards filled the country with physicians who had received mediocre or poor training. The reputation of medical practitioners was further diminished by constant professional infighting.

In the post-Civil War period, the national ethos of progress reached even into the field of medical science. In a utilitarian society that was interested not in identifying causes but, rather, in finding cures, medical research was not supported until such discoveries as insulin and sulfa demonstrated to the public the pragmatic, beneficial implications of medical investigation. Under the influence of Sir William Osler, medicine began to seek identification of specific etiological agents of disease in order to then develop controls for disease. Support of medical research grew as continued progress, especially in the field of infectious diseases, gained momentum and led to improved treatment and control of disease.

As the United States entered the twentieth century, medical research was becoming generally accepted as a valuable pursuit. The milestone *Flexner Report* in 1910 further substantiated the scientific basis of medicine and led to the improvement of medical education by placing the medical school in the university, which, it asserted, was the proper home for medical education and research.

In the era that followed the *Flexner Report,* more important medical discoveries, better organization by the medical profession, and legislation of controls over the licensing of medical practitioners led to greater public respect for the medical profession. As their professional status became more secure, medical men grew increasingly more preoccupied with expansion and improvement of medical knowledge and techniques. Greater emphasis was placed on the objective, scientific nature of medicine, less on the supportive role of the doctor. This process perpetuated the problem-solving approach of seeking causes, controls, and cures for disease. As its scientific foundation took shape, medicine became ever more rational and objective. The growth of medical research activities, particularly after the Second World War, was accompanied by an enormous surge of medical knowledge, the development and refinement of medical and surgical techniques, and revolutionary advances in medical technology. In recent decades, the advances have accelerated, producing reverberations of profound ethical and social dimensions in the study and practice of medicine.

The impact of medical progress is clearly illustrated by changing patterns of mortality and morbidity. In the past, actue infectious diseases such as malaria, influenza, and polio were major causes of death and permanent disability. With the development and distribution of vaccines, penicillin, sulfa drugs, and antibiotics, most of these diseases can now be controlled or prevented; and the threat of others such as smallpox and diphtheria has virtually been eliminated.

While the prevalence of severe, acute illnesses is declining, physicians must increasingly deal with chronic illnesses, which have become the chief causes of morbidity and death. In treating chronic diseases like cancer, heart disease, or diabetes, the physician may be unable to cure the patient in the traditional sense. Instead, his major role is helping the patient restore and maintain his physical and psychological equilibrium. The physician can save the patient's life with digitalis, insulin, or other chemotherapeutic agents; but management of patients with heart disease or diabetes requires extensive and often elaborate treatment over a long period of time.

The ability to manage chronic illnesses for long periods of time has had complex social and ethical ramifications. Scientific advances that have created the possibility of heart transplants and artificial kidney machines have raised critical questions regarding the determination of death and criteria for determining who among the many desperately in need will or will not receive new, artificial, or mechanical organs.

Prolongation of life has also created a generational crisis at the distant end of the age scale. A large and growing population of elderly persons is facing poverty, loneliness, and misery in a society that is wholly oriented toward youth. The aged often find themselves rejected by their own families as well as by the rest of society, and are confined to nursing or rest homes or golden age ghettos.

Unfortunately, advances in science and technology have not been accompanied by progress in humanistic, organizational, and economic aspects of medical care. The great emphasis in medicine remains on the diagnosis and treatment of symptoms. While this is unquestionably an essential approach, it is geared toward responding to the overt demands of the sick patient, while it neglects his unspoken needs. The rational, scientific orientation of physicians has made doctors both perpetrators and victims of what Roszak (1969) calls the "myth of objectivity," that is, so great a concern for the scientific and rational aspects of disease that much of health and illness that lies outside the realm of medical science is ignored.

The rise of the hospital as medical center is an apt illustration of the sacrifice of humanistic medical values on the altar of medical science and technology. As new medical knowledge became overwhelming in scope, doctors began to specialize in narrower areas so that they would be more knowledgeable about a particular field. Because most severe illness cases were generally found in the hospital, these specialists tended to congregate in the hospital, which became the center of medical research and education, in affiliation with university-based medical schools. Moreover, the prohibitively high cost of technical equipment for diagnostic tests and therapeutic management restricted their availability for doctors with private practices in the community. But hospitals had large budgets and better facilities, could purchase these machines and materials, and could provide them to the many doctors on their staff.

Concentration of manpower and technology further attracted physicians to hospital-based or hospital-oriented specialty practice. As centralization increased, the number of hospital-based specialists also rose, while the number of family physicians and other primary care physicians—the doctors who provide first contact for their patients with the health care system—declined drastically. People who could not find or afford primary care elsewhere looked to the hospital for it, especially to the hospital emergency room. Other medical and medically related services subsequently became concentrated in the hospital as well.

But these changes were for the most part unplanned, and hospitals are not adequately organized or equipped to handle the various demands made on them. They continue to be clinical institutions suited to the needs of the medical professions rather than to those of the sick patient. Today's hospital-trained physicians frequently find themselves unprepared to deliver medical care in the ambulatory setting of their offices when they start to practice. They may feel more confident in the hospital, and may hospitalize their patients unnecessarily to satisfy their own anxieties, giving little consideration to the emotional and financial stresses that hospitalization may place on the patient and his family.

The alienation and impersonality that characterize contemporary society are intensified in the large modern hospital, at a time when the individual may be in greatest need of personal attention and emotional support. Once in the hospital, particularly in a public or teaching hospital, the patient virtually loses his identity and becomes a "case," presenting certain common, classical, or unusual symptoms. If he has an unusual or medically interesting condition, he may become a victim of what Greenburg (1965) calls "assembly-line medicine," a process which may begin even before he enters the hospital, in which he is examined by a series of consultants and specialists and handled by a variety of other medical personnel. Each consultant is paid on a fee-for-service basis, and any kind of personal relationship between doctor and patient in this setting is usually lacking or transient. The physician views the patient as a person with symptoms that indicate a problem within his range of expertise. To the patient, his physician and consultants are scientific technicians who represent more tests and more bills, as the traditional role of the doctor as comforter has been superseded by the physician as an objective—and expensive—clinician.

Skyrocketing costs, decreased quality and availability of general medical services, and dehumanization of medical care have touched off a consumer rebellion against the medical profession and the present health care delivery system. The disparity between health needs and medical services has led to public demands on the medical establishment to shift its emphasis from medical science to medical care. The people are rejecting the fragmented system of hospital-based, disease-oriented, assembly-line medicine. They are demanding a "repersonalization" of medical care. Whereas recent generations of physicians have had little social or community orientation and have provided medical care as a privilege to those who could afford it, consumer activism and political agitation are forcing doctors to acknowledge health care as a right and to reassess and broaden their concepts of medical practice.

THE CONCEPT OF FAMILY MEDICINE

Family medicine is a new concept in medicine, designed to meet the health care needs of the public in a more responsive and responsible manner. The physician trained in family medicine assumes primary responsibility for both the acute medical care and the continuing health maintenance of the family. By treating family units as well as individuals and by practicing continuous and primary health care, the family physician personalizes medical care and can be more effective and far-reaching in treating not only the demands of illness but also the patient's frequently unspoken needs. And by the practice of this kind of medicine, which includes and emphasizes preventive techniques and early detection and treatment of disease, he is able to reduce the need for hospitalization.

Family medicine departs from the traditional approach which is limited to diagnosis and treatment of symptoms. The family physician is oriented more positively to the prevention of disease and the maintenance of good health. He thinks of health not simply as the absence of disease, but rather, as defined by the World Health Organization, as the optimal state of physical, mental, and social health. Included in his view of health care are the knowledge and application of medicine for physical ailments, behavioral science for emotional problems, and community dynamics for social aspects of health and disease.

The family physician deals with his patients as members of family units, viewing the family as the basic unit of social organization, the functional interdependent group with which the individual establishes primary relationships. The organizational form of the family varies and may have a nuclear, extended, communal, or other type of structure. Nevertheless, as the source of the individual's primary relationships and interactions, the family is naturally the primary unit of health management.

The family doctor takes a holistic, patient- and family-centered approach in delivering health care. He views his patients as unique individuals, greater than the sum of their complaints and symptoms. Whereas other specialties deal with specific problem areas or age or sex groupings, family medicine trains physicians who do not differentiate and limit their patient populations by such criteria. Education in family medicine is designed to prepare the physician for medical practice by combining hospital training with extensive training in ambulatory care. For although the family physician needs to have the knowledge gained by hospital experience, most of the problems brought in to his office are not life-threatening or serious enough to require hospitalization. It is more important that the family physician be a competent diagnostician and have a functional knowledge of epidemiologic methods to determine the frequency of common diseases in his patient population, for he must be an expert in the management of common illness. Family medicine also attunes the physician to the interrelatedness of biological, social, and emotional components of health and illness, and provides him with problem-solving techniques for handling undifferentiated or nonspecific illnesses and for psychosomatic conditions.

This perspective enables the family physician to recognize historical, environmental, or other nonclinical factors that a specialist might not uncover. The family doctor can also assist the specialist in the long-term management of a patient, complementing the specialist's occasional patient contact through his long-term relationship with the patient.

In the case of a patient with a chronic disease, for example, the specialist may prescribe medication and therapy to treat the patient's physical complaints. The illness may be controlled and the risk of disability reduced, but not without considerable economic and emotional strain on the patient and his family. For the patient with a chronic condition, and in some cases for his family, guidance for social and psychological adjustment may be as important as, or more so, than guidance for physical treatment and adaptation. The interrelationships of the social, emotional, and biological components of disease are never more evident than in the case of a patient dying of cancer or that of a small child with a congenital defect struggling to adapt to his condition and his environment. The family physician is specifically trained and prepared to help his patient through this lengthy and difficult process.

This broad-based approach is essential for the practice of comprehensive care, which is the responsibility of the family physician. Comprehensive care involves concern both with demands, for which the patient seeks care, and with needs, of which the family or individual may be unaware. The degree of "comprehensiveness" is the extent to which the needs as well as the demands are met. To achieve this, the family physician works with other professionals

Table 4-1   Components of Family Medicine*

	Discipline	Specialty	Practice
Where based	University	Profession	Community
Who involved	Allied professions	Certified M.D.'s	Practitioners
To whom responsible	Academy	Specialty organizations	Public (licensure)
What concern	Study and education	Standards of training	Needs and demands
Level of education	Undergraduate and postgraduate	Graduate (vocational)	Continuation
Reason (why?)	Creativity	Interest	Service

* From Lynn P. Carmichael, "A Department of What?" *Bulletin of the New York State Academy of General Practice*, **22**:9–13, September 1970.

in health related fields as part of an interdisciplinary health team, which works cooperatively to provide services for the patient's total health needs.

The family physician, with his concern for comprehensive, ongoing health care, differs from the general practitioner, who gives episodic treatment for disease without regard to age, sex, or organ system. General practice is a method of delivering medical care rather than a medical discipline or specialty, while family medicine involves an academic discipline, a medical specialty, and a form of practice (see Table 4-1).

PRACTICE OF FAMILY MEDICINE

In the past, a doctor might become a family physician through experience gained in the general practice of medicine or pediatrics. The primary care physician still frequently "evolves" into a specialist in family health care as he begins to practice in his community. The process generally starts with the inauguration of a continuing relationship with his patients when they return to him periodically with different complaints and illnesses. As he becomes increasingly more familiar with the individual family members that he cares for, the physician begins to see the family as more than simply a collection of individuals. Instead, he becomes aware of the unique interactions and dynamics within each family, and he soon realizes that the family is a living unit and the basic social group. Consequently, he also finds that proper management of a patient's health problems requires the involvement and participation of his family.

As their relationship develops, the physician comes to know the families more intimately. Their trust and confidence in him gradually move their relationship beyond the usual fee-for-service, episodic type of doctor-patient contact to the establishment of a continuous relationship in which the physician assumes ongoing responsibility for the health of the family.

Finally, as the practitioner begins to see his families on a regular basis, he starts to view them as more than just patients requiring episodic attention. He becomes increasingly interested in preserving their physical and emotional health, and possibly uses the illness visit as an opportunity to practice preventive medicine. His concern becomes the total management of the patient's and the family's problems, as he completes the transition from general medical practitioner to family physician. The knowledge of such "transformed" practitioners is now being organized and systematized as the discipline of family medicine, offering physicians formal training in the areas previously accessible only through personal experience.

The practice of family medicine requires training and skills in areas other than those of the internist or pediatrician. The skills important for treating disease are the cognitive and manipulative or motor skills, i.e., the application of knowledge about a given disease process in order to diagnose, treat, and rehabilitate. But the family physician also sees patients in times of health and in the early stages of disease as well as during acute episodes of illness. He also needs highly developed perceptive skills in order to recognize subtle changes in an individual or a family, to understand nonverbal communications, and to detect environmental or behavioral conditions which may have a deleterious effect on health. An even more important skill that the family physician must cultivate is the affective skill, or the ability to alter behavior, which requires the use of the doctor-patient relationship.

The doctor-patient relationship exists on three levels. The first, or *activity-passivity* stage, involves a passive patient and an active doctor. This is usually the relationship between the patient who undergoes a surgical procedure and the surgeon who performs the operation. The second level is the stage of *guidance and cooperation,* in which the physician gives instructions which the patient follows. The physician's instructions usually involve medication schedules or other simple tasks, and the patient's response is usually automatic. This is the level of most doctor-patient relationships. The third level, that of *mutual cooperation,* is more difficult to achieve and requires more direct participation and responsibility on the part of the patient. This type of relationship is more mature and complex and prevails over a longer period of time than the others. The physician recognizes the dignity inherent in each individual and helps the person to help himself.

An essential element in developing the affective skills necessary for a good doctor-patient relationship is a strong background in behavioral and social sciences. In order to be of help to his patient, the family physician needs to know about the person, his family, culture, and community. He must be able to adjust scientific medical findings to the individual circumstances of the patient, i.e., to integrate the opinions and prescribed regimens of other physicians who may be consulted and to design and coordinate a suitable health care plan for the patient. This presupposes familiarity with the concepts of health ecology and the various components of health and illness.

Because he is concerned with the total health maintenance of his patients, the family physician knows how to effectively use and coordinate the interdisciplinary health team, including nurses, psychologists, social workers, technicians, and various paramedical personnel. As a leading member of the health team, the physician can attend to the medical needs of his patients while seeing to it that the nonmedical needs are also met. Familiarity with medical economics; organization of health care delivery; and available community resources, services, and agencies also facilitates his efforts to help his patients restore and maintain health. He tries to maintain health and prevent disease through specific prevention techniques and health education, both in regard to any current problems and in anticipation of any that are likely to occur.

It is important that the family practitioner provides an environment in which the patient feels free to state his thoughts and feelings honestly without fear of judgment or condemnation. He must develop acuity in interviewing skills which help him elicit information about the patient's feelings as well as his physical complaints. He must try to communicate his own interest and compassion to his patients in order to gain their confidence and to establish a comfortable personal relationship.

The family doctor needs to possess an extensive knowledge of human behavior and development in order to recognize early signs of deviation. In his position as physician of primary, long-term contact, he can notice signs as they begin to manifest. Prompt diagnosis and treatment, particularly in cases of mental illness or emotional disorders, can frequently mean more effective results.

The doctor of family medicine is prepared to deal with the major life events of the individual and the family (birth, death, marriage, pregnancy, divorce, and so on) because he follows families as they grow and develop. He must understand the critical periods that are common to all family life cycles and be able to distinguish healthy deviations from those that may be destructive to the family unit or its individual members. He must have a comprehensive knowledge of human sexuality and family dynamics, an understanding of illness behavior and the limitations illness places on the family, and an awareness of the differences in expectations of doctor and patient.

The importance of behavioral and social sciences as they relate to medicine has continued to increase as the effects of environmental, behavioral, and socioeconomic factors on health and illness have become more evident. The study of cultural attitudes as they relate to health and disease has led to greater interest in illness as a cultural phenomenon, as in alcoholism or drug abuse or nutritional deficiencies. The relation of interpersonal dynamics to health and illness has also been shown. Alvin Toffler (1970) has spoken of "future shock" as it affects a person's mental and physical stability. He points out that in today's mechanistic, fast-moving world, the failure of traditional support-giving institutions, the consequences of frequent sudden changes in all spheres of life, and the proliferation of choices that constantly bombard the individual have led to crises and dislocations that take a heavy toll in mental and physical problems.

Perhaps it is within this milieu that family medicine should be viewed. It is not so much a creation of the medical profession as a response by the profession to the needs of society. In this view, family medicine assumes the continuing responsibility for the health maintenance of the family. While the physician's agreement to accept this challenge is an essential ingredient, the participation of the other health professions, such as nursing, is just as necessary if our society is to receive the full benefits of health.

BIBLIOGRAPHY

Carmichael, L. P.: "A Department of What?" *Bulletin of the New York State Academy of General Practice,* **22**:9-13, 1970.

Greenberg, S.: *The Troubled Calling: Crisis in the Medical Establishment,* New York: The Macmillan Company, 1965.

Roszak, T.: *The Making of a Counterculture,* New York: Doubleday & Company, Inc., 1969.

Toffler, A.: *Future Shock,* New York: Random House, Inc., 1970.

Chapter 5

Law and the Family

Jed B. Maebius, Jr.

The purpose of this chapter is to acquaint the nurse with several common legal problems which are faced by families of all socioeconomic levels. Whether the nurse is working in a hospital, a doctor's office, or the community, he is bound to encounter families with some of these problems. A basic introduction to such problems will help the nurse better understand how the family unit functions. In giving nursing care to a patient, the nurse's assessment of the patient's family situation should reflect the family's legal problems.

The laws dealing with family problems emanate primarily from court decisions and state statutes. As such, these laws vary from state to state. Therefore a general statement of the law will be given, with occasional references to specific statutes. The reader should keep in mind that in any particular state the law may be different from statements made in this chapter.

The scope of this chapter will be limited to a discussion of family legal problems. There will be no discussion of the legal aspects of nursing, although the bibliography at the end of this chapter supplies several helpful references in this area.

LEGAL ASPECTS AND PROBLEMS OF THE FAMILY

Marriage

The couple, composed of husband and wife, or the group, composed of husband, wife, and children, constitutes the family. The relationship begins with the marriage; this can be accomplished by a ceremony performed upon the issuance of a marriage permit after certain legal prerequisites have been met. The marriage relationship, with all its legal implications, can also exist without formal entry into a marriage contract according to law. Certain marriages are prohibited according to laws of the various states. A person may not marry any close blood relative. A person may not marry if he or she has not dissolved a prior marriage. There are also minimum age requirements in all states for males and females; the age requirement is usually lower for females.

Many centuries ago husband and wife legally became "one person" by marriage, and the entire legal status of the woman was completely incorporated into that of the husband. However the evolution of the law has seen the emergence of the separate legal existence of the wife and her property. The relationship of husband and wife imposes on each of them certain legal marital rights and duties. Each spouse has a right to the support, company, affection, and service of the other. If either party fails to live up to these obligations of the marriage contract to the extent that the purpose of the marriage is defeated, the law will allow the innocent party to dissolve the marriage contract.

In addition to divorce, the family relationship is terminated by the death of one spouse if there are no children or by annulment. The family unit continues after death if there are children and after the divorce for the spouse who retains legal custody of the children. All states have laws prescribing grounds for having a marriage annulled. Typical of these is the situation where one party was under the influence of drugs or alcohol at the time of the marriage and has not voluntarily cohabited with the other party since the marriage; impotency of either party; marriage by inducement by fraud, duress, or force; mental incompetency of one party; and others.

A parent is under an obligation to furnish support for his or her infant children. If the parent neglects that duty, any person who supplies items such as food and clothing is deemed to have an implied promise to pay on the part of the parent. The reasoning behind this rule is the inability of the child to care for himself and the public policy of not leaving such care in the hands of the state, except as a last resort.

Divorce

The state statutes providing for divorce specify the grounds for which a divorce can be granted, and include such grounds as cruelty, adultery, conviction of the other spouse of a felony, abandonment, etc. Traditionally, divorce has been handled as any other lawsuit is handled in our adversary system. Our adversary system of justice operates on the premise that if each side to a lawsuit has an attorney and prepares its case in the best possible way to promote that side's "best interests," the judge or jury will be able to choose from the best of both sides. In this way, a just decision can be reached.

A divorce suit is instituted in the following manner. One party files a petition for divorce, in the name of John Smith versus Mary Smith, alleging that the other party has been cruel or alleging any other legal basis for the divorce which may exist. The other party may or may not hire an attorney to contest the divorce.

Many state statutes have a mandatory waiting period after the petition is filed for the divorce hearing, such as 60 days. The theory behind this waiting period is that the two parties will have time to think about what they are doing and perhaps reconsider. The setup of our system usually results in a court having to find one of the parties to blame for the failure of the marriage. The other party is then granted the divorce.

In addition to granting the divorce, the court must also divide the parties' property equitably between them. In many, but not all, states, the court must prescribe alimony payments for the husband to make to the wife. All states provide for child support, and the husband is usually required to make support payments for the children who are in the wife's custody.

Child Custody

It is the general rule that, if for any reason a husband and wife have divorced or legally separated, the court has the power to determine which parent shall have the custody of the children. It is the court's duty in such cases to place the best interests of the children above the rights of either parent and to make provisions for their care and custody as will best serve their welfare.

It is within a court's power in making such a determination to award custody to neither parent, but rather to a third person, if the best interests of the child so dictate. A parent who is not awarded custody still has the right of reasonable visitation with such child, and some divorce decrees will enumerate specific times at which the parent can visit with the child, such as every other weekend from Saturday morning until Sunday evening and one month each summer. Many times divorce decrees provide simply for "reasonable visitation" by the parent who does not have custody. Such language can lead to a conflict between the parents over the meaning of "reasonable."

Adoption

The family unit can be legally expanded by adoption of a child as well as by the birth of one. However adoption poses questions relating to the legal status of the child and his new adoptive parents as well as that of the child and his natural parents. Generally the adopted child and his new parents take on the same legal relationship of a natural child and his parents. The legal relationship between the adopted child and his natural parents is severed.

The law has not always been this way, and adopted children were often denied the rights of natural-born children in many situations, such as not being given the right to inherit from their adoptive parents. Most courts and state legislatures have attempted to give the child the rights and obligations that a natural child has. Some states have enacted statutes which allow an adopted child to inherit through his adoptive parents as well as from them. [A recent Wyoming statute provides that an adopted person can inherit from all relatives of his new parents, just as a natural child, and all of his parents' relatives can inherit from him (Wyoming Laws of 1969, Chapter 74).] Many states however still have statutes which do not allow a child to inherit from relatives of his adoptive parents. For example, if a grandparent in such a state leaves his property in a will to his "grandchildren," only his natural-born grandchildren would inherit. In order for his adopted grandchild to inherit, his will would have to specifically mention the adopted grandchild.

The adoptive process generally takes 1 or 2 months from the time the petition for adoption is filed. Many states have statutes requiring a specified waiting period before the court can hear the adoption. During this time the child may live with his prospective parents. Also during this period, many states require that a social worker be appointed by the court to make an investigation of the family and of the child's background to see if they are suitable for each other. The social worker then recommends to the court whether or not the adoption should take place.

The Battered Child

One of the most difficult family problems to deal with from a legal standpoint, as well as medical and sociological standpoints, is that of the battered child. States statutes require child abuse cases to be reported by health care workers to public agencies or law enforcement agencies. The statutes are designed to prevent further abuse to children. In addition, statutes provide criminal penalties for parents who are convicted of inflicting physical injury on their children.

The responsibility of parenthood carries with it the duty to train and educate children. Involved in the execution of these duties is the right of the parent to exercise reasonable control over the child in the form of discipline. The right to discipline children is based on the premise that a certain amount of discipline is in the best interests of the child. The limits of reasonable discipline are determined according to standards which foster the best interests of the child. A parent is allowed to inflict such punishment and to use such force as is reasonable under the circumstances. The circumstances which determine what is reasonable are age, sex, physical condition, and other characteristics of the child.

The legal machinery presently existing to deal with the problem is inadequate in many areas. The statutes requiring reports of child abuse are lacking in many particulars. One problem is that the only requirement is that a report be made, and, once the report is made, there is little assurance of a follow-up. In many areas, there is also no centralized reporting. This means that a parent who has been guilty of child abuse more than one time can go to a different hospital in his city each time and avoid discovery of previous incidents (Grumet, 1970, p. 306).

Criminal prosecution of the parents has proved to be ineffective. In the first place, it is very difficult to obtain convictions. Even if a conviction is obtained and a sentence is imposed, the problem itself is not being solved. Often criminal prosecution destroys the possibility of being able to work with the parents (Grumet, 1970, p. 307). Some courts have taken custody of children away from parents in these circumstances, and it appears to be necessary in many cases.

Even in the most extreme cases, it is difficult to obtain convictions. An example is the case of *State v. England* [349 P. 2d 668 (Ore. Sup. 1960)]. The defendant was charged with involuntary manslaughter of his twelve-year-old son. The father was accused of striking his son about the head and face with such force and violence that the injuries eventually caused his son's death. The manslaughter statute of Oregon contained a provision which stated that the killing of a human being is excusable when it is committed by accident or misfortune when lawfully correcting a child or in doing any other lawful act, by lawful means with usual and ordinary caution and without any unlawful intent. In this case, the father was not convicted, because the court held that the evidence showed that the death resulted from the negligence of the father while he was correcting the child.

It would seem that health care workers, lawyers, law enforcement officials, and social workers will all have to work together to bring about the best possible solutions for child abuse cases, for both the parent and the child. It is obvious that a family with such a problem is undergoing a volatile and stressful period.

Juvenile Courts

There are many definitions of the term *juvenile delinquency,* but, generally, it can be said to mean conduct of a child which would be considered criminal if he were an adult. Many states have established juvenile courts by statute to administer the problems of juvenile delinquents. Such courts can also be empowered to handle dependent, neglected, and abandoned children.

These are special courts designed to deal only with the problems of juveniles. The justification for such courts is that a juvenile delinquent should not be considered as nor treated as a criminal, but rather handled as a person requiring care, education, and protection.

Incompetent Persons

All states have laws providing for the care, treatment, and commitment to institutions of persons (either adults or minors) who are mentally ill or mentally retarded.* Legal proceedings for the commitment of such a person can be instituted by the state upon motion or information filed by an adult stating that the person in question should be committed. Often an affidavit from a family member is filed stating that it would be in the best interest of such a person for him to be committed. Traditionally, these legal proceedings have been adversary in nature, with the state attempting to show that the person should be committed by means of medical testimony from one or two doctors. The person who is the subject of the commitment proceedings can have an attorney, and in many states the court is required to appoint such an attorney to undertake his defense. In actual practice, it is doubtful that such a system results in serving the best interests of the person who is the subject of the commitment proceedings in all cases.

Traditionally, the only alternatives open at such a hearing are either total commitment or total freedom. Often a statute requires commitment for a temporary period before there can be an indefinite commitment. There are likewise statutory provisions for commitment of habitual drunkards and sexual psychopaths.

Death

In addition to being a very emotionally upsetting experience for the family unit, death of a family member has several immediate legal implications for the family. The most immediate legal problem facing the family unit is disposal of the body. The disposal of the dead has such a relation to public health that the state has the power to regulate such disposal, as an incident of its power to provide for the public health of the people. There may be laws and regulations providing for cemetery locations, burial permits, and many other necessities. Most cities have ordinances stating that there can be no

---

* For a thorough treatment of the laws relating to and the legal problems of mentally ill and mentally retarded persons, see Allen, Ferster, and Weihofen, *Mental Impairment and Legal Incompetency*, Prentice-Hall, Inc., Report of the Mental Competency Study: An Empirical Research Project Conducted by the George Washington University Institute of Law, Psychiatry and Criminology (1968).

burial of a body within the city limits until a permit has been issued by the proper city authority. Generally, on the death of a husband or wife, the surviving spouse is the person in charge of making the necessary legal arrangements for burial. Otherwise the next of kin has the duty and right.

Additional laws which come into immediate effect at the death of a family member are those relating to the disposition of his property. If the deceased person has written a valid will in accordance with the law, his property passes under the terms of the will, but only after the will has been admitted to probate in the particular state where the deceased resided.

If there is no will, state statutes contain rules of descent and distribution and designate the persons who are to take the deceased's property; it is usually on the basis of closest relatives first, such as spouse and children, parents and grandchildren, brothers and sisters, etc.

A person's debts must be paid at his death, and his property is subject to being sold to satisfy all such debts and taxes. If the debts of a decedent are not paid before his property passes to his surviving heirs, or devisees, his creditors may sue the heirs in order to be paid upon a valid claim. Whatever remains after debts have been paid is distributed to the heirs, or devisees.

The rules governing who should take a decedent's property become complicated in certain situations. If a person lives in Iowa, owns land in Iowa and Minnesota, and dies without a will, which state laws control how his land is divided? Iowa law might provide that his land should go to his surviving spouse. Minnesota law might provide that his land should go to his surviving children. It is the general rule that the state where the land is located has the paramount interest in having its laws regulate land in that state. Therefore, in the above example, the surviving spouse would inherit the Iowa land, and the children would inherit the Minnesota land.

Even if a person dies without having executed a will, there can be an administration of his estate in the probate court if the necessity exists. In such a situation, the court would appoint some person or some institution as administrator to take charge of the assets and to administer the decedent's estate. Sometimes, if the deceased had no debts and no substantial assets, there will not be a necessity to have an administration of any kind. It may be necessary to prepare an affidavit, however, to indicate the heirs. Such an affidavit would be filed in the county records to show the "chain of title" of any property the decedent did have.

An additional problem affecting the family unit with children at death is that of the necessity of appointing a guardian for the estate of the children. If a deceased person dies leaving property to his children while they are minors and did not make special provision for the care of that property, the laws of most states require that a guardian be appointed. This property is called a minor's estate, and the guardian serves until the minor reaches maturity. Court supervision over a minor's estate is felt to be necessary in order to protect minors from family members or others who might take advantage of them. Of course, the surviving parent or other family member of age can apply to be appointed guardian for the minor children's property, but he or she must account to the court for all actions taken with regard to such property. Ordinarily a guardian must post a bond, guaranteeing the faithful performance of his duties.

SOLUTIONS TO FAMILY LEGAL PROBLEMS

The above outline of some of the legal aspects and problems of the family is intended to give the nurse an idea of the effect that such aspects and problems have on the well-being of the family unit. It can be seen that when the family unit faces a problem such as divorce, death, or possible commitment of one of its members, a great amount of emotional stress can result. Perhaps the adversary process of solving such problems as divorce and commitment adds to the trauma facing the family unit. In recent years, new legislation and court opinions have reflected a different attitude of our society to the solution of such problems. The examples of divorce and commitment will be discussed as illustrations.

When a husband and wife are having marital problems, and one of them has reached the point of filing a suit for divorce, the adversary process requires that the husband and wife be pitted against each other in a "legal battle." Much harm to the family, especially to the children, can result from these battles (Hawke, 1970).

In 1969, the Texas legislature passed the Texas Family Code which establishes a new direction for handling divorce. A divorce petition in Texas is not now entitled Mr. Smith versus Mrs. Smith, but rather the petition is entitled "In the Matter of the Marriage of Mr. & Mrs. Smith" (*Texas Family Code Annals,* 1969). Although the traditional grounds for divorce, such as cruelty, adultery, abandonment, or conviction of a felony exist under this new code, an important new ground has been added. On the petition of either party to a marriage, a divorce may be granted without regard to fault if the marriage has become "insupportable" because of discord or conflict of personalities which destroys the legitimate ends of the marriage relationship and prevents any reasonable expectation of reconciliation (*Texas Family Code Annals,* 1969).

The importance of the new grounds of "insupportability" for divorce is that the statute makes legal the reasons that are actually the basis for most divorce suits. In most divorce situations, there is simply not one party who is the sole blame for the divorce. Prior to the new code, it was necessary to allege cruelty in most divorce cases in order to get the divorce granted. If there was any chance of reconciliation, such allegations would certainly not help the possibility. In many cases, there were simply not facts supporting cruelty, and the parties were forced to exaggerate and say things that were not necessarily true in order to get a divorce.

Another section of the statute provides that after a petition for divorce is filed, the court may, in its discretion, direct the parties to counsel with a person or persons named by the court who shall submit a written report to the court stating his opinion as to whether there exists a reasonable expectation of reconciliation, and, if so, whether further counseling would be beneficial (*Texas Family Code Annals,* 1969).

Other states have also adopted such statutes. Some states have established family clinics in an attempt to provide counseling service for persons with marital problems (Hawke, 1970). The importance of these changes is an attempt to provide a basis for the solution of a problem without directly pitting the husband and wife against each other.

Another area of the law in which a change of direction can be seen is in the commitment of mentally ill or retarded persons. As stated previously, the courts traditionally have approached the solution to the problem as being one of either total commitment or total freedom. In a recent case, the United States Court of Appeals for the District of Columbia illustrated a new approach to this problem [*Lake v. Cameron,* 364 F.2d 657 (Dist. Col. Cir. 1966) *cert. denied,* 382 U.S. 863 (1966)]. The court in this case recognized that there are other alternatives to commitment and freedom. These people are not criminals, and the primary purposes of any type of commitment should be treatment and rehabilitation. The court stated in its opinion as follows:

> Proceedings involving the care and treatment of the mentally ill are not strictly adversary proceedings. . . . The Court may consider, e.g., whether the appellant and the public would be sufficiently protected if she were required to carry an identification card on her person so that the police or others could take her home if she should wander, or whether she should be required to accept public health and day care services, foster care, home help aid services or whether available welfare payments might finance adequate private care. Every effort should be made to find the course of treatment which appellant might be willing to accept.

The court has recognized not only that the state has the burden of showing whether the person is mentally ill or mentally retarded, but also that it has the burden of finding what the best solution is for the problem. Neither total commitment nor total freedom may be the best answer in a particular case. This decision recognizes the fact that family problems such as possible commitment should be treated differently from an ordinary civil lawsuit or criminal lawsuit. The opinion recognizes the fact that an interdisciplinary approach to solutions of such a problem may be in the best interest of both the individual involved and the society.

SUMMARY AND OBSERVATIONS

It is hoped that this chapter has provided the nurse with some small insight into the vast area of legal aspects and problems of the family. The well-being of the family is greatly affected when it faces emotionally upsetting and stressful situations such as divorce, commitment, or death. Perhaps the traditional legal approach to the solution of these problems adds to the trauma of the family. Changes in the approach of legislatures and courts to solutions of these problems, such as were discussed, should help to reduce the trauma of these problems. A basic understanding of the legal aspects and problems of the family unit should help the nurse make a more meaningful assessment of the patient and his family.

BIBLIOGRAPHY

Allen, R., E. Ferster, and H. Weihofen: *Mental Impairment and Legal Incompetency,* Prentice-Hall, Inc., Report of the Mental Competency Study: An Empirical Research Project Conducted by the George Washington University Institute of Law, Psychiatry and Criminology, 1968.

Anderson, B.: "Orderly Transfer of Procedural Responsibilities from Medical to Nursing Practice," *Nursing Clinics of North America,* 5(2):311-319, June 1970.

Creighton, H.: *Law Every Nurse Should Know,* Philadelphia: W. B. Saunders Company, 2d ed., 1970.

Curran, W.: "Public Health and the Law," *American Journal of Public Health,* 60:2400-2401, December 1970.

Grumet, R.: "The Plaintive Plaintiffs: Victims of the Battered Child Syndrome," *Family Law Quarterly,* Section of Family Law, American Bar Association, 4(3):296, September 1970.

Hawke, L.: "Divorce Procedure: A Fraud on Children, Spouses and Society," *Family Law Quarterly,* 3:240-253, 1969.

Kempe C., F. Silverman, B. Steele, W. Droegemueller, and H. Silver: "The Battered Child Syndrome," *Journal of the American Medical Association,* 181:17-24, 1962.

Parker, S.: "Lake v. Cameron: Involuntary Civil Commitment Storm Warnings," *Family Law Quarterly,* Section of Family Law, American Bar Association, 4(1):81-89, March 1970.

Sadusk, J.: "Legal Implications of Changing Patterns of Practice," *Journal of the American Medical Association,* 190:1135-1136, 1964.

Springer, E.: *Nursing and the Law,* Pittsburgh: Health Law Center, Aspen Systems Corporation, 1970.

State v. England, 349 P. 2d 668 (Ore. Sup. 1960).

Texas Family Code Annals, 1969.

Willig, S.: *The Nurse's Guide to the Law,* New York: McGraw-Hill Book Company, 1970.

Wyoming Laws of 1969, chapter 74.

Chapter 6

Sociological Aspects of Parenthood*

Gerald Handel

Sociology,[1] like psychology and psychiatry, is concerned with understanding human behavior, thought, and feeling. Its distinctive task, however, is to understand how these phenomena are shaped by group life, a term whose scope encompasses a range from society in the large to two-person or dyadic relationships. Whereas psychology differentiates and elaborates upon the components of personality, studying behavior as the outcome of interrelationships among these components, sociology differentiates and elaborates upon the components of group life. To be sure, psychology attends to and investigates factors or environmental conditions that shape personality components,

*Reprinted from E. J. Anthony and Therese Benedek (eds.), *Parenthood: Its Psychology and Psychopathology*, Little, Brown and Company, Boston, 1970, pp. 87–105.
[1] Sociology shares an indistinct boundary with social psychology. I have tried to adhere to a strictly sociological presentation in order to highlight the effects of large-scale social forces on parenthood. For this reason and also because of space limitations, I do not discuss many topics which form part of the sociology of parenthood and which are of a more social psychological nature. For one approach on the other side of the boundary see G. Handel (Ed.), *The Psychosocial Interior of the Family* (Chicago: Aldine, 1967). Thanks are expressed to my wife, Ruth D. Handel, for editorial suggestions which have helped to sharpen the presentation.

but it is not systematically concerned with the order that obtains among these extrapersonal conditions, treating them, rather, as discrete variables. In contrast, the guiding conception of sociology is that man lives in a socially ordered world, and that behavior is to be understood as a product of that order.

Sociologically considered, parenthood is a position in a social structure. To say this is immediately to state that it is tied to other positions in a set of interconnected groups of institutions. To be a parent is to occupy a position that is connected in socially defined ways to such other social positions as parent of the opposite sex, child, neighbor, teacher, pediatrician. Each position is socially defined in terms of a set of expectations. The expectations that define a position in one group differ from those that define the same position in another group. Thus, for example, a teacher in a school serving a working-class neighborhood is expected by the parents to be more of a disciplinarian than is the case among parents in an upper-middle-class neighborhood. The latter, being generally more articulate and better educated, expect to have more influence in the curriculum content than would working-class parents. More generally, upper-middle-class parents expect to exert more direct influence on their children's schooling than do working-class parents.[2]

From this illustration it can be seen that parenthood is definable not only in reference to such institutionalized positions as teacher but also in terms of more embracing, though noninstitutionalized, aspects of social order such as social class. The way in which the position of parent is enacted is shaped, then, not only by the expectations deriving from other institutionally based positions but, more importantly, by more pervasive aspects of the social order. The structure of the society as a whole is one such pervasive shaping factor. Thus, in an industrial society, a father does not typically teach his son an occupation. In an agricultural society, a father who is a farmer will teach his son to earn his living by farming. In the two types of society, the position of father is defined by different expectations concerning preparation of the child for an occupation.

While the structure of society as a whole sets certain general expectations, no society of any size is homogeneous. It is, rather, differentiated into a variety of different kinds of segments, of which the most significant are social class and (in our society) ethnic group. Other segmentations which have some importance are religion, occupation, and type of community (e.g., suburban vs. urban). These social segmentations cut across each other in multi-

---

[2] The author has studied one school system in which upper-middle-class parents succeeded in pressing the Board of Education to provide foreign language instruction in elementary schools in upper-middle-class neighborhoods, over the opposition of the Board's own professional staff of educational administrators. The administrators spoke more approvingly of parents in lower-middle-class and working-class neighborhoods who "support" the schools but don't "interfere."

farious ways, and one task of sociology is to identify what kind of importance each type of segmentation has upon the way in which parenthood is performed. This task has not yet been carried out so comprehensively and systematically that we can, say, differentiate the parental performance of the upper-middle-class, Irish Catholic, suburban mother married to a professional man from an upper-middle-class, Irish Catholic, suburban mother married to a businessman, or from an upper-middle-class Negro or Jewish mother married to either a professional or businessman and living in either a suburb or in a city. In other words, each of these segmentations (social class, ethnicity, religion, community type) has been shown to have some effect on how parenthood is performed, but not enough work has yet been done to provide a comprehensive and composite picture of how they all interact. In addition, it must be noted that the significance of each type of segment changes through time so that the relative importance of different kinds of segmentation changes. Thus, for families of a given social class level, but diverse in ethnic origin, who have moved to the suburbs, the fact of being suburban probably has a greater effect on how parenthood is enacted than the fact of being Irish or Swedish in ethnic origin. A conclusion of this kind, is, however, somewhat inferential, based on the general knowledge that ethnic origin among whites is somewhat less important in the suburbs than it was in the areas of earlier settlement in the city.

So far as the study of parenthood and child-rearing is concerned, more concentrated attention has probably been given to the importance of social class than to other types of social segmentation. This is due, in part, to the fact that attention was emphatically drawn to the existence of social classes in America by a series of researches during the 1930s, particularly those conducted by W. Lloyd Warner and his associates. Although Warner's particular approach to social class became the subject of some dispute, sociologists thereafter generally had no difficulty recognizing the importance of this type of segmentation in America. Even so, the emphatic enunciation of the existence of social classes in the United States challenged the vague but prevalent ideas of universal equality of opportunity. If social classes exist, children start out in life with systematically different preparation. Indeed, the notion that children were starting out in life with equal opportunity to participate in a wide-open race in which they were all running had to be modified in two major respects. Investigation began to suggest not only that they did not start out with equal opportunity but that they were not even being prepared for the same race. It became evident, rather, that parents in each social class were primarily preparing their children to become adult members of the same social class into which they were born, rather than to compete in a kind of free-for-all in which the members of each succeeding generation would sort themselves out independent of their origins.

Prior to Warner's work, students of child development had discovered that children's mental development was affected by their socioeconomic status. But these earlier studies did not examine parental behavior, attitudes, and values. Two of Warner's principal co-workers, Allison Davis and Robert J. Havighurst, applied his concepts of social class to the study of parental behavior [6]. This study stimulated various efforts first to replicate it, then to improve upon it, and thus played an important part in setting the problem for a whole series of later studies.

Over time, the most sustained attention, then, has been given to social class as a factor influencing parental performance. This dimension has emerged as the most enduringly significant large-scale social influence on parenthood in the United States. The importance of rural-urban differences has shrunk, in view of the increasing urbanization of the American people. With the decrease in immigration, ethnic differences became less important, the principal exception to this being the Negro-white difference, which is partly a social class difference. Religion as a segmenting factor retains some importance, as will be suggested, but its significance is attenuated. In any case, it has not attracted the same concentration of interest that social class has. For these reasons, the reader will find more frequent references to social class than to other large-scale social factors in the balance of this chapter. However, it should also be noted that as knowledge has grown, some efforts have been made to draw distinctions within social class and also to locate smaller-scale social groupings that mediate the effects of social class.

THE SOCIOLOGY OF REPRODUCTION

No society commits suicide. Every society seeks in various ways to maintain itself, to preserve its continuity. It does this by such means as fashioning legends of its past which it then cherishes and transmits to its young. It seeks to preserve its territorial boundaries against encroachment from other societies. Not the least important, it recruits new members through reproduction. Parents are, then, society's agents for replenishing its population. Society reveals its interest in this process through various official means which encourage or discourage the rate of reproduction: programs to limit family size when overpopulation threatens, programs to stimulate reproduction when the net reproduction rate is insufficient to maintain the population at its existing size or to sustain a desired growth rate. Most fundamentally, society declares its interest in reproduction by establishing norms for the legitimacy of unions and their offspring. Certain unions and their offspring are defined as illegitimate; these are, at the very least, denied the honor that society accords to legitimate unions and births. Often, illegitimacy is subject to additional penalty beyond dishonor. Various legal and social disabilities still attach to illegitimacy; efforts to moderate or abolish these continue in the United States at the present time. The social significance of illegitimacy is highlighted in these observations by Vincent:

> Because of their greater visibility, and consequently their greater threat to the value judgments sustaining marriage, illicit births are given far greater attention than is given to the more generic problem of *unwanted pregnancy*—licit and illicit. Not all illicit births are unwanted and pose a social problem; and not all licit births are desired and problem-free. This becomes evident when we consider whose value judgments determine which births are unwanted by whom. *Illicit pregnancies* may be unwanted by the mothers and society, as in cases of rape and incest; they may be wanted by the mothers but not by society, as in some cases of very low-income unwed mothers receiving public assistance; and they may be unwanted by the mothers but highly desired by other couples, as in cases of unwed mothers who release their children for adoption and enable childless couples to establish families. Similarly, *licit pregnancies* may be unwanted by the mothers and society, as in cases involving severe genetic abnormalities or economic deprivation; they may be unwanted by the mothers but desired by childless couples, as in the case of the estimated 15% of adoptions that involve children relinquished by married couples; and *licit pregnancies* may be wanted by the mothers but not by society, as in some cases of extreme economic deprivation, or unwanted by the mothers but wanted by society as in some cases of affluent and brilliant parents. . . .
>
> The far greater public concern about illegitimacy than about the more generic problem of unwanted pregnancy is consistent with the value judgments and social mores involved in the following: (1) The amount of public (and research) interest in a social problem is closely related to the visibility and public expense of the problem; unwed parenthood not only is the most visible of the various alternatives in coping with unwanted pregnancy, but in cases of very young and poor females it imposes the greatest cost upon the public. (2) The "principle of legitimacy" is maintained by censuring the unwed mother. . . . Censuring her is believed to serve as an object lesson to prevent these mores from "dying out in the conscience" of society. (3) The greater concern with illegitimacy is also consistent with the mores which prescribe that the sexual relationship be a private, covert experience [18].

Vincent's analysis of the statistical data on rates of illegitimacy reveals that, contrary to widespread belief, the rate of increase in illegitimacy between 1938 and 1963 was far greater in age groups over 20 than among teen-agers.

The biological route to parenthood is the same for all parents, but the social route is not. Whether or not an act of sexual intercourse that has a high probability of resulting in a pregnancy will occur is influenced by various social factors which operate at various junctures in the time sequence between mental concept and biological conception. The most comprehensive study of this problem is that by Rainwater; in what follows we draw upon his study except where otherwise indicated [13]. The study is of interest also because it reveals the complex interplay of social factors in parenthood.

The general problem to which Rainwater addresses himself is that of family size—how families come to have the particular number of children that they do. As Rainwater phrases it: "Each couple is confronted with the twin goals (and necessities) of having 'enough' children and not having 'too many.'" Most generally, the number of children that a couple has is a function of (1) the number of children that they desire, and (2) the effectiveness with which they practice contraception. The first, second, third, or nth child may be the result of a planned effort to conceive in order to realize some ideal concerning family size or it may be the result of failure in the use of contraception and thus a defeat in the effort to realize a goal. The inquiry follows out these two proximate determinants of family size to *their* determinants; that is, the study investigates the factors influencing number of children desired and the factors influencing effectiveness of contraceptive practice. From a summary of some of the main findings of the study, it will be evident that conception has social as well as biological and psychological determinants.

The research is based on interviews with 409 persons—152 couples plus 50 men and 55 women not married to each other. The sample includes members of four social classes—upper-middle class, lower-middle class, working class, and lower class; it also includes Catholics and Protestants, and whites and Negroes, since it was anticipated that family size would reflect these three aspects of social segmentation. Since the investigator was interested not simply in showing the existence of a relationship between these large social groupings and family size but also in indicating how membership in such groupings was related to marriage, the data gathered included information on conjugal role relationships [3] and on sexual relations. These five major factors—social class, religion, race, type of conjugal role relationship, and social psychological aspects of sexual relations—significantly affect the number of children a family will have, because they affect both the number of children desired and the effectiveness with which contraception is practiced.

The Rainwater study yields a great number of specific findings which are not readily summarizable in brief compass. A short statement of certain

---

[3] This concept was introduced by Elizabeth Bott in *Family and Social Network* (London: Tavistock Publications, 1957). As adopted by Rainwater, it refers to "those aspects of the relationship between husband and wife that consist of reciprocal role expectations and the activities of each spouse in relation to the other." Three types of role relationship are distinguished: (1) *Joint:* the pattern is one in which most husband-wife activities are either shared or interchangeable; (2) *Segregated:* husband's and wife's activities are separated and different, sometimes carried out with minimum, day-to-day articulation, sometimes fitted together to achieve coordination; (3) *Intermediate:* sharing and interchangeability of task performance are valued, but more formal division of household tasks is maintained than in the joint conjugal role organization.

highlights will, however, indicate the complex interplay of social determinants of parenthood: Protestants tend to want fewer children than do Catholics at all social class levels except the lower class, where there is no difference between the two religious groups. (In a study of the effects of religion on family life, Lenski found that Protestant mothers are somewhat more likely than Catholic mothers to feel that children are burdensome [11].) Family size preferences tend to shift during the course of marriage, with middle-class couples often wanting fewer children than when they were first married and lower-class couples wanting more (as a passive adaptation to the larger number actually born to them because of ineffective contraception). But within the middle class, couples who have a joint conjugal role organization, with much husband-wife sharing and interchanging of activities and responsibilities, are more likely to want a small family than couples with a lower level of husband-wife involvement. But irrespective of social class or religion, large families tend to be more often desired by those couples in which both members consider sexual relations very important than by those couples in which one or both partners say sexual relations are not very important.

Effective use of contraception (regular and consistent use of a method that has a high degree of effectiveness when used appropriately) varies according to the same general factors as does desired size of family. To begin, middle-class Protestants are more optimistic than other groups studied that the size of family they want can be achieved. Middle-class Catholics and working-class whites and Negroes are hopeful but less confident. Lower-class whites and Negroes are passive and fatalistic; they do nothing because they do not think anything will help, or they go through the motions of using a method in which they have little confidence and thus do not use it consistently. As would be anticipated from such basic attitudes, among the middle-class Protestants alone, of the groups studied, is there much serious discussion of family planning between husband and wife early in the marriage. Not surprisingly, middle-class Protestants are most likely to use effective contraceptive practices before the birth of the last child they want. After the birth of the last wanted child, this contraceptive superiority is maintained by the middle-class Protestants, although an increased number of couples in all groups learn to use the methods more effectively (98 percent of middle- and working-class Protestants; 73 percent of middle- and working-class Catholics; 50 percent of working-class Negroes; 33 percent of lower-class Protestants, and 13 percent of lower-class Negroes and Catholics use contraception effectively after the birth of the last wanted child). Within the lower class, after the birth of the last wanted child, effective contraceptive practice is more likely in couples maintaining joint or intermediate conjugal role relationships than segregated, and in couples in which the wife finds sexual relations gratifying and important to the marriage.

It can be seen from the summary of Rainwater's study that the likelihood of a couple's becoming the parents of yet another child is not a chance event but is influenced by the particular position of the parents in the social structure. Conception of a child has societal determinants as well as biological and psychodynamic ones.

INFANT CARE AND CHILD REARING

From a sociological point of view, the principal task of parents is to prepare their children to become adult members of society. This involves various kinds of care, the inculcation of values and norms, training in certain specific kinds of behavior, provision of models of adult roles upon which the child can draw in forming his concept of himself and his place in society, and the fostering of appropriate self-regard—all of which are summed up in the concept of socialization.

Although socialization begins with the birth of the child, the earliest days of life have been little, if at all, studied by sociologists; the field has essentially been left to psychologists and psychiatrists, so that we do not as yet have a sociology of the neonate. Sociological attention has been directed to that point in the infant's development at which the explicit imposition of "discipline" begins. The control of feeding has been regarded as the first major socializing experience, followed by toilet training. Recognition of the importance of these activities had been stimulated by psychoanalysis, and efforts were then made to place their significance in a larger social context.

The Davis-Havighurst study mentioned above aroused particular interest. The studies which followed in its wake resulted in various findings which seemed incompatible. Bronfenbrenner has endeavored to integrate results obtained from fifteen studies done over a 25-year span from 1932 to 1957 [3]. Over time, he finds that whereas the middle-class mothers were previously more strict than working- and lower-class mothers, they have become more permissive. Middle-class mothers, in contrast to their earlier practice and in contrast to working- and lower-class mothers, now more often allow self-demand feeding and wean later from the bottle, although breast-feeding is apparently becoming less common in all social classes. As part of the same overall trend toward increased permissiveness, middle-class mothers at the end of the period reviewed were instituting bowel and bladder training later than were working- and lower-class mothers, reversing the situation that existed at the beginning of the period.

The basic trend that Bronfenbrenner identifies is an increase in middle-class permissiveness, although he finds also a less marked trend in the same direction for the working and lower classes. An interesting aspect of his analysis is his relating of his survey to Wolfenstein's survey of successive editions of the U.S. Children's Bureau bulletin on infant care [19]. Her study showed that over substantially the same time period the advice issued by this publication changed from an emphasis on dominating and "taming" the child to an emphasis on meeting his needs. Research has indicated that middle-class mothers have been more likely to read not only this bulletin but other child-care literature such as Spock's *Baby and Child Care*. Bronfenbrenner concludes: "Taken as a whole, the correspondence between Wolfenstein's data and our own suggests a general hypothesis extending beyond the confines of social class as such: *child rearing practices are likely to change most quickly in those segments of society which have closest access and are most receptive to the agencies or agents of change (e.g., public media, clinics, physicians, and counselors)*. From this point of view, one additional trend suggested by the available data is worthy of note: rural families appear to lag behind the times somewhat in their practices of infant care" [3].

Bronfenbrenner finds similar trends in the training of children beyond the age of 2. In the 1930s and 1940s, the middle-class mother was more restrictive of freedom of movement; since then, less so. Also, since World War II, the middle-class mother has become more permissive toward the child's expressed needs and wishes in such diverse areas as oral behavior, toilet accidents, dependency, sex, aggressiveness, and freedom of movement outside the home. At the same time, however, the middle-class mother has higher expectations for the child with respect to independence and achievement.

Methods of discipline were found to differ. Working- and lower-class mothers are more likely to use physical punishment, while the middle-class mothers use more symbolic and manipulative techniques such as reasoning, isolation, and appeals to guilt. But over the 25-year period surveyed, the overall parent-child relationship in the middle class was reported as being more acceptant and egalitarian than in the working class, which is more oriented toward maintaining order and obedience.

THE NATURE OF SOCIAL CLASS DIFFERENCES

The differences in the parent-child relationship between the middle class and the working and lower classes arise from systematically different life experiences which, in turn, lead to differences in basic outlook and life style. Rainwater, Coleman, and Handel found these important characteristics of the working-class mother: Central to her outlook is her underlying conviction that most significant action originates from the world external to herself rather than from within herself [15]. Further, she sees the world beyond her doorstep and neighborhood as fairly chaotic and potentially catastrophic. She feels she has little ability to influence events, and her outlook is shaded by a fairly pervasive anxiety over possible fundamental deprivations. Similarly, she feels it is difficult to influence the behavior of her children. The study found that "the middle-class woman is more likely to perceive her child's behavior as complex, requiring understanding. The working-class mother is more likely to see her child's behavior as mysterious, beyond understanding. The latter, consequently, looks for rules or authoritative guidance which she hopes will work and take hold on the child." Middle-class mothers want to give their children "worthwhile experiences" to make them well-rounded; working-class mothers want their children to grow up to be moral, upright, and religious-minded.

How can we explain the apparent contradiction resulting from our finding that working-class mothers want specific rules or authoritative guidance in dealing with their children and Bronfenbrenner's finding that middle-class women are more attentive to child-care experts and literature? Kohn argues—substantially correctly, we believe—that middle-class parents' attentiveness to experts and other sources of relevant information represents not a search for new values but for better techniques of realizing the values they already have [9]. He believes that middle-class values have remained substantially the same over the period surveyed by Bronfenbrenner, but that the attentiveness of middle-class parents to expertise stems from greater readiness to accept innovation in the service of their unchanging basic goals and from the fact that these parents regard child-rearing as more problematic than do those of the working and lower classes. His interpretation that the middle class is not only more receptive to—but also more in search of—innovation than the working classes and lower classes is borne out by much research. However, the conclusion that basic middle-class values have not changed over 25 years is somewhat more open to question. It does not seem sufficient to say that earlier middle-class rigidity and more recent middle-class permissiveness are simply two different techniques in the service of the value of self-direction. Various social analysts have noted, for example, a change from production-oriented to consumption-oriented values. Insofar as such a shift in value emphasis has occurred, the increased permissiveness in child-rearing documented by Bronfenbrenner may derive from a more general acceptance of impulsivity in the middle class.

Kohn believes that sociological emphasis on child-rearing techniques is somewhat misplaced, and he seeks to redirect attention from specific techniques to the larger question of how the social structure influences behavior. His analysis takes the following general form: Values (conceptions of the desirable which influence choices) are products of life conditions. Middle-class and working-class parents live under different conditions; they therefore have different values, although they also have some values in common. The value differences result in differential parental behavior in the different social classes. To understand parental behavior one must know what their values are, particularly those concerned with child-rearing.

Filling in the specifics of his analytic model, Kohn notes that the significant value difference is that working-class and lower-class parents want conformity to external proscriptions while middle-class parents want their children to become self-directing. The life conditions which most directly determine these values are occupational, educational, and economic. Middle-class occupations deal more with manipulation of symbols, ideas, and interpersonal relations; working-class occupations, with manipulation of things. Middle-class occupations are more subject to self-direction, and getting ahead in them depends more on the individual, whereas working-class occupations are more subject to standardization and direct supervision, and getting ahead in them depends more on the collective action of labor unions. The greater income and higher educational preparation of middle-class parents enables them to be more attentive to motives and feelings, including their children's. Thus, in disciplining them, middle-class mothers are more concerned with the child's intent; working-class mothers are more concerned with the overt consequences of the child's act. A more general consequence of the value difference is that middle-class mothers tend to feel a greater obligation to be supportive of their children, whereas working-class and lower-class mothers are more attentive to the parental obligation to impose constraints. In keeping with this, middle-class mothers want their husbands to be supportive of the children, especially the sons, but do not expect them to impose constraints to any great extent. In the working class, the reverse holds: the wives expect their husbands to be more directive and look less to them to give emotional support to the children. However, Kohn finds that while middle-class fathers' own role expectations for themselves accord with what their wives expect, this is not as frequently true in the working class, since the working-class father believes that the most important thing is that the child be taught proper limits, and it doesn't much matter who does the teaching. He would rather not be bothered, and expects his wife to take major responsibility for child care.

A few years ago, after some 10 or 15 years of postwar growth in affluence, there was a growing belief that "now everyone is middle class." This notion proved to have a rather short life, since it was followed by the "rediscovery of poverty." During the interim of popular illusion, however, some research was directed to this question, particularly since it was unmistakable that some working-class families were moving to suburbs and an increasing number of their children were going to college. The fact that suburbanization became a mass phenomenon during the 1950s lent credence to the illusion. Berger, however, studied a new tract suburb settled largely by working-class families and found that the increased level of material comfort had not resulted in any significant shift in outlook or life style as compared with their life before the move to the new suburb [2]. Berger's basic conclusion is that the fact of being of the working class was more influential than the fact of having moved to a suburb. Berger's results are understandable in terms of Kohn's analysis, since the men remained in working-class occupations. At the same time, it should also be said that Berger's study was done only two and one-half years after the settling of the new community, perhaps too soon for any suburbanizing effects to become evident. Even so, residence basically follows from occupational level, rather than the other way around, so that the "working classness" of a working-class suburb is likely to remain more consequential than its "suburbanness."

Handel and Rainwater also studied the question of change in the working class and found it useful to distinguish between a traditional and a modern working class. Nonetheless, the basic difference in values between middle class and working class endures, although some changes in outlook occur. For example, the growing working-class interest in a college education for their children is largely focused on their sons, for whom it is seen as a means to a better-paying job rather than as a means of personal inner growth. College education for girls is discouraged unless the girl has a definite vocational objective such as becoming a nurse or a teacher; a year or two of college that does not lead to a definite vocation is seen as wasted [8].

FATHER ABSENCE AND UNEMPLOYMENT

Until now, the parental differences we have sketched assume intact families. They assume further that the father is engaged in some kind of gainful work. The presence or absence of the father in the home has significant consequences. The kind of work he does—or his lack of work—is scarcely less consequential. It is therefore useful to indicate here some facts concerning father absence and unemployment, particularly their uneven incidence. Clausen observes that the 1960 U. S. Census reports that 11 percent of all American households with children under 18 had only one parent present; the absent parent was usually the father [5]. Moynihan, in his summary of statistical data pertaining to Negro families, states that 36 percent of Negro children are living in broken homes at any give time [12]. In addition, he reports an estimate that only a minority of Negro children reach the age of 18 having lived all their lives with both parents. More than 20 percent of Negro households are headed by a female, as compared to 9 percent of white households. [4] Moynihan shows that over a period of years from 1951 to 1963 the number of broken Negro families rises and falls with Negro male unemployment.

[4] A social psychological analysis of the lower-class female-headed Negro family is presented by L. Rainwater in his "Crucible of Identity" [14].

Although both series of statistics show a long-run rising trend, there are numerous fluctuations during the period; an increase in unemployment tends to be followed a year later by an increase in separations, and a decrease in unemployment by a decrease in separations. In 1960, Negro unemployment was double that of whites; even so, as Moynihan points out, the usual way of reporting unemployment understates the problem. The average monthly Negro unemployment rate for males in 1964 was 9 percent, but during 1964 some 29 percent of Negro males were unemployed at one time or other.

The father's occupation is obviously of enormous significance for parenthood. When the father has no sustained gainful occupation, the consequences for the family can be devastating. The discrimination in education and employment directed to the Negro male plays a significant part in undermining the Negro (particularly lower-class) family. The destructive effects of unemployment on the family, now most clearly evident among Negroes in American society,[5] but also apparent wherever unemployment is pervasive and long-enduring, were epidemic during the Great Depression [1,10]. The amount of evidence accumulated to date is substantial: Long-continued unemployment among males, especially fathers (though also among young unmarried men), is one of the most important causes of pathological conditions within the family, with far-reaching consequences for both parents and children, as well as for the entire society.

STRUCTURED STRAIN IN BECOMING A PARENT

The traditional interest in the study of parenthood, in sociology as in psychiatry and psychology, has been to ascertain the consequences of different kinds of parental performance on the child. In concluding this chapter, it is appropriate to take note of a relatively new line of sociological inquiry, the socially structured strains in becoming a parent, particularly in the middle class and particularly for women. This problem has been addressed most directly by Alice Rossi, who argues that the transition to parenthood is more difficult in American society than either marital or occupational adjustment[6] [16]. She notes Therese Benedek's point that the child's need for mothering is absolute, while the need of an adult woman to mother is relative. Mrs. Rossi then observes: "Yet our family system of isolated households, increasingly distant from kinswomen to assist in mothering, requires that new mothers shoulder total responsibility for the infant precisely for that stage of the child's life

---

[5] For a comparable picture among Appalachian whites, see Caudill's *Night Comes to the Cumberlands* [4]. The way in which family relationships are affected by larger social forces has seldom been more effectively traced than in this beautifully written book.

[6] I wish to express my thanks to my colleague Dr. Betty Yorburg for bringing this article to my attention.

when his need for mothering is far in excess of the mother's need for the child." Thus, she continues, what is often interpreted as an individual mother's failure to be adequately maternal "may in fact be a failure of the society to provide institutionalized substitutes for the extended kin to assist in the care of infants and young children." Rossi notes these additional strains in the transition to parenthood: (1) There is great cultural pressure on growing girls and young women to consider maternity necessary for individual fulfillment and adult status. (2) Pregnancy is not always a voluntary decision, but society does not allow the termination of unwanted pregnancies. (3) First pregnancy is now the major transition point in a woman's life, because of the spread of effective contraception. This is a change from the past, when marriage was the major transition and first pregnancy followed closely upon marriage. (4) Parenthood is irrevocable, since society allows one to be rid of wives and jobs but not children, and one consequence of this social fact for women with unwanted children is that "the personal outcome of experience in the parent role is not a higher level of maturation but the negative outcome of a depressed sense of self-worth. . . . The possibility must be faced, and at some point researched, that women lose ground in personal development and self-esteem during the early and middle years of adulthood, whereas men gain ground in these respects during the same years." (5) American society does not provide adequate preparation and training for the role of mother. (6) The period of pregnancy does not allow adequate training, unlike the period of anticipatory socialization for marriage (i.e., engagement). (7) Finally, the transition from pregnancy to motherhood is abrupt; it does not allow for a gradual taking on of responsibility, as is true in a professional work role.

Thus, Rossi seems to be describing two main kinds of strain: (1) American culture presses many women into maternity who are not very maternal and perhaps should not become mothers and (2) motherhood in America is difficult because the role demands exceed woman's capacity to meet them adequately and, further, because the social structure provides no built-in surrogates to help the mother, particularly right after delivery but also throughout the rearing of the young.

Rossi's analysis of the strains in the transition to motherhood locates them in the basic structure of American society rather than in any particular segment of it. Some questions arise. Her argument turns to some extent on characterizing our family system as consisting of isolated households which thus deprive the new mother of kinswomen to help in mothering. However, some sociologists have conducted studies which show that the nuclear family is not nearly so isolated as had been commonly supposed. Sussman is most closely identified with this line of inquiry [17]. But while this work shows that there is much more help among kin (including that of parents to their married children and to their minor grandchildren) than had been supposed, the findings are not specific enough to confirm or disconfirm Rossi's specific claim that basic mothering is a solitary task rather than one shared with others, as formerly. Another source of doubt: perhaps Rossi's analysis holds for the middle class but not for the working class. Numerous studies have shown that working-class married women in several societies retain close ties with their own mothers and other kin. A brief overview will be found in Gans's study of working-class Italians [7]. The evidence would seem to suggest that Rossi's analysis may be less tenable for the working class, though again the evidence is not in a form that permits a confident confirmation or disconfirmation of her analysis.

What about the abruptness of full-scale mothering responsibilities in the middle class? Rossi's strongest case would seem to be located here, but numerous questions will have to be laid to rest before it can be accepted. For example, many young newly delivered mothers hire a practical nurse to live in for at least a week after returning home from hospital confinement; others have their own mothers visit and help out. We do not know how widespread such practices are in the middle class. Perhaps this is true in only a small "deviant" group of middle-class mothers. Or perhaps Rossi's mothers constitute the small deviant group rather than the basic pattern to which the middle class is tending. Another informal observation: rooming-in arrangements in maternity hospitals seem to be growing in popularity. If this is a demonstrable fact, how does it fit with Rossi's analysis?

Rossi offers her paper to raise questions and to stimulate rethinking of important issues rather than to provide answers. The largest question she raises is that of the goodness of fit between psychological propensities and the social arrangements which channel wishes, motives, and behavior. This is one of sociology's enduring questions, one that follows close on the heels of the master question: How does society structure wish, motive, and behavior?

BIBLIOGRAPHY

1 Angell, R. C.: *The Family Encounters the Depression,* New York: Scribners, 1936.
2 Berger, B. M.: *Working-Class Suburb: A Study of Auto Workers in Suburbia,* Berkeley: University of California Press, 1960.
3 Bronfenbrenner, U.: Socialization and Social Class Through Time and Space. In E. E. Maccoby, T. M. Newcomb, and E. L. Hartley (Eds.), *Readings in Social Psychology* (3d ed.). New York: Holt, Rinehart and Winston, 1958.
4 Caudill, H.: *Night Comes to the Cumberlands.* Boston: Little, Brown, 1963.
5 Clausen, J.: Family Structure, Socialization and Personality. In M. Hoffman (Ed.), *Review of Child Development Research,* Vol. II. New York: Russell Sage, 1967.
6 Davis, A., and Havighurst, R. J.: Social class and color differences in child rearing. *Amer. Sociol. Rev.* 11:698–710, 1946.

7 Gans, H. J.: *The Urban Villagers: Group and Class in the Life of Italian-Americans.* New York: Free Press, 1962. Pg. 238 ff.

8 Handel, G., and Rainwater, L.: Persistence and change in working class life style. *Sociol. Soc. Res.* **48**:280–288, 1964. Reprinted in A. Shostak and W. Gomberg (Eds.), *Blue-Collar World.* Englewood Cliffs, N.J.: Prentice-Hall, 1964.

9 Kohn, M. L.: Social class and parent-child relationships: An interpretation. *Amer. J. Sociol.* **68**:471–480, 1963. Reprinted in B. Farber (Ed.), *Kinship and Family Organization.* New York: Wiley, 1966.

10 Komarovsky, M.: *The Unemployed Man and His Family.* New York: Dryden, 1940.

11 Lenski, G.: *The Religious Factor: A Sociological Study of Religion's Impact on Politics, Economics and Family Life* (rev. ed.). Garden City, N.Y.: Anchor, 1963. P. 221.

12 Moynihan, D. P.: *The Negro Family: The Case for National Action.* Washington: Office of Policy Planning and Research, U.S. Department of Labor, March, 1965. Pp. 6, 9. Reprinted in L. Rainwater and W. L. Yancey, *The Moynihan Report and the Politics of Controversy.* Cambridge, Mass.: Massachusetts Institute of Technology Press, 1967.

13 Rainwater, L.: *Family Design: Marital Sexuality, Family Size and Contraception.* Chicago: Aldine, 1965.

14 Rainwater, L.: Crucible of identity: The Negro lower class family. *Daedalus* **95**: No. 1 (Winter), 1966. Reprinted in G. Handel (Ed.), *The Psychosocial Interior of the Family.* Chicago: Aldine, 1967.

15 Rainwater, L., Coleman, R., and Handel, G.: *Workingman's Wife: Her Personality, World and Life Style.* New York: Oceana, 1959; paperback ed., Macfadden, 1962.

16 Rossi, A. S.: Transition to parenthood. *J. Marriage Family* **30**:26–39, 1968.

17 Sussman, M. B.: The Isolated Nuclear Family: Fact or Fiction? *and* The Help Pattern in the Middle-Class Family. In M. B. Sussman (Ed.), *Sourcebook in Marriage and the Family.* Boston: Houghton Mifflin, 1963.

18 Vincent, C. E.: Teen-age unwed mothers in American society. *J. Soc. Issues* **22**:22–23, 1966.

19 Wolfenstein, M.: Trends in infant care. *Amer. J. Orthopsychiat.* **23**:120–130, 1953.

Chapter 7

Economics and the Family

Michael A. Viren

The word *economics,* like the word *engineering,* has been so commonly misused that its true meaning has become lost. From the economist's view, economics is a very general science which yields implications about many specific areas like the stock market, finance, government spending, taxes, money, income, consumption, and so on, that have become synonymous with the term economics. This chapter addresses the more general and theoretical aspects of economics and the family, leaving to others the more specific aspects of family finances, income, and consumption.

Economics, to simplify, is involved with the concept of supply and demand. This concept holds that there is, at some price, a point of equilibrium where the demander will demand exactly the same amount of a certain good or service that the supplier will supply. However, this view of economics is too simplistic and yields too few fruitful implications. Thus what this chapter attempts to accomplish is to develop economics in a manner more complex than simply supply and demand and then see what implications it might have for the family.

The available literature on the economics of the family is primarily discussed in terms of financial aspects of family behavior. In addition most literature on the subject tends to treat the family as some kind of whole. This macroscopic view, along with limiting the analysis to only the financial aspects of the economic behavior of the family, has tended to create in the literature gross generalization and value judgments—thus resulting in very few fruitful implications about family economic behavior. This chapter hopes to overcome this problem by viewing the family in the microscopic, i.e., as a collection of individuals. Viewing the family at the micro level yields two sets of implications. The first set pertains to individual and collective decision making by the family, and the second pertains to the distribution of income among family members.

Before proceeding it might be important to explain why implications of family economic behavior are important to health professionals involved in a helping relationship with families. The reason is simple and straightforward. Decisions of families and members of families may seem irrational when viewed as an outsider. However, when the set of assumptions upon which a family makes a decision is known to the outsider, the seemingly irrational decision often becomes logical. Hopefully the economics developed below will allow the health professional to more clearly understand the process by which individuals and families make decisions.

INDIVIDUAL BEHAVIOR

Economics assumes that the world is made up of agents. An agent is either an individual, a productive organization (i.e., a company, corporation, farm, store, or business), or a government. Each agent performs two activities: (1) consumption and (2) production. All agents, whether they be individuals or large corporations, consume; and they all produce. An individual produces a supply of labor. He uses the proceeds from his labor for consumption. The productive organization (and government) consumes labor and other inputs (like land, capital, and raw materials) and produces the goods and services that are consumed by the individuals. Thus all the individuals in a society, in their efforts to consume, generate a *demand* which is fulfilled by the *supply* of goods and services that were produced through the use of labor and other inputs supplied by the individuals and society. This dual behavior of all agents is the essential basis of an economic system.

To further complicate the matter, goods and services are a large bundle consisting of commodities, services, experiences, happenings, and so on. For example, a boat trip down the Green River in Utah is considered a good or service, so also is a picnic in the park, even though it may not cost anything to visit the park. The point being made here is that the concept of goods and services is an all-encompassing term used to describe all possible items that an agent may want to demand or supply. To complicate the matter still further, agents of an economy must choose among not only a large variety of goods and services, but also the quantity of each good and service he wishes to consume and produce.

Individual agents make these decisions with the guidance of a utility or preference function. Other agents in the economy have different methods for making decisions. For example, corporations have the profit motive to guide their decision making. However, since we are only concerned with the family which is made up of individual agents, we will simply assume that other agents exist, but they will not be discussed. This function is a system of values which allows individual agents to rank all possible bundles of goods and services that he could possibly consume or produce. For example, suppose an individual has before him three bundles each with the same three kinds of goods, but in varying amounts (i.e., bundle one contains two cans of beer, one sandwich, and three boiled eggs; bundle two contains one can of beer, two sandwiches, and two boiled eggs; and bundle three contains three cans of beer, three sandwiches, and one boiled egg). It would seem reasonable that it would be possible to rank the bundles as to which was preferred the most, the next best, and the least. However, we still do not have sufficient information to make a decision as to which of the three bundles to consume. As stated above, each individual must produce as well as consume; i.e., the individual most likely produces labor. In other words, he works or sells skills for which he derives an income. Now, combining the fact of the existence of a preference function and the existence of an income gives sufficient information for an individual to make a decision. The decision would be to choose the most preferred bundle the individual can afford. In other words, individuals will choose a bundle of goods and services that has the highest preference ranking subject to the constraint that the bundle does not cost more than his income.

We can now introduce slightly more complexity by acknowledging the fact the income constraint is not the only constraint that may keep an individual from choosing his highest rank bundle. This can be understood by considering that the act of consumption also requires the use of time and energy. Thus the price of each good or service in a bundle has three components: the money price, the time price, and the energy price. This implies that it might not be possible for a person to purchase the most preferred bundle of goods and services; i.e., he may have sufficient income, but in fact chooses a less preferred bundle because the most preferred requires the use of too much time or energy.

We now have sufficient information to draw some implications about individual economic behavior. This can be done by keeping in mind that all individuals are not equally endowed with talent, intelligence, physical stamina, and emotional stability. These inequitable endowments imply that individuals have different endowments of the resources of income, time, and energy. Thus each individual goes about choosing his most preferred bundle of goods and services subject to different constraint levels. These different constraint levels can be used to draw implications about the behavior of individuals.

Health Care: Want Versus Need

The idea that there is a difference in understanding between the economist and the health professional over the meaning of demand was first suggested by Boulding (1966). He introduced the idea that demand was a collection of wants and needs. He stated that the behavior of individuals toward their wants could be explained by economic reasoning but that needs were more basic and were beyond economic reasoning. As could be expected this idea was well received among health professionals and not so well received by economists. In order to maintain economics as a useful tool in the solution of health problems, Jeffers et al. (1971) pointed out that need was a technically defined concept. That is, the amount of goods and services that are needed for the maintenance of health is defined by the health professional. The amount of health goods and services that an individual will consume depends upon his resources and income; time and energy; and the price of health goods and services in terms of money, time, and energy. The amount of goods and services supplied depends upon the amount of revenue derived from selling the goods and services. This is to say, the higher the money price of goods and services, the greater the supply of health goods and services. Since there is no relationship between the technically defined quantity of health care and the quantity demanded and supplied, the actual quantity of health care goods and services delivered would equal the amount *needed* only by accident. If somehow individuals changed their demand for health goods and services as they became more educated, the economic mechanism would bring about an equilibrium between what is demanded, what is supplied, and what is needed. However, if the technology base the health professional uses to define need is expanding faster than the education of health consumers, equilibrium will not be reached. There is considerable evidence to indicate that this is the case.

A better understanding of why consumers do not consume what they *need* can be obtained by referring back to the individual, his preference function, and his resource constraints. Note that the preference function is a value system that allows an individual to rank all choices before him. The goods and services that are *needed* to maintain health are in a sense competing with other goods and services. Assume that an individual has sufficient resources to purchase the needed amount of health care. Let the other goods and services in his consumption bundle be classified as *wants*. If by consuming less health goods and services than he *needs* the individual's resources are also sufficient to purchase the goods and services he *wants,* and if the *wants* are valued sufficiently high by the individual's preference function, he will trade off *needed* health goods and services for the goods and services that he *wants.*

This seemingly irrational behavior is observed with great regularity. The classic example is the family on welfare who has barely sufficient funds to buy food, yet purchases a color TV set. However, when viewed from the prospective of the individual's value system, i.e., his preference function, the choice he makes is perfectly logical.

Present Versus Future Consumption

Before concluding the discussion of the behavior of individuals, the relationship between present versus future consumption should be highlighted. Just as the individual's value system allows trade-off between wants and needs, it is possible to make trade-offs between present and future consumption. This is particularly easy in the United States economy with its large system of retail credit and savings institutions.

Basic to the relationship between present and future consumption is, that for two identical goods or services, the one consumed now is valued higher than the one consumed in the future. A second devaluation of future consumption occurs when there exists a lack of knowledge as to the benefits from the consumption of goods and services. The reverse is true, of course, for goods and services that are detrimental to the individual.

The effect on individual behavior is even more pronounced when considering the consumption of health promotional goods and services. Individuals tend to undervalue the benefits of health promotional goods and services because of the two reasons cited above but also because resources must be expended now in order to receive the benefits (i.e., the value of the consumption of health promotional goods and services) in the future. Take for example the decision-making process that a pregnant woman uses in deciding to expend resources in order to obtain a program of prenatal care. The benefits from the program are mostly in the future, and therefore, the benefits to her now are some discounted value of her future benefits. Secondly, since she lacks perfect knowledge as to exactly what the benefits of prenatal care are, she may tend to underestimate the future benefits. This does not deny the possibility that out of ignorance and optimism she could overestimate the future benefits of prenatal care. Finally, since the value of the consumption of prenatal services is separated in time from the expenditure of her resources on the purchase of prenatal services, she must also forego the consumption of some other goods and services while waiting for the value of prenatal care to be received in the future.

The last point to be made about individual behavior pertains to an economic explanation of a statement that poor health creates poverty and that poverty creates poor health. The definition of the level of consumption of health goods and services that is *needed* to maintain an individual at some minimum level of health is independent of his endowment of resources. That is, if a person *needs* 2,000 calories per day to keep in health, that amount would not change if he became wealthier.

This in general causes poor individuals to spend a higher proportion of their income in just meeting needs. Further, this causes a consumption of wants in the present over future consumption of wants and needs to be valued more highly than the same comparison made at higher levels of endowed resources. A person on a $3,000 income values the consumption of wants in the present at a higher level than he would if he earned $10,000. This phenomenon manifests itself in the inverse relationship that exists between the interest rate individuals will pay in order to consume a product. Individuals from poor urban communities are willing to borrow from "loan sharks" and finance companies at high interest rates; and high- and middle-income individuals will borrow on their life insurance policy at low interest rate. Thus, when faced with a choice of either purchasing health promotional services or consuming *wants* in the present, the individual with a low endowment of resources chooses to sacrifice health goods and services, which may result in declining health. A reduced level of health in turn impairs the individual's earning capacity. The cycle again repeats itself with individuals choosing to meet present needs over future health promotional goods and services.

It is important to note that these conclusions do not depend upon rich and poor individuals having different value systems, but simply on having different levels of endowed resources.

COLLECTIVE BEHAVIOR

Up until this point we have been discussing the individual's economic behavior. We now develop the economic behavior of the family. Again, it must be remembered that we are discussing the economics of the family, not the finances of the family. The family behavior will be based on the same general theory of value that guided the individual in his decision-making processes.

In order to view the family in perspective with the individual, it is important to visualize a hierarchy along a continuum. At the beginning of this continuum is the individual. He must make the decision as to what and how much of a good or service he wishes to consume, given that he knows the price of that good or service. The goods consumed by individuals are called *private goods*. All the decisions are single-person decisions. This constitutes the first level of the hierarchy.

With the next level of the hierarchy we enter the world of public goods. That is, at this level a collective of two individuals must make the decision of how much and what kinds of good and services will be consumed at the prevailing price. All decisions at the second level of the hierarchy are *two-person public goods*. (Using this terminology consistently a private good should be called a *one-person public good*.) The third level of consumption is that of the three-person public goods. The hierarchy continues in increasing numbers of persons forming collectives in order to make consumption decisions about higher-level public goods. As the number of individuals increases, we see the formations of neighborhoods, communities, towns, cities, counties, states, and nations.

The family is a collective formed to make consumption decisions about two-person and larger public goods. Please note that we are discussing the economic basis of family behavior; there clearly are other social and physical reasons for forming the family. In this respect there is nothing special about the family. It is not the foundation of a society. In this framework the individual is. As will be discussed below, the family is the first step in the hierarchy of collective decision making. All the problems of decision making at the national level can also be found at the family level of the hierarchy.

Public Goods and Services

Before proceeding we must be sure that the concept of public goods is understood. The family must make a collective decision as to the amount and kind of good or service they wish to consume. This implies that in making the decision to consume a five-bedroom house, or a 17-inch TV set, each member of the family must consume the same amount of the public good. That is, if the family's collective decision is to buy a 17-inch TV, then all members must watch the same size TV set. Whereas, if the same decisions were made by all members of the family as individuals, then each member could purchase the size of television that would be consistent with his preference function and the endowment of resources. It is clearly more economical to consume a television as a public good as opposed to a private good provided a collective decision can be made. The making of the collective decision is much more difficult than the making of an individual decision. The problems of such a decision-making process will be developed below.

A second aspect of public goods and services is derived from the fact that the consumption by one individual in the collective does not prohibit another individual from also consuming the public good. For example, a show being watched on a 17-inch TV set by one individual does not interfere with another individual watching the same show. Whereas, an individual eating an apple precludes another individual eating the same apple. Private goods, like apples, have the property of exclusion, whereas public goods are only exclusive between the collective groups. That is, one family may view their TV set as a public good but exclude their neighbors from using it. In like manner two families may view the streetlight in front of their houses as a two-family or neighborhood public good. But because of the distance, the neighbors down the street are excluded from use of it.

It is hoped that the above discussion of public goods and services has added another dimension to the concept of a good or service. Originally, when there were only individuals who had to make decisions about consumptions, the only dimension we were concerned with was quantity. As we introduced the collective nature of society, we added a *publicness* dimension to the nature of good and service. A TV set might be described as having a quantity measure of 17 inches and have a publicness measure of being a family public good. An apple might weigh 13 ounces and be a one-person public (private) good. The classic example of a nation-level public good is national defense. The quantity dimensions of national defense might be measured by the 2.7-million man army, and its publicness dimensions might be described as a 200-million-person (national) public good.

Collective (Family) Decision Making

One of the distinguishing aspects of public goods is that the quanitity consumed by each member must be the same. Yet a family is made up of individuals with individualistic preference functions, i.e., different value systems. It seems reasonable to ask whether family consumption decisions can be made on the same rational, nonconflicting basis that individuals use. To answer this question, we find that conflict is a natural phenomenon in family decision making, and it can only be avoided by establishing rigid family structures that minimize the degree of democracy and freedom of the individuals within the family (or for that matter individuals of higher-order collectives, i.e., the city, state, or nation).

To help support this conclusion, let us return for a moment to a society of only individuals. If we assume that this society is free of monopolies, then certain other assumptions hold. [These assumptions are not important to the present discussion, but for those more interested they may consult any intermediate microeconomic text, such as Ferguson (1969).] Then each individual with his initial endowment of resources (wealth) and guided by his preference function (value system) will engage in a decision process that will allocate his initial resource bundle in such a way that his final consumption bundle will be his best choice and that society as a whole cannot be made better off by any other reallocation of original endowments. When such a phenomenon occurs, it is referred to by economists as the *Pareto optimal state* of the economy. Any attempt to improve the position of one individual in society would result in someone else being made worse off. It should be noted that it is possible for a society to reach many different Pareto optimal states, depending on the original allocation of wealth to each member of society. The important point here is that it is theoretically possible for a society made up of only individuals who consume only private goods to reach the Pareto optimal state.

Now, as we expand the definition of goods and services by adding a publicness dimension to them, we find in general that it is not theoretically possible for just any initial endowment of wealth to reach a Pareto optimal state. In order to achieve a Pareto optimal state, the most desired state of all possible Pareto states must be selected, and the initial endowment of resources must be allocated in such a way as to ensure that the desired Pareto optimal state will be achieved. The process of selecting the best of all Pareto optimal states develops the majority of fruitful implications about family economic behavior.

Professor Kenneth Arrow presented in *Social Choice and Individual Values* (1963) several conditions that must exist in order for the selection of the best of all Pareto optimal points to somehow reflect the values of all individuals in a society (or a family). Arrow found that there existed no way to select the best state and still have it reflect individual values. However if those conditions were weakened sufficiently, they would allow for the existence of (1) social customs and religious dogma; (2) a dictatorial decision maker; or (3) a special case of item (2) where individuals through conflict inform others of the strength of the value they place on certain states of the world (or family) and in turn, through conflict, are receptive to the strengths of the value that others place on alternative states of the world (or the family).

A casual tracing of the historic changes in family style will show that all three of these above exceptions to Arrow's conditions were used in directing individuals toward the Pareto optimal state (of their family).

To see this, let us break the dynamics of family decision making into three discrete periods. The first period involved the family in a struggle for survival against predators. Examples of this period occurred many times in the history of man, i.e., the Dark Ages, settlement of the New World, times of war.

The second period involved the family in a struggle for physical survival. During these periods the families' objectives were to ensure an adequate supply of food and shelter. Examples of such periods in Western civilizations were the Renaissance and the first half of the twentieth century.

The third period might be described as the modern period of the family. It is the time when the struggle against predators and for physical survival was no longer necessary.

During the first period the sheer struggle against predators required the family to have a head, a dictator, usually a man, who imposed his value system on the rest of the family. He made the ethical decision as to which Pareto optimal state was best for the family. He then allocated the family resources in such a way as to achieve the desired state of the family.

As man mastered his predators, he turned his attention to his physical needs. This lessened the need for the family to have a dictator to make its ethical decisions. As the dictator rule faded, it was replaced by strong social customs and religious dogmas. These dogmas defined for the family the Pareto optimal state it *should* obtain. The family then allocated its wealth in such a way that the desired state was obtained.

In the third period, succeeding in the struggle against predators, and the achieving of physical security also ended the role of man as a dictator of the family and ended the influence of social customs and religious dogma in the decision-making process of the family. Herein lies the final and maybe the most important economic implication for the modern family behavior. We are now only left with conflict if we wish to reach a Pareto optimal state.

This period has also seen the woman's role in the family change, and her role in society has become more significant. Along with this there has come an increasing amount of conflict within the family structure. This conflict has been interpreted by others to mean the signaling of the end of the family as an institution within society. This author, however, places a different interpretation on this sign. It seems more reasonable to view the increasing conflict as a natural process of weighting individual values within the family such that the best Pareto optimal state can be decided upon.

Having lost the basis for assuming dictatorial power over his family, man has had to accept the competition of the woman in her desire to make decisions that would improve her state of being. In addition, they have both been freed of the strong religious dogma and social customs that had previously made the ethical decisions. Thus, both individuals in the family (a man and a woman) must select the Pareto optimal state of their family with equal representation of both of their value systems. The use of the word "equal" does not mean the resources, or the goods and services, that are produced will be divided equally but instead that the values of individuals have equal weight in the process used to select the Pareto optimal state of each family.

Herein lies the naturalness of conflict as a process of deciding on the Pareto optimal state. When two (or more) individuals consider themselves equals, the expression of their values about various states of nature (or the family) can result in conflict. This conflict allows the expression of the strengths of each individual's value system. The strength of each individual's value system *equally* considered could then lead to a Pareto optimal state.

It is still possible to argue that this conflict will divide the family. This is particularly true when one individual is trying to find the Pareto optimal state through a dictatorial decision or religious dogma and the other individual considers her (or his) value system of lesser importance.

Opposing the pressure to divide the family is the economics of consuming public goods. Also, the increasing awareness of the fact that we live on a finite planet might begin to lay the economic foundation for the explanation of the increasing occurrence of group marriages and multinuclear families. In addition, with a society such as ours with its ever-increasing use of public goods as opposed to private goods, the collective nature of the family might have to be expanded, not contracted, to allow for collections of families in order that decisions can be made about higher-level public goods.

CONCLUSIONS

The important conclusions of this paper can be summarized in the following statements. (1) Individuals through the guidance of their preference functions and by their constraints of limited resources are willing to make trade-offs between their wants and their needs. On the surface these trade-offs may appear to outsiders as being irrational, but when viewed within an economic framework, these decisions are founded in logic. (2) Families cannot, by the independent action of their individual members, reach the optimal state of well-being; and in our modern society conflict may be a very rational process by which individuals within a collective arrangement, i.e., a family, can decide upon the optimal state.

BIBLIOGRAPHY

Arrow, K. J.: *Social Choice and Individual Values,* 2d ed., New York: John Wiley and Sons, Inc., 1963.

Boulding, K. E.: "The Concept of Need for Health Services," *Milbank Memorial Fund Quarterly,* **44**:202-223, 1966.

Ferguson, G. E.: *Microeconomic Theory,* 2d ed., Homewood, Ill.: Richard D. Irwin, Inc., 1969.

Jeffers, J. R., M. F. Bognanno, and J. C. Bartlett: "On the Demand Versus Need for Medical Services and the Concept of 'Shortage,'" *American Journal of Public Health* **61**(1): 46-63, 1971.

Chapter 8

Game Theory as a Conceptual Framework for Nursing Practice

Mary Reardon Castles

The task of this chapter is to identify a particular theory in the behavioral sciences which can be useful to the nurse oriented toward the perception of the family in its entirety as a responsibility of nursing care. The theory of games offers a framework which appears especially useful.

BACKGROUND

Any attempt to identify one particular behavioral science framework as a model for nursing is automatically subject to at least two criticisms: (1) the new conceptual framework is an exercise in semantics, saying in different words what is equally well described another way; and (2) there is a better model to be derived from another source. Both criticisms are true as far as they go. Any accurate description of an empirical situation is likely to bear some resemblance to any other accurate description of the same situation, in that the salient relationships among variables will hold whether they are described in terms of status and role, input and output, lines of communication, or formal and informal groups. How well any model fits depends to a large extent on the frame of reference of the modeler. However, it should be remembered that neither immortality nor universality are necessary characteristics of a useful model; the closer and more accurate the representation of immediate concrete situations, the more ephemeral and narrow the model is likely to be, and for any given frame of reference any one model may be better than any other. The model is judged on its usefulness.

Folta and Deck (1966, p. 11) point out, when they make explicit their own commitment to symbolic interactionism as a conceptual framework for nursing, that there are many ways of seeing; most theories in sociology are more or less relevant to the nursing goal.

THE SICK ROLE

The behavioral science approach to the circumstances surrounding illness behavior is heavily influenced by Parsons's (1951) concept of the sick role. Most writers accept his view of illness behavior as a special case of deviant behavior. The sick person is considered to have certain rights and responsibilities: he has the right to be excused from normal duties, and to claim assistance from others; his responsibilities are to want to get well as quickly as possible, to seek help from a competent source, and to cooperate in his treatment.

Wilson (1963) discusses the Parsonian concept of the therapeutic relationship. He indicates that while the patient and the child are not the same, "the process of inducting an individual into society and of returning him to a full and sanctioned functioning in society are remarkably parallel" (1963, p. 289). The subordinate position of the patient is expressed in his catalog of the four major features of the therapist-patient relationship (1963, p. 287) as they are singled out for analysis. Since these summarize effectively a point of view which is still current, they are presented in toto.

> *Support*　The therapist expresses his obligation to be of assistance, to provide a stable figure on whom the patient may lean. He will be available, helpful, nurturant toward the patient's needs for dependency. It is understood, however, that the support is temporary and contingent on the patient's continuing efforts to get well.
>
> *Permissiveness*　The therapist allows the patient to express feelings and indulge in actions which would not be acceptable in a nontherapeutic relationship. Again the dispensation is temporary and rooted in the idea that patient or child is for the moment unable to adhere strictly to ordinary norms of social intercourse. Permissiveness is granted with the justification that the patient, by reason of his illness, "can't help" doing certain things and cannot be held to usual expectations of responsibility.

Manipulation of reward The therapist exerts leverage on the ill person by controlling certain rewards which are especially significant to the dependent party. As in child-rearing, the primary reward is probably approval, which can be offered or withheld at the discretion of the socializing or therapeutic agent. Rewards are given for doing the "right thing," for trying to "grow up," or to "get well."

Denial of Reciprocity The therapist, as a condition for granting of support and permissiveness, withholds from the patient his own full interpersonal responsiveness. He keeps the relationship asymmetrical by refusing either to feel all the patient feels or to allow the patient access to his, the therapist's, true feelings. He will not meet fire with fire, irritation with irritation, adoration with adoration; for to do so would be to sacrifice the independent terrain on which he stands, and with it the potential for helping the other.

The concept of rights and responsibilities inherent in the sick role is not in itself derogatory in its assumptions about the patient and his family; however somewhat disparaging inferences are frequently drawn.

Parsons (1951), in his conception of the sick role, models the doctor-patient relationship on the child-parent relationship. Both children and sick people lack the capacity to perform the functions of adults in everyday life, both are dependent and rely on the stronger, more adequate physician or parent. Parsons and Fox (1952) in a later article suggest that because of this close correspondence between the sick person and the child, it is important to have the major part of an illness dealt with outside the family.

Extrafamilial care of the sick is considered to be positively functional for American society, because it protects the family against the disruptive effects of the illness of its members; it provides some of the positive functions of the sick role as a mechanism of social control; and it facilitates the therapeutic processes, both motivationally and technologically.

This view of the vulnerability of the American family may be sociologically sound; however, any practitioner of nursing is able to offer empirical evidence that suggests that it may be the *institutionalization* of the sick person which is frequently extremely disrupting. While the therapeutic process may be facilitated in technological terms (certainly it is more economical of professional time and effort to have all the patients in one place), it cannot truly be said to be facilitated in any other way. With the possible exception of a mental illness in which the family may have explicit etiological significance, it is unlikely that the stress involved in hospitalization contributes to therapeutic efficacy in any illness.

There is no doubt that it is usually extremely inconvenient and frequently impossible for a patient to be cared for in his home. There may be no room; there may be no caretaking person; the environment, because of extremes of temperature, lack of food, the presence of vermin, etc., may be inimical to his recovery. These are problems of the health care delivery system, and need not be all met by immediate institutionalization. Even if the home stresses are such that the patient must be removed from that environment, the therapeutic efficacy of institutionalization can be questioned. Whether institutionalization is necessary to protect the family against the "disruptive effects of the illness" can also be questioned by health care practitioners. Whatever psychological dynamics are involved, the literature provides evidence that care of a patient in the home by his family can be extremely rewarding.

Parsons and Fox (1952, p. 359) argue that the tendency to remove the patient from the home is only partly due to technological development; they believe that "certain features of the American urban family in their impact on the personalities of its members have tended to push the sick person out of the home." This article is not recent. It is discussed here in such detail because this concept of the sick person as passive, dependent, and childlike, and of the family as particularly vulnerable to his illness and needing to be protected by his institutionalization, continues to be pervasive not only in social science, but in nursing.

PSYCHOSOCIAL CONCEPTS OF ILLNESS BEHAVIOR

Coe (1970, pp. 107-111), in his chapter on the response to illness, presents a chronological progression of psychosocial concepts of illness behavior, in which each episode of illness is viewed as involving a series of stages or phases. Barker et al. (1946), in a work antedating Parsons's, described the patient's reduced mobility and reduced interaction with others, and indicated the sick person is characterized by egocentricity, regression, and apathy. Convalescence is described as a period in which to test returning skills as an adult. Lederer (1958) added to a set of similar stages the period of becoming sick, and discussed the patient's reaction primarily in psychological terms.

The most recent formulation of the stages of illness is provided by Suchman (1965):

Symptom experience   This is the stage in which the individual perceives that something is wrong, evaluates the degree of severity and responds emotionally to the evaluation.

Assumption of the sick role   In this stage the individual decides to adopt the sick role and seeks agreement from significant others that he is ill. Provisional validation of the sick role by the family leads to the stage of medical care contact.

Medical care contact   This is the point of contact with the professional care system when the individual seeks both treatment and validation of his assumption of the sick role.

Dependent patient role   The decision to undergo treatment for his illness makes the sick person a patient.

Recovery and rehabilitation   In this stage, the patient "must renounce any pleasures attained from being dependent on others" (Coe, 1970, p. 110) and leave the sick role or be classed as a malingerer. With the accomplishment of a cure, the patient regains health and adulthood.

It is to be noted at the same time that, in spite of the apparent perception of the patient as childlike in his dependence, and his need to be coaxed and coerced into "proper" behavior, the patient and his family are explicitly seen as decision makers. In Coe's terms (1970, p. 111), "entry into and exit from each stage involves decision making on the part of the sick person and those around him."

Szasz and Hollender (Bloom, 1963) also accept the Parsonian sick role in their description of three types of doctor-patient relationships: *activity-passivity,* which is compared to the parent-child relationship, and in which treatment takes place regardless of the patient's contribution; *guidance-cooperation,* which is modeled on the parent-adolescent relationship (guidance is provided by the therapist, cooperation by the patient). Bloom (1963, p. 41) says, ". . . the patient . . . is capable of following directions and of exercising some judgment. . . . When the approach is geared at this level, the patient is expected to look up to his physician and obey him." And finally *mutual-participation,* which is modeled on an adult-adult relationship. According to Bloom (1963, p. 41), in this model "the physician helps the patient to help himself. Since it requires a complex psychological and social organization on the part of the patient it is rarely appropriate for children or for people who are mentally deficient, very poorly educated, or profoundly immature." The author indicates that one model is not better than another, only more appropriate in diverse situations. However, guidance-cooperation is perceived as the most usual model, with very few patients (or doctors? or nurses?) able to sustain a mutual-participation relationship.

Mechanic (1968) enters a slight caveat to the general acceptance of the implications of the Parsonian construct.

> The concept of the "sick role" is an ideal-type in the sense that it is a theoretical model that attempts to depict the patient's behavioral orientations when he seeks medical care, but is not itself a description of empirical reality. It thus constitutes a perspective for viewing patient behavior (1968, p. 173).

Mechanic's criticism is not of the theoretical model of the sick role developed by Parsons, but rather of attempts to use it as a description of empirical reality. He says:

> Some of the popularizers of the sick role have applied the concept too glibly without an awareness of the many nuances that affect the behavior of the patient (1968, p. 174).

The antitherapeutic stress provided both by assuming the characteristics of the sick role and by hospitalization receives some recognition. Croog (1963, p. 254), in his article on interpersonal relationships, says, "Moving into the alien atmosphere of the hospital away from the familiar things of home and family represents one sort of strain. The requirement of adopting the dependent, infantilized behavior patterns which are forced upon adults who become hospital patients represent another." Luke Smith (1966, p. 133), although believing that the patient is a social deviant, and that the hospital has the latent therapeutic function of making him desire to return to conformity, recognizes that the hospital is essentially an economic rather than a therapeutic device. Coe (1970, p. 291) recognizes that hospitalization of an ill member may change the balance of relationships in the family; for instance, institutionalization of the aged can cause emotional as well as financial strain in the family group.

The Parsonian concept of the sick role is not, of course, the only way of perceiving the patient, but it is omnipresent. Attention is directed to it here because its more pernicious implications about the patient and his family are widespread in nursing.

Empirical evidence obtained by an informal canvass of the nursing divisions of a general hospital indicates that clinical practitioners in nursing are not at all uncomfortable with the concept of the patient as dependent, passive, and childlike. A young nursing student admitting an elderly woman to the division calls her by her first name. A practical nurse giving a bed bath to a middle-aged man is visible from the hall. She washes his exposed buttocks vigorously while carrying on a conversation with the patient in the next bed. The medication nurse says to an adult woman, "Now let's take our medicine, we want to get better, don't we?" Nurse clinicians and educators may deplore but are unable to prevent such practices. When nurses unconsciously assume patients are indeed dependent, passive, and childlike, the usual rules of modesty and courtesy between adult and adult are apparently not considered applicable. Leonard (1966, p. 75) has observed that the patient's motivation to participate in the health care system is likely to be neglected. He says, "Among professionals and staff there is a tendency toward a 'take it or leave it' attitude. It seems assumed that the patient will do what he is told without question. . . ." Dorothy Smith (1966, p. 59), in discussing medical organizations, concurs, "The patient's role involves being there to be treated and cooperating with the physician and the nurse in treatment procedures."

Directly related to this view of the patient, and as ubiquitous in the literature, is the Parsons and Fox statement of the danger to the family inherent in the care of the sick member in the home. However, in spite of its perceived vulnerability to the disruptive effects of illness, the United States family is apparently resuming some function in the care of the sick. Robert Bell (1966, p. 188) points out that "it appears that increasingly the family is expected to handle a greater amount of illness and that increasingly this is becoming a part of the 'professional' role of the wife-mother." He sees this involvement as meeting medical needs rather than family needs, and also asks whether the family really provides the best setting for handling illness. He feels, however that health workers must focus on the family, since it is the basic social unit, in order to understand the total impact of illness. Folta and Deck (1966, p. 50) are in agreement that "the return of the patient to his home and community is gaining in impetus. Medical care is making the full cycle back to the home."

Although the social scientists appear to accept the implications of the Parsonian sick role, it is interesting to note that even when the patient is being regarded as dependent and regressed, and the family as vulnerable and non-therapeutic, the sick situation and illness behavior are likely to be described in terms of conflict, decision making, and negotiation. As Coe (1970, p. 290) points out, "At several points in time during the development of an illness, the individual must make certain choices or decisions with respect to his behavior." Mechanic (1968, p. 2) presents a perspective of illness behavior and reactions to the ill as "aspects of a coping dialogue in which the various participants are often actively striving to meet their responsibilities, to control their environment, and to make their every day circumstances more tolerable and predictable."

In a society in which civil rights are considered the prerogative of all members of the social group, and in which the consumer of products and services begins to wield a powerful influence over the provision of those products and services, the patient remains an object of patronage. At best in the therapeutic situation he is perceived as a child, to be guided back to health by his firm but loving professional parents. At frequent worst he is an object upon whom others work their skills, to be cured in spite of himself.

GAME THEORY

The game theory orientation to be presented here is in strong contrast to this patronizing view of the patient. It provides a conceptual framework for health and illness which allows the patient and his family the dignity of equality in the strategies devised for his return to health. Its use makes it possible to think of the family as Bell (1966, p. 181) does when he says that in the family adaptation to the illness of one of its members, it is possible to think in terms of alteration rather than disorganization.

The theory of games provides a methodology for decision making in situations of conflict in which information may not be complete, and none of the persons making the decisions are in complete control of the events. The decision makers may have different goals, and there are many possible outcomes in the situation, all of which have different values to each player. The outcome may be positive or negative for any number of players. Shubik (1964) describes it as follows:

> Game theory is a method for the study of decision making in situations of conflict. It deals with human processes in which the individual decision-unit is not in complete control of other decision-units entering into the environment. It is addressed to problems involving conflict, cooperation or both at many levels. The stage may be set to reflect primarily political, psychological, sociological, economic or other aspects of human affairs.
>
> The essence of a "game" in this context is that it involves decision makers with different goals or objectives whose fates are intertwined. The individuals are in a situation in which there may be many possible outcomes with different values to them. Although they may have some control which will influence the outcome, they do not have complete control over others (1964, p. 8).
>
> A game is described in terms of the players, or individual decision makers, the payoffs, or values assigned to the outcomes of the game, and the rules, which specify the variables that each player controls, the information conditions, and all other relevant aspects of the environment (1964, p. 11).

The patient, the patient's family, the doctor, and the nurse may all be defined as players in the game of ill health. Each player is in control of some resources, and the rules of the game specify how the resources may be utilized. All four players will interact in the game situation, each utilizing different resources. The strategies involved may be medical, emotional, rational, physical, mental, financial, or any and all combinations of these and other categories.

The theory of games was developed by Von Neumann and Morgenstern (Shubik, 1964) in the field of economics. Behavioral scientists in other fields of endeavor have adapted the model to their own areas of practice and research.

Gaming is not referred to in its usual sense, but refers merely to a set of frameworks for interdependent behavior in which the consequences for each participant depend to some extent on his own behavior, but also on the behavior of others over whom he exercises little or no control. At least some interests will conflict, and situations in which there are both cooperation and conflict are the subjects of analysis. When gaming is considered in this manner, nursing activities may be viewed in the context of a game situation.

A factor of gaming which is likely to go against the mystique of feeling which is a part of nursing sentiment is the factor of detachment as distinct from commitment, which is an integral part of the games orientation. Wohlstetter (1964, p. 222) indicates this is also true in other areas of behavioral science, where there is frequently hostility to the concepts of gaming. He believes this is derived in part from "distaste for coolness, detachment and calculation (all of which are connected with games) as against warmhearted-ness, commitment and intuition. . . . In the extreme, these critics may stress the importance of being committed rather than right."

In spite of the feelings which may be generated in nurses by these characteristics of the gaming framework, game theoretic distinctions can be useful both in conceptual analysis of the basic concepts of family nursing and in empirical study. Nursing care is based on what nurses believe about the patient. If he is perceived as "difficult," nursing interactions will be geared to that expectation. As Bloom (1963, p. 36) points out, "Rather than perceiving patients as they are, the doctor (or nurse) views the patient according to preconceived attitudes of how 'good' patients should behave." If the nurse believes that a patient should be dependent and manifest regressive tenden-cies, then the patient who retains his adult expectations of himself, and demands to be treated as an adult by the persons caring for his physical needs is only too likely to be considered recalcitrant. When the family is considered unable to care for the patient, it is easy for the nurse to perceive them as merely being in the way.

It is an important part of the nursing responsibility to encourage the patient to do what he can for himself and by himself and, equally, to encour-age his family both to support him in his independence and to participate as necessary in his care. Therefore, it appears detrimental to the nursing process to think of the patient as dependent and childlike, a social deviant who must be "returned" to the assumption of adult role requirements. The concept of the family as needing to be protected from the psychological dangers inherent in patienthood for one of its members also has a less than ideal effect on the nursing process. While there is no doubt that dependency and regression characterize some patient behaviors, and that some families are less able to adapt to illness than others, why should not nursing explicitly draw on the strengths of both the patient and his family, while protecting them as neces-sary and as possible from their weaknesses?

The theory of games provides a conceptual framework for the delivery of nursing care which allows for the recognition of strength and permits the patient and his family to continue in an adult status, in spite of the illness. Game theory makes assumptions about behavior in illness which anticipate a certain amount of rationality, rather than complete dependency. Most important, the game orientation gives equal status to all players. In this view of the health game, the strategies of the family, the patient, the doctor, and the nurse are equally important. The framework is oriented toward decision making in a situation of conflict, rather than toward regression, dependence, and vulnerability, and allows for strength as well as weakness. This orienta-tion necessarily takes into account the consumers as well as the providers of care, and gives them equal status as players in the game, rather than as counters to be manipulated.

THE HEALTH GAME

Game theory is not necessarily limited to the concept of rational players using optimal relevant information to make ideal decisions. The techniques are designed to accommodate the fact that the rules of rational behavior must provide for the possibility of irrational moves by the other players. Health gaming can be considered as "free," or open, gaming (Goldhamer and Speier, 1964, p. 261). This kind of gaming is exemplified by political games, and is contrasted with formal games where all rules are assumed to be specified and known in advance.*

The two-person nonconstant sum game, in which there are many different interrelationships between the strategies and objectives of several decision makers, is probably the best games model to use to describe the professional and lay behavior surrounding illness.

A person is defined as either an individual or a set of individuals who have coincident interests. These "two persons" could be the doctor and the patient, the family and the patient, the nurse and the patient, the nurse and the family, etc., or any combination of these players, since, although the model is described for two persons, it can be generalized for any number. Chance is also recognized as a player, and can be exemplified in the illness situation by the disease process.

Nonconstant is defined as a lack of dependability of commitment to any one strategy by any player.

A *sum game* is one in which the amount that one player wins is not exactly equivalent to the amount that the others lose; that is, there can be a time when everyone wins a little or loses a little. These can be described as *cooperative solutions*. The fundamental idea behind cooperative solutions is that in general there are gains to be had from cooperation, and rational individuals will realize these gains. They will argue only about their shares.

Strategies can be defined generally as a plan of action containing instructions as to what to do in every contingency.

The essential features of the sick situation may be described by the essential features of a bargaining situation:

> Parties perceive that there is the possibility of reaching an agreement in which each party would be better off or no worse off than if no agreement is reached.

* The gaming concept is not entirely foreign to nursing. An article in the May-June 1971 issue of the *NLN News* reports a health game developed by a nurse and others at Hunter College in which the goal is to raise the level of health of the citizens of a mythical community.

Parties perceive that there is more than one such agreement which could be reached.

Parties perceive each other to have conflicting preferences or opposed interests with regard to the different agreements which might be reached (Deutsch and Krauss, 1964, p. 325).

Dorothy Smith (1966, p. 56) agrees with this; she believes that a negotiation between the doctor and the patient terminates the sickness.

As Deutsch and Krauss (1964) indicate in their discussion of interpersonal bargaining, it is necessary to beware of the possibility that shared purpose may not develop nor agreement be reached even when cooperation would be mutually advantageous. Their discussion is directed toward an overt bargaining situation, but the participants in the health game also may have mutually exclusive goals and mixed feelings toward one another. The doctor-nurse relationship is not always harmonious; the techniques of cure frequently interfere with the techniques of care. The patient may manifest extreme ambivalence in his feelings about the doctor, the nurse, and his family. It is not always easy to be grateful, and he is in a position in which the norms demand gratitude as the appropriate feeling. The doctor who is curing his body of disease is not interested in his damaged body image, nor his nonphysiological problems, and is charging what appears to be an astronomical sum for the cure. The nurse who has taken such good care of him is associated with embarrassed memories of catheters and bedpans and having to do as he was bid. His family is too impatient for him to be well and does not understand how debilitating his illness can be. The family, expecting gratitude and an effort to get well from the patient, and understanding from the nurse and the doctor of the problems involved in having a sick family member, may perceive the patient as angry and difficult, and the professional members of the team as disinterested.

In the health game, as in other bargaining situations, ". . .bargaining is by manuever as much as by words, communication is poor, legal enforcement unavailable and the participants make irreversible moves while they bargain, are uncertain about each others' values and have some power to inflict gratuitous damage on each other" (Schelling, 1964, p. 315).

There is never a time in which the illness situation is not a stituation of conflict and negotiation. Even when there is complete agreement between a patient and his family on the strategies to be employed and the values of the possible outcomes, the basic conflict between the patient-family coalition and chance (exemplified by the disease process) exists; and, indeed, complete agreement between patient and family on outcome value is unusual. There is always the conflict engendered by the monetary cost of illness. The values assigned to time on the kidney dialysis unit for one child as opposed to a college education for the others cannot be easy to designate.

The values attached to the various outcomes by the professional players in the game are also likely to be incongruent with the values attached to the same outcomes by the lay players. For instance, the nurse's recognition of the fact that hygiene, both personal and environmental, is likely to be more important to her than it is to many of her patients in the lower socioeconomic group can improve her strategies of care. Particularly in terms of prevention and rehabilitation, Simmons's (1966, p. 39) statement that "readiness to sacrifice the present for some possible gain in the future may not be nearly so pervasive a pattern among lower status people, who may accord priority to immediate rewards" is relevant to this incongruence in type and magnitude of professional and lay values. Health workers frequently make the assumption that their goals for health care are shared by their patients when they are not. Even when they realize that values are different, they are prone to consider their professional values the "correct" ones.

NURSING STRATEGY

Given the assumption that a model for nursing is appropriately derived from a theory of decision making, the question arises as to how to apply game theory to the concrete situation of illness. Consideration of the strategies open to all the players is the necessary first step in any game, with attention given to the possibility of chance events.

It is, of course, impossible to list all the options open to all the players in any game. However, some estimate of the possible actions which are both highly possible and relevant must be made. The probability and the relevance of events are questions of judgment, a judgment which the nurse would have to make in any case, before she devises her plan of care. Along with her estimate of which strategies are likely to be employed by the other players, either individually or in coalition, must be an estimate of the various outcomes resulting from the strategies, and the values for each player associated with each outcome. Strategies involved may be pure strategies (that is, a single strategy for one play in the game) or mixed strategies (the overall game strategy, which can consist of any number of pure strategies). How well the game is played is synonomous with which strategies are chosen.

Nursing strategies are implicit in the nursing care plan; they are probably not based on a consideration of all the options which are open to the players. Nursing decisions have a tendency to be heuristic in nature, growing out of information concerning the patient, and goals for his recovery, plus evaluation of immediate nursing responsibilities for other persons. Medical strategies impose certain explicit constraints on nursing strategies, since the rules of the game specify that the doctor's orders should be carried out. (The curative medical strategies are likely to be laid out on the order sheet; the strategies employed by the doctor to protect his time from the demands of the patients and their families are less obvious but must be considered).

It is apparent that patient strategies exercise little effect on nursing strategies, since the caring techniques take a poor second place to both curative procedures and professional convenience. Getting the work done on time and meeting hospital schedules obviously have higher payoff values to most nurses than the meeting of intangible patient needs. Family strategies (for instance, spending the night with the patient) are likely to be seen merely as an infringement on the nurse's ability to care for the patient, rather than as lay therapeutic ploys. In an atmosphere in which a patient has bathroom "privileges," and "admits" or "denies" past illnesses, it is not easy for health workers to allow equal status to lay players. It is more comfortable for the nurse in such an atmosphere to assume the role of a mother surrogate, loving but authoritarian, than to encounter patients who are equal players with other goals and other values.

How the game will terminate depends upon two things: the strategies which are employed by each player, and the occurrence of those events beyond the control of any player. The problem of making choices between known alternatives is compounded by misperceptions, partially known goals, inconsistent payoff values, and outcomes subject to chance. Although, in cooperative solutions, individuals with parallel interests can almost always gain by joint action, situations can be wrecked by misperception. Nursing strategies must take into consideration the uncertainty and lack of knowledge about what is at stake manifested by the lay players.

Ideally, in the health game the conflict is between a player called nature (exemplified by the disease process) and a coalition of lay and professional players dedicated to the patient's return to health. Actually, this is seldom the case. The transient cooperations and shifting coalitions among the players in the health game make it obvious that interests seldom coincide completely.

The nurse must also consider that the patient is playing more games than the one he is playing with her. Any player in the complicated health game may in fact be a pseudo-player. When the quality of patient care is poor, it may be because the nurse is only pretending to play in the patient's game of health. Her visible behavior may reflect the strategies she is planning or carrying out in another game, one she plays with the doctors or her nursing colleagues. The patient may be a counter or a strategy in such a game, or he may be only an object who interferes somewhat with her review of last night's social game. On the other hand, the patient or his family may also be only pretending to play, and opt out of any strategic behavior. The current concept of the behavior appropriate to the sick role encourages them to do so.

There are many questions of information and misinformation, perception and misperception, and values which are not comparable between players which arise. In spite of these, the game theory orientation is useful to nursing. It provides a framework for interaction with the elements of the nursing situation in a way which systematically, explicitly, and necessarily makes the patient and his family active participants in the return to health. It provides for the constant evaluation of the somatic and psychological strategies the nurse employs in the nursing care plan. What is perhaps equally important, it is a framework which demands explicit statements of the assumptions from which she proceeds.

In nursing as in other areas of behavioral science, numerical manipulation of data depends on the ability to assign reasonably accurate values to various outcomes. There seems to be no reason to assume that this cannot be accomplished in nursing, at least at the ordinal level. In order to make nursing care plans, it is necessary to evaluate the various outcomes which are the result of nursing interventions, and to assign a value to those outcomes. Where there is nursing consensus as to which outcomes are poor, fair, good, and best, a computer program of different nursing interventions, combined with relevant physiological, psychological, and sociological patient and family data, can be devised. When nurses are asked "What is nursing?" a computer printout of appropriate nursing strategies to be applied in various health games may provide a tangible answer.

BIBLIOGRAPHY

Barker, R. G., Beatrice A. Wright, and M. R. Gonick: "Adjustment to Physical Handicap and Illness: A Survey of the Social Psychology of Physique and Disability," New York: Social Science Research Council, Bulletin 55, 1946.

Bell, R.: "The Impact of Illness on Family Roles," in J. R. Folta and E. S. Deck (eds.), *A Sociological Framework for Patient Care*, New York: John Wiley & Sons, Inc., 1966, pp. 177–190.

Bloom, S. W.: *The Doctor and His Patient*, New York: The Free Press of Glencoe, Inc., 1963.

Coe, R. M.: *Sociology of Medicine*, New York: McGraw-Hill Book Company, 1970.

Croog, S. H.: "Interpersonal Relations in Medical Settings," in H. Freeman, S. Levine, and L. G. Reeder (eds.), *Handbook of Medical Sociology*, Englewood Cliffs, N.J.: Prentice-Hall, Inc., 1963, pp. 241–271.

Deutsch, M., and R. M. Krauss: "Studies of Interpersonal Bargaining," in M. Shubik (ed.), *Game Theory and Related Approaches to Social Behavior*, New York: John Wiley & Sons, Inc., 1964, pp. 324–337.

Folta, J. R., and E. S. Deck, (eds.): *A Sociological Framework for Patient Care*, New York: John Wiley & Sons, Inc., 1966.

Goldhamer, H., and H. Speier: "Some Observations on Political Gaming," in M. Shubik (ed.), *Game Theory and Related Approaches to Social Behavior*, New York: John Wiley & Sons, Inc., 1964, pp. 261–272.

Lederer, H.: "How the Sick View Their World," in E. Gartly Jacob (ed.), *Patients, Physicians, and Illness,* New York: Free Press, 1958, pp. 247-256.

Leonard, R. C.: "The Impact of Social Trends on the Professionalization of Patient Care," in J. R. Folta and E. S. Deck (eds.), *A Sociological Framework for Patient Care,* New York: John Wiley & Sons, Inc., 1966, pp. 71-82.

Mechanic, D.: *Medical Sociology: A Selective View,* New York: The Free Press, 1968.

NLN News, **19**(3); May-June, 1971.

Parsons, T.: *The Social System,* New York: The Free Press, 1951.

────── and R. C. Fox: "Illness, Therapy and the Modern Urban American Family," *Journal of Social Issues,* **13**:31-44, 1952.

Schelling, T. C.: "Experimental Games and Bargaining Theory," in M. Shubik (ed.), *Game Theory and Related Approaches to Social Behavior,* New York: John Wiley & Sons, Inc., 1964, pp. 311-323.

Shubik, M. (ed.): *Game Theory and Related Approaches to Social Behavior,* New York: John Wiley & Sons, Inc., 1964.

Simmons, O. G.: "Implications of Social Class for Public Health," in J. R. Folta and E. S. Deck (eds.), *A Sociological Framework for Patient Care,* New York: John Wiley & Sons, Inc., 1966, pp. 35-42.

Smith, D.: "The Role of Sociology in Medicine," in J. R. Folta and E. S. Deck (eds.), *A Sociological Framework for Patient Care,* New York: John Wiley & Sons, Inc., 1966, pp. 53-62.

Smith, L. M.: "The System-Barriers to Quality Nursing," in J. R. Folta and E. S. Deck (eds.), *A Sociological Framework for Patient Care,* New York: John Wiley & Sons, Inc., 1966, pp. 134-144.

Suchman, E. A.: "Stages of Illness and Medical Care," *Journal of Health and Human Behavior,* **6**:114-128, 1965.

Wilson, R. N.: "Patient-Practitioner Relationships," in H. E. Freeman, S. Levine, and L. G. Reeder (eds.), *Handbook of Medical Sociology,* Englewood Cliffs, N.J.: Prentice-Hall, Inc., 1963, pp. 273-275.

Wohlstetter, A.: "Sin and Games in America," in M. Shubik (ed.), *Game Theory and Related Approaches to Social Behavior,* New York: John Wiley & Sons, Inc., 1964, pp. 209-225.

Chapter 9

The Nurse and Cultural Barriers

Carol Taylor

The anthropologist can help the nurse, or any other person in a helping profession, to recognize cultural barriers and to work around them rather than against them. In this chapter this author will show how the nurse can use anthropological information to improve nursing practice, but first an exotic example.

Some years ago a nurse from Australia described a unique nursing problem. Apparently an acute and chronic problem in bush hospitals is keeping the aborigine in hospital beds. In their natural habitat these nomadic people sleep clustered in groups on the ground. During the rainy season they build shelters with branches and leaves, and in the cold season they sleep in circles around fires. The nurse said, "They leave a nice, clean hospital bed and you (the nurse) spend half the night with a torch (flashlight) in the bush looking for them." She also talked about the difficulties of getting aborigine patients to take proper nourishment.

It seemed that patients accustomed to sleeping in clusters on the ground might not feel safe and comfortable in nice, clean hospital beds. When the

119

author discovered that the proper nourishment provided was Australian rather than aborigine, it was suspected that an alien diet might be a factor contributing to the proper nourishment problem. And I suggested, as tactfully as possible, that something might be done about beds and diets. The nurse raised her eyebrows, pursed her lips, and said, "The proper place for patients is hospital beds."

Possibly because these suggestions would not be used to change the nursing practice in bush hospitals the author began to use this example of two cultural barriers which seemed to interfere with nursing care when lecturing the nursing students. Some years after this particular story was no longer used to explain how anthropological findings might be useful to nurses, a nurse approached me with the following report.

She had spent several years nursing for the military in foreign countries; and, during this stint of duty, she had been assigned to a hospital which, in addition to caring for base personnel and their families, cared for sick natives. Ten to twelve beds routinely were occupied by members of the indigenous population. She said:

> I remembered the aborigines and hospital beds. Fortunately for me an anthropologist was studying the tribe out of which our patients came and he described their way of life to me. Between us we decided on three changes.
>
> 1 To get patients from his tribe off beds onto floor mats, their way of sleeping.
>
> 2 To provide them with the diet to which they were accustomed.
>
> 3 To see to it that minimum communication, in the native tongue, was established between these patients and staff members.
>
> Target number three was simple. With the aid of an interpreter I learned to ask and understand the answers to basic questions—Do you hurt? Where? And so forth. Then I translated this set of questions and possible answers into a phonetic version of the native tongue which I then translated into English. The how-to-say-it what-does-it-mean approach. This communication system was painted onto the wall of the ward reserved for native patients. Beds and diet were changed in a less straightforward fashion.
>
> The head of the hospital agreed with my rationale for requesting change and admitted that the changes suggested would be desirable. But he said, "My hands are tied by army regulations." He suggested that I talk matters over with the supply officer and the head of dietary. And he dismissed me by saying, "I'd go to the supply officer first."
>
> The supply officer said, "Good thinking. The problem is that as long as we have enough beds to go round everyone, including natives, must be put into beds. That is what we have to do something about: enough beds to go 'round." Systematically, and over a relatively short period of time, the maintenance crew, armed with sledge hammers, saw to it that the supply of usable beds was sufficiently decreased to permit native-style sleeping.

The head of dietary couldn't see the sense of providing a special cuisine for natives. He said, "Much better off on a balanced diet." But, when it was pointed out to him that the patients didn't even appreciate the expensive and superior diet they were offered, he said, "Then they don't deserve anything better than they're used to." And he arranged to feed them native style.

Anthropologists are best known for their work on small preliterate societies and, as the account above suggests, anthropological information can be put to productive use by a nurse working with exotic peoples whose cultures differ so dramtically from the culture in which the nurse grew up and became a nurse. The question is, has the anthropologist anything to offer the United States nurse caring for her fellow countryman? The answer to this question is two yeses. The first yes concerns ethnic pockets in our population—groups of people who, for one reason or another, are not being assimilated rapidly into the mainstream of our society. These groups have been studied in considerable detail by anthropologists, and the anthropological information about them should be useful to nurses intending to practice on Indian reservations, in Spanish-American communities, and in other ethnic pockets. The second yes has to do with the various subcultures which, on the surface at least, seem to be melting into what most of us think of as the American way of life. Here again anthropologists have provided information that can be used by the nurse. Esther Lucille Brown had the nurse in mind when she provided thumbnail sketches of Italian, Chinese, Mexican, and other ethnic subcultures in our society (1964). And in the author's book for students in all health-related professions, a subculture, the "Cracker" (a disparaging term for poor whites), not included by Brown, was used in order to add to the literature information that would be pertinent to nurses who might not realize that there are significant cultural differences among people who consider themselves everyday Americans (Taylor, 1970).

In my opinion the anthropologist can most help the nurse when he or she turns an anthropological eye on America's mainstream-related subcultures. In part because culturally conditioned biases and blindnesses in the nurse are most acute when dealing with the cultural mainstream and its fringe elements, and in part because the anthropologist's holistic approach to culture yields detailed information about everyday life styles. A culture is how people eat, sleep, work, play, and relate to their mothers-in-law, as well as their values, beliefs, and superstitions. Down-to-earth information of this sort can be most useful to the nurse. Here is an example of how the anthropological eye can be used to make nursing everyday Americans more productive.

Some years ago a public health nurse had a problem. She was working with white, lower socioeconomic families. The nurse had succeeded in teaching her notions of proper infant care to about half her mothers. The other half could not seem to understand that smothering infants in oil was bad for them. And she had come to the conclusion that these mothers were stupider than the mothers who learned about oil. To an anthropologist this conclusion does not make sense. If all mothers were capable of learning everything about infant care except the proper use of oil, an anthropologist would wonder why only some of the mothers refused to change their infant oiling patterns, particularly when the person demanding this change could remove infants she considered unsatisfactorily cared for from their homes.

In this case it was found that coating the skin of young infants was part of the folk tradition in all families. This fact suggested that the refusal of some mothers to abandon this practice might be tied in with their belief systems. On investigation it was discovered that all the refusing mothers attended the same church and that the complying mothers either attended other churches or did not go to church. The minister of the offending church was cooperative. He said, "The Bible teaches that annointing with oil is efficacious. Your problem is that this practice has got out of hand. I will preach on the subject and, in the future, annointing will be limited to a drop of oil on the head."

Some weeks later the nurse reported that her problem had been solved by the preacher and that she had identified other oil-related problems which also had been solved by him. A woman with an infected leg was not responding to treatment, and the nurse was puzzled by this lack of response. Suddenly and rapidly the leg began to mend. The lady said, "I stopped rubbing it (the wound) with oil. Preacher said it was sinful to do so." And the lady's ten-year-old son said, "The thing God gets behind is a reverent drop on the forehead. More than that is a waste of oil and makes God mad."

A hospital nurse said, "I'm doing my best but in three days I cannot give her the help she needs. That's what's so frustrating about this place (the hospital); we get lots of cases like this." Cases like this were: unmarried mothers who rejected their infants, refused to allow them to be adopted, and forced their grandmothers to care for them. When an anthropological eye was turned onto this problem it was discovered that the nurse was nursing a problem which did not exist. It also was discovered that society was creating a problem for itself.

The nurse had been culturally conditioned in a subculture where the mobile nuclear family—mother, father, and offspring—was considered normal and where grandmothers were mothers-in-law who should not be allowed to interfere with the rearing of their grandchildren. In this particular subculture unwed mothers customarily delivered their young secretly and arranged for them to be adopted by strangers. In the case of legitimate births the custom was to begin the name-choosing ritual well in advance of birth.

The patients in question came out of a subculture in which the child of an unmarried woman is not stigmatized and in which it is customary for the young to be reared by the mother's mother. In this particular subculture the mother does not name her child. The mother selects a female relative of her own mother's generation as namer of her child. The namer names the infant during a feast to which the entire extended family and close friends are invited. The namer assumes specific responsibilities for the child she names; she becomes a combination of godparent and backup grandmother. For economic reasons birth and funeral feasts frequently are combined. When a child is named at a dual-purpose feast, one of the given names, as distinct from the family name, of the dead person is given to the child even when the dead person and the young infant are different sexes.

This subculture is matrifocal, one in which the adult male tends to be an in-and-out member of the family. The adult male is expected to contribute to the support of the matriarchy of his origin—his grandmother, his namer, his mother, his sisters and their children—as much as, if not more than, to the support of his own offspring and their mother. In this particular subculture stable common-law marriages are the rule rather than the exception, and it is common practice to legalize, from the point of view of the larger society, these unions when the children are grown and a marriage feast can be afforded. In short, the couple does for itself what the parents of the bride are expected to do in the subculture from which the frustrated nurse came.

The nurse had identified a problem that, under similar circumstances, would have occurred in her own subculture. A member of the nurse's subculture would have felt ashamed and guilty at having a baby out of wedlock. If she planned to keep her child, she would have concocted a cover-up story to protect both the infant and herself, and she would have entered the hospital with both male and female names already selected. Culturally conditioned to think to this fashion, the nurse knew that her patients were in serious trouble. They had what she called denial symptoms. They did not express guilt and shame, and they made no attempt to keep their birth-giving a secret. From her point of view the patients were denying the reality of the situation by not responding to it in the way she herself would have responded to a similar set of circumstances. In addition to denial symptoms, these patients also had proved to the nurse that they had rejected their young. This fact was attested to not only because they had come to the hospital to give birth unprovided with names for the child about to be delivered, but also because they expected the infant to be reared by their own mothers as if they were producing siblings rather than children. The nurse said, "Just think about what havoc can be wreaked by this sort of burden in the subconscious." When the cultural context within which her patients would view their situations was explained she said, "If you're right there's nothing to worry about." However, she did not seem entirely satisfied and although she did not say so I suspect she thought that I did not know what I was talking about.

The name-choosing practices of the subculture from which this nurse's patients come must make it difficult for the society to identify at least some of its members. In our society births must be registered; and the registration document demands a first, or Christian, name for the child. Unless they were stillborn, infants may not leave hospitals without names, and in most cases the nurse is expected to secure a name. As this particular nurse said, "With these patients there is no guarantee that they'll even remember the name they agreed to. Probably a lot of the kids grow up with names different from those they were born with." Observations support this conclusion.

The family structure in the subculture described above is characteristically found at lower socioeconomic levels in our society. And, because nurses frequently work with families structured in this fashion, let us look at traditional health care which has been designed by middle- and upper-middle-class WASPs and see what can happen when these health practices are imposed on the members of matrifocal families.

According to WASP tradition, the person caring for the infant and young child is its mother, and the health of young children can be improved by teaching mothers to do a better job of childrearing. In dominant segments of our society teaching mothers works because mothers rear their own young. In a matrifocal family the outcome is somewhat different. In most cases this is what happens. The grandmother is not taught childrearing techniques because she should not, according to WASP tradition, be rearing the young. The mother is taught how to rear her young according to the latest childrearing formula, and she is put under pressure not only to rear her own infants and young children but also to see to it that her own mother does not interfere in this process. Under these circumstances the nurse tends to become a social reformer. The nurse's need to shape up the mother so that she, the child's mother, fits a WASP stereotype can be both strong and stubborn. In extreme cases, documented by the author, children have been removed from their homes and placed in foster homes not because of failure to thrive but because the child's mother refused to shape up.

When a child from a matrifocal family is hospitalized, a similiar problem may arise. Hospitals and those who work in them expect parents to care for and be responsible for their children. The doctor talks to the mother and in some cases the father, and it does not occur to him that it might be more productive to talk to the child's maternal grandparent. The nurse cares for the child and, if it is necessary to do so, instructs the mother about caring for the child after the return home. The nurse rarely thinks to ask who will be caring for the patient at home. If the hospital considers it desirable for parents to stay with their hospitalized children, the mother of the child is expected to want to do so. If the grandmother who routinely cares for the child volunteers to stay during hospitalization, she is considered an unsatisfactory substitute. In this situation the rapid turnover of hospital patients does not allow time for social reform. As one hospital nurse said, "We don't have time to work on mothers who won't look after their own kids."

During labor and delivery the matrifocal family may produce a more complex problem. In some hospitals fathers are expected, or permitted, to stay with the mothers during labor. The theory is that the fathers support the mothers during this particular crisis. In a number of matrifocal communities, any male, including the father of the child, would be contaminated by being physically present in the labor room. In some of the communities the author studied, the father supports the mother but in a somewhat different fashion. His knife is placed under the mattress to cut pain and his hat is placed on the mother's abdomen to give her strength. In the traditional situation, which in the case of most of our matrifocal subcultures was birth at home with a midwife in attendance, the mother of the woman delivering, or a female relative of that generation, was present both to support the birthing woman and to assist the midwife. Mothers from these subcultures do not expect the fathers of their children to sit with them during labor, but they would welcome and receive support from the presence of their own mothers or from suitable substitutes. My own observations suggest not only that hospitals do not permit the presence of this natural source of support, the patient's mother, but also that the conscientious nurse sometimes substitutes for support attempts to solve problems which may not exist. One nurse said, "If we're not busy, I work on their psychosocial problems during labor. Believe me, they really have them (presumably this sort of a problem), particularly the un-weds."

Another area in which the anthropological eye might be useful to the nurse is in identifying and characterizing the natural clustering behavior of families from different subcultures during sickness, dying, and death. Hospital visiting rules are designed for nuclear families who consider it reasonable and satisfactory to visit the sick and dying in small groups (no more than two at a time). In many of our subcultures visiting the sick and dying in a pattern reminiscent of Noah leading the animals onto the Ark is most unsatisfactory both to the patient and to his family and friends. As one nurse said about the visiting behavior of people from nonnuclear subcultures, "They don't even know how to behave in hospitals; visitors pour in by the carload." Another nurse said, "They won't even let them die in peace; as soon as your back is turned, they sneak back in. I've seen as many as sixteen people in the room with a terminal (dying patient). That's no way to die." According to conversations with those guilty of this sort of behavior, some people do consider a crowd around the bed the right way to die. One man put it bluntly, "Dad is too far gone for the nurses to take it out on him because they're mad at us. So nobody's going to stop us seeing him out proper." In this case, the wake which followed seeing Dad out proper also upset the staff. One nurse said, "I know a wake is part of their grieving process, but they ought to control themselves until they get out of the building." Most hospitals are not designed to accommodate this sort of clustering and other behavior, but the extended family's attempts to behave in what to them is a natural way might be more readily tolerated if it were better understood.

While different subcultures may speak the same language, a single word might have different meanings. The consequence of this state of affairs is miscommunication. For example, in the days when the most frequent failure of the birth control pill was due to a miscount of days, a nurse said to a repeater, "What happened, did you lose count of the days?" This cause for failure was denied, and on further investigation it was found that the patient did not know that when instructed to take a pill one is supposed to put it in the mouth and swallow it. She had assumed that the pill was to be applied to the part of her body being protected from becoming pregnant, and she had conscientiously attempted to do so. The nurse said, "It never occurred to me that there was anyone in the world who could misunderstand when told to take a pill. Now I demonstrate as well as tell." As far as the patient was concerned, it was customary to take a poultice for the chest and ointment for the elbow so the way she took her birth control pills made sense to her. And an anthropologist who knew anything about the subculture in which she was reared would have been aware of the fact that the instructions about the pill would be misinterpreted.

Another communication hazard is caused by differences in verbal style. For example, misunderstandings sometimes arise when a nurse encounters a person who comes from a subculture in which long pauses punctuated by single words or short phrases are considered good conversation. This verbal style is found among mountain folk and in some rural areas. The nurse comes from and is accustomed to a highly verbal environment, and, when she encounters the naturally nonverbal patient, she tends to leap to the conclusion that the patient is depressed and needs cheering up. In one case, a patient who did not talk was put through a series of diagnostic tests to find out what was wrong. No one asked whether he could talk; it was assumed that if he could, he would. No physical cause was found. Shortly after the tests had been completed, two carloads of relatives and close friends visited the patient; and to the staff's amazement the patient talked to them without apparent difficulty. The staff developed a psychological explanation of the rapid recovery. This theory was abandoned when, in response to the physician's comment that they had been concerned because the patient could not talk after his accident, the patient's brother said, "Wouldn't, not couldn't. Doesn't like strangers." And the patient's father said, "Should have asked the boy."

In this chapter the author has attempted to show how cultural barriers can prevent the care given by nurses from being as effective as it might otherwise have been. The anthropologist is in a position to provide information which will make nurses aware of the cultural barriers they encounter in their patients. These barriers are to be anticipated not only in exotic peoples and ethnic groups but also when dealing with everyday Americans. The greatest contribution the anthropologist can make to nursing is to make nurses aware that, like all other human beings, nurses leap to culturally conditioned conclusions. It is the author's hope that the nurses who read this chapter will ask a man who doesn't talk whether he can talk rather than start to work on the assumption that if he could he would.

BIBLIOGRAPHY

Brown, Esther L.: *Newer Dimensions of Patient Care: Patients as People,* part 3, New York: Russell Sage Foundation, 1964, pp. 56-86.
Taylor, Carol: *In Horizontal Orbit: Hospitals and the Cult of Efficiency,* New York: Holt, Rinehart and Winston, Inc., 1970, pp. 151-162.

Section A
Beliefs of the
Mexican-American
Family

Ora Prattes

Because of the numerous religious and ethnic minorities that comprise the population of the United States, it is virtually impossible for a nurse to practice in any part of the country and avoid contact with people in one or more of these groups. The care the nurse renders her patients may depend on her understanding of beliefs and a subculture foreign to her own. As an example of this type of challenge to health care delivery, the Mexican-American family has been selected.

Acculturation and assimilation of a large number of Mexican-Americans have been retarded for certain social reasons. One of the most important of these is their segregation in slums or ghettos called *barrios.* In this isolated environment, many folk beliefs of Spanish or Mexican origin persist, and modern medical knowledge and health practices cannot be transmitted. As their economic situation improves, Mexican-Americans tend to move out of the barrios into middle-class neighborhoods and are then replaced by newer immigrants from Mexico.

The poor and poorly educated Mexican-Americans are isolated in the barrios because they can afford the cheap housing there and do not have to learn English. Since the United States and Mexico share an 1,800-mile open border, the Mexican ways remain powerful influences upon these Mexican-Americans. A plentiful supply of Mexican literature, movies, material goods, and radio programs further entrenches Mexican culture.

FOLK BELIEFS

Many Mexican-Americans in the barrios—especially those who are educated and have had positive experiences with modern health care practices—have accepted the ideas and practices of scientific medicine and allow their children to become immunized, to attend clinics, and to have professional medical care. But many Mexican-Americans from the barrios have their own set of folk beliefs about illness and its treatment which they practice in addition to or before seeking medical care. Many times when a patient is brought to a clinic or hospital with an illness that seems to have been neglected, he is asked why he did not seek medical care earlier. It is probably because he has attempted to cure his illness with folk remedies.

The folk beliefs of Mexican-Americans about diseases and their cures are derived from experience and experimentation and handed down from generation to generation. Often, two or more cures may be recognized for a single ailment. Clark, (1969, p. 164) who investigated folk medicine in California, has identified two categories of folk disorders—those of emotional origin and those of magical origin.

Martinez and Martin (1966), who carried out a study of seventy-five Mexican-American housewives living in a public housing project in a Southwestern city, found that relief from ailments recognized in folk medicine is rarely sought from physicians. Healers are relied upon instead. Several women in this study cite instances in which they or others had sought treatment from physicians without disclosing the folk diagnosis. Two-thirds of the women believe that medical doctors do not know how to treat folk disorders because they lack either faith or knowledge and understanding.

Superstition and the Supernatural

Among the unenlightened Mexican-Americans, there is no distinction between the natural and the supernatural, the scientific and the superstitious. Their folk beliefs are not a separate entity but a part of their daily living. If a folk remedy works, no one is surprised; but, if it does not, the failure is rationalized and some other cure tried. The younger generation of Mexican-Americans is becoming more skeptical of the traditional superstitious and supernatural beliefs of their people.

It is common for Mexican-Americans to believe that illnesses are caused by external forces. Many think that they are victims of evil forces in the environment or sometimes of the malicious behavior of others. This superstition applies particularly to mental illness. The afflicted (for example, an epileptic) may have had a spell or curse put on him. The belief in *brujas* (witches) is widespread, and even though the majority of the people will admit to knowing someone who is thought to be a witch, they will admit to consulting one only to have a hex or spell cast on a friend or relative removed.

Illness may also be a punishment for sin. If this is believed to be the case, the afflicted will go to confession and carry out his penance. Long pilgrimages to certain religious shrines are often undertaken to bring about a cure for a certain illness. The wearing of a habit exactly like that of a certain saint or virgin for a prescribed number of days is also believed to bring about a cure, particularly if the sick person has sinned.

A few years ago, it was believed that by promising not to cut an infant boy's hair until he reached the age of five, the parents could save their baby's life during the first year if he became severely ill. These young boys with long hair were very often mistaken for girls, but if *una promesa* (a promise) had been made to the Virgin it was kept until the time was up. Any embarrassment or ridicule was accepted as part of the agreement. Today, with the trend toward long hair for boys and men, this practice would not seem so odd.

HEALERS

Espiritistas (spiritualists) practice in the barrios. Not all of them are Mexican-Americans; some claim to be from India, Puerto Rico, and other countries. The main reason for consulting an espiritista is to communicate with a dead relative, particularly one who died suddenly. The prestige of the spiritualists is not very high among Mexican-Americans, partly because of the high fees they charge, which must be paid before each séance.

The *curandero* (male folk healer) or *curandera* (female) is the healer most often sought. Most of these healers will not deal with the supernatural or with diseases believed to be caused by spells or hexes, but they will treat for simple *susto* (fright) or *susto pasado* (passed fright) and for evil eye. The *curandera* usually sets up practice in her own home. Usually she has installed a small altar in a hall in her house. A statue of a favorite saint and lighted candles adorn the altar. *Curanderas* usually do not charge a set fee but merely ask for donations. Most of them are very religious and prescribe prayers, the wearing of certain religious medals or charms, herbs, baths given with certain herbs, and poultices or teas made with a large selection of herbs.

A respectable *curandera* will not attempt to cure a person that she knows is critically ill. Fearing an investigation by the legal authorities should the patient die in her care, she will usually advise the family to seek professional medical care instead.

The *curandera* consults with all members of the family who are present and attempts to elicit as much information as possible about the patient's daily habits and what the family and the patient think about the illness. She is courteous, attentive, and warm toward her clients, and involves the whole family in her treatments, as the following narrative illustrates:

> A middle-aged woman, accompanied by one son, one daughter, and her daughter-in-law, sought the services of a *curandera*. The woman's chief complaints were loss of sleep and appetite because she had not heard from another son in over 6 weeks. He had been in trouble with the law before this time, and she was afraid that he was in trouble again. The *curandera* asked the woman about her son's habits and listened attentively while the woman explained what a good son he was and that he had just gotten into bad company. She seemed to be deeply depressed about him, even though she had four other sons and three daughters, who were all living either in her home or very near her home. The *curandera* gave her some herbs, telling the daughter-in-law how to fix the tea and when to administer it. She gave the woman a charm and told her to say certain prayers every night. She asked the son if it was possible for the whole family to take their mother to the park or for a walk every day and recommended some warm baths with a certain herb at least two evenings a week. The *curandera* did not guarantee that all this would help the woman to hear from her son; the only thing she promised was that the tea would help her appetite and the exercise and baths would help her sleep. The prayers would be the answer to her main problem. The woman appeared to be more relaxed and serene as the family left, leaving two dollars at the altar.

A few *curanderas* in the barrios combine the usual folk remedies with magical or supernatural rituals:

> A young girl whose engagement had been broken was experiencing severe loss of appetite—she could not eat at all. A *curandera* was recommended to her, and she went to see her. The *curandera* told her to rub herself all over with a raw egg for the next three nights and to repeat a certain prayer three times. She was instructed to then return to the *curandera* and bring the egg. When the girl completed the treatment, she went to see the healer, who took the egg and broke it on top of a newspaper on the floor. Inside the yolk the *curandera* found a dead worm wrapped in some hair. She told the girl that the worm was what was making her sick. Then the healer asked for five dollars and told the girl that she was cured. The girl's appetite improved immediately.

FOLK AILMENTS AND THEIR REMEDIES

Evil Eye

The disease known as *mal de ojo,* or evil eye, is very prevalent. Of magical origin, the effect is most common among infants and children. The belief is that if a person, especially a woman, admires someone else's child and looks at him without touching him, the child may fall ill of the evil eye. Any person who has *vista caliente* (hot vision) is capable of inflicting evil eye, even though he may not be aware of having this power. If possible, the person who inflicted the evil eye should perform the curative treatment.

An object such as a vase or a breakable glass is also capable of having the evil eye cast on it by a person (not the owner) who admires it. Thus, because of the evil eye, a vase or some such object can break even when no one is handling it.

Any nurse who works with Mexican-American families should know about their belief in the evil eye. If she admires an infant or a child, she should touch his head, tousle his hair, run the palm of her hand over his face, or touch him in some other manner. This practice will prevent anyone from believing her responsible for giving the child the evil eye.

The evil eye is diagnosed by some or all of the following symptoms: fretful sleep, vomiting, fever, diarrhea, excessive crying. It can be cured by any person who knows how to cure, not necessarily just a *curandera*. The healer is sometimes an older family member, usually a grandmother or an aunt, or someone in the neighborhood.

First the stricken child is rubbed all over with a whole raw egg. He is rubbed in the sign of a cross, two strokes down from head to foot and two strokes across from left to right; prayers are said. The egg is broken and placed in a small saucer under the child's bed. In the morning or after a set period of time (preferably overnight), the egg is examined for signs of an "eye" (a spot, usually white, in the center of the yolk). If the egg appears cooked or a white film has formed over the yolk, the cure is believed to have been doubly effective, the egg supposedly having drawn out all the illness.

The evil eye can also occur in other groups, particularly attractive young females, as the following account illustrates:

> A twenty-year-old girl working as a nurse's aide had gone to work one day with her hair fixed in two long braids (she normally wore it pulled back in a bun). Everyone admired her braids and commented on how cute she looked. When she got home that evening, she complained to her mother of having had a severe headache all afternoon. Her mother asked her if the girls at work had touched her braids. Her answer was that some had, but she was not sure if everyone had done so. Her mother told her to lie down, and she proceeded to treat her daughter for the evil eye. The young girl took a nap and when she woke up, her headache was gone.

Susto

Susto (fright) is caused by a frightening or traumatic experience. Being scared by a dog or involved in a traffic accident (not necessarily getting physically hurt, just frightened) is enough to cause symptoms of *susto*—excessive nervousness, loss of appetite, and loss of sleep.

Simple *susto* can be cured by a member of the family who is familiar with its diagnosis and cure. The afflicted person is placed on the floor in a reclining position, or on a low cot, and is covered with a sheet. Then he is swept in the sign of a cross with palm leaves or a broom while certain prayers are repeated. Afterward the patient is given a drink of water. Usually this procedure suffices to make the person well. In the case of a child, the emotional support, attention, and feeling of importance he derives during this ritual is bound to be beneficial psychologically.

If simple *susto* is not taken care of immediately, it can become *susto pasado* (passed susto), which usually needs the services of a professional folk healer.

The following narrative illustrates this malady:

Three little girls aged six, eight, and ten had been riding in the back of a pick-up truck with their father when one of the tires blew out. The father managed to maneuver the truck to the side of the road without an accident. After checking to see if the girls were all right, he proceeded to change the tire. When they got home, the man told his wife what had happened and stated that even though the girls had been frightened, they had not cried. Late that night one of the girls woke up screaming. The other two, who slept in the same bed with her, also woke up and started to cry. Immediately a diagnosis of *susto pasado* was made. The father's older brother and his wife and their five children, who lived next door, were awakened and asked to come over for a family conference about what to do for the girls. It was decided that the uncle should go down the street and ask the *curandera* to come and treat the girls for *susto*. When the healer came, she first asked about everyone's health and was served a cup of coffee. After a brief social visit, she inquired about the girls, chatting with all members of the family and agreeing with their diagnosis. The *curandera* was then taken to the bedroom to see the girls. All the family members followed her into the bedroom, standing quietly along the wall. She covered the girls with the bedsheet and proceeded with her treatment, the girls giggling with delight at the attention they were receiving. As the *curandera* left, the father gave her a couple of dollars from his pocket in payment.

This example of a woman afflicted with *susto pasado* did not end so fortunately:

One cold morning a woman went to visit her neighbor a few houses down the street, leaving her four children in the care of the oldest girl, who was nine. The others were seven and five years and eighteen months of age. The infant was strapped in a highchair. While the mother was gone, the fire in the family's wood-burning stove began to die out. When the nine-year-old child put more wood in the stove, the fire appeared to go out completely, so she drenched the fire with kerosene kept in a can beside the stove. As she did so, flames shot out of the stove. The girl dropped the can, spilling the rest of the kerosene on the wood floor. The flames started spreading, and the children ran out of the house screaming, leaving the infant strapped in the highchair. The infant died in the burning house. The mother never got over this tragic experience. She was taken to numerous folk healers in the area but continued to be depressed. She could not eat and lost a lot of weight. Folk healers could not bring about a cure for what was believed to be *susto pasado,* and the woman was finally taken to a local hospital. There the diagnosis of pulmonary tuberculosis was made. She had gone without medical help for almost 2 years and died a few months later in a tuberculosis sanatorium.

Sereno

Another common illness is caused by *sereno* (dew or draft). *Sereno* is thought to be produced by some types of evil spirits which live in the night air. Because of *sereno,* a young child is never taken outside in the evening, even in the summer, without first being covered. Exposure to the evening dew may cause a cold or symptoms such as vomiting, diarrhea, and fever. Usually these symptoms go away by themselves, or the services of a *curandera* are sought. She may treat this illness with teas made out of herbs, mainly *ruda* (rue).

Mollera Caida

Mollera caida (fallen fontanel) is a common disorder in very young Mexican-American infants. Two main folk causes are recognized. One is a fall suffered by the infant—it is believed that the impact of the fall causes the anterior fontanel to cave in. The other folk cause, which is the more common, is pulling a nipple out of a baby's mouth too vigorously. It is thought that this practice causes the fontanel to be sucked down into the palate of the baby's mouth. The most easily recognized symptom is the infant's inability to suck the nipple. He cannot grasp it, and the sucking reflex is very poor and weak. Other symptoms of *mollera caida* are irritability, crying, diarrhea, sunken eyes, and vomiting.

There are several folk cures for *mollera caida.* One is to insert a finger in the child's mouth (while holding the infant by the feet with his head down) and exert pressure on the palate. Another is to apply to the soft spot a poultice made of soap shavings. Another mixture used for a poultice is egg white mixed with soap shavings.

Most of the babies with a fallen fontanel who are brought to the hospital have a history of diarrhea and show some evidence of the soap poultice having been applied to the soft spot. It is when these remedies have not worked that the parents bring the infant to the hospital. They usually do not mention the treatments they have tried, even though the evidence is very apparent. Once a young intern asked a mother what that "stuff" was on the baby's head. When the mother replied that it was egg white mixed with soap, the intern told her that it would have done the baby more good if she had fed the egg to the baby because the reason for the fallen spot was hunger and malnutrition and not some superstitious belief. Some of the hospital employees, nurses included, thought this remark was very funny. The mother smiled and agreed with the intern even though she was very embarrassed.

Rather than try to "educate" these parents, it is better to institute a program for postpartum mothers to teach them causes and symptoms of diarrhea, inability to suck, and a sunken soft spot, showing actual photographs or films of infants with a fallen fontanel and calling it by its Spanish name, *mollera caida*. Another part of this program could be to show the women how hydration of the infant after intravenous fluids are given "pushes" the fontanel back into place. Their own cures, along with modern medical practice, will assure these parents that everything possible is being done to help their child. The nursing staff should also be cautioned about pulling a nipple out of an infant's mouth with too much force, particularly in the presence of the mother.

Resfriado and Catarro Constipado

Catching a cold or getting chilled *(resfriado)* from exposure to a cold draft or from getting wet and not changing into dry clothing right away is usually treated by applying mentholatum to the patient's body and covering him with warm blankets. For *catarro constipado* (chronic head cold or sinusitis) a mixture of *poleo* (pennyroyal), *mastranzo* (round leaf mint), and *alhucema* (lavender) is made with boiling water. The remedy is sniffed up into the nostrils, where it will supposedly clear the head and open the nose.

Empacho

Empacho is caused by a bolus of poorly digested food sticking to the stomach lining. This condition may occur at any age. The symptoms are loss of appetite, vomiting, diarrhea, stomach ache, fever, excessive crying, and restlessness. The folk treatment is rubbing and pinching the back, or rubbing the stomach. The pinching process involves grasping a fold of skin, pulling it up, and releasing it. This procedure is done with both hands and repeated three times *or* until an audible pop is heard, which means that the food bolus is dislodged. A tea may be given after the rubbing. It is usually made of *estafiate* (larkspur), *hojas de senna* (senna leaves), and *manzanilla* (camomile).

Cleft Palate and Hydrocephalus

There are no acknowledged folk cures for cleft palate and hydrocephalus, but superstition still surrounds these congenital anomalies. A pregnant woman may wear a metal key on a string around her abdomen to prevent cleft palate in her unborn infant, believing the anomaly to be caused by an eclipse of the moon. Plastic surgery is an acceptable cure.

A few Mexican-Americans still believe that hydrocephalus is caused by a precious rock inside the child's head. This rock is thought to be very valuable. If the infant dies, most parents refuse to give permission for an autopsy. They believe the doctors remove this rock right after the infant's death and sell it to become rich. The success of surgery, particularly on young infants, in arresting the growth of the head has managed in large part to dispel this misconception. It is still common, though, for Mexican-American parents to believe that they are directly responsible for this affliction—that it is a punishment for some indiscretion or sin.

Pain

Pains in various parts of the body are treated by *ventosas* (cupping). A candle, mounted on a coin, is placed over the painful spot and lighted. A small jar is then placed over the lighted candle. When the air is exhausted, the skin is pulled up by the vacuum inside the jar. A prayer is recited during this procedure: *En el nombre de Dios, que salga este dolor* (In the name of God, draw out this pain). The jar is moved around over the entire back. Finally, the patient's back is massaged with *accite de volcanico* (volcanic oil).

Infant Health Problems

The cutting of a baby's fingernails or toenails with a metal instrument such as scissors is believed to cause near-sightedness. So, instead of trimming the baby's nails, a mother may make cotton drawstring mittens and place them over her infant's hands to prevent him from scratching his face. It is also believed that a copper penny hung on a string around the infant's neck will prevent painful teething.

NURSING IMPLICATIONS

The nurse who works with Mexican-Americans should always try to involve the entire family when teaching about health care, and should include all the family members close to the patient when giving nursing care. All the relatives in a family usually live close to one another, so this is not difficult to do.

Tolerance of the superstition and folk beliefs of some Mexican-Americans is very important. It *is* easy to become dismayed and exasperated at their failure to see the benefits of scientific health care practices, such as having children immunized against communicable diseases and consulting a physician in the early stages of illness. But it must be remembered that scientific medical care is often not available to these people in a form that is meaningful to them, and many of them have seen little evidence of the benefits of modern medicine and nursing.

BIBLIOGRAPHY

Clark, M.: *Health in the Mexican American culture,* Berkeley and Los Angeles: University of California Press, 1959.

Martinez, C., and H. Martin: "Folk Diseases among Urban Mexican Americans," *Journal of American Medical Association,* **196**(2):147–150, 1966.

Section B
The Mexican-American
Family and the
Mexican-American Nurse

Maxine Cadena

What would the difference be if the word Mexican-American were deleted and the title read, "The Family and the Nurse"? Should not the same considerations be taken into account regarding family differences when any nurse is working with any family? It is readily agreeable that the answer would be yes. But it is believed that there are characteristics, though common to many groups of various national origins, that require particular consideration when the nurse is working with the Mexican-American family.

The Mexican-American people have a rich culture. It is not the purpose of this chapter to discuss the culture of the Mexican-American but to discuss specific cultural factors that are distinct to the Mexican-American family and that have an influence on the nursing situation.

There are many generalizations about the Mexican-American family. The term *Mexican-American* refers to people living in the United States who are of Mexican origin, or whose parents or grandparents were of Mexican origin. They either speak or understand Spanish, and/or the Spanish language was a language of their parents or grandparents. They continue to practice or identify, in some way, with specific customs of their ancestors. Because a large percentage of Mexican-Americans are on the lowest of economic, educational, and social levels, many times it is believed that the Mexican-American is inferior. He is thought to be illiterate, lazy, and unable to learn. It is assumed that he does not want to work, he is very passive, and he has a philosophy of *mañana*. *These are generalizations believed by a vast majority of the United States population, and they are fallacies.*

THE MEXICAN-AMERICAN NURSE

The term *Mexican-American nurse* refers to a person who has been prepared for either vocational, technical, or professional nursing, as defined by the ANA position paper on nursing education. This person also is of Mexican origin, or her parents or grandparents were of Mexican origin. They either speak or understand Spanish, and/or the Spanish language was a language of their parents or grandparents. In an effort not to be identified with this group and these generalizations, the Mexican-American nurse may deny cultural factors that have been a part of her family background. Attempting not to be identified with this group, she may at times work with the Mexican-American family in a manner that is most ineffective and works directly against cultural influences. Or she may be working with a Mexican-American family that denies any cultural factors that are Mexican, and the nurse will be just as ineffective by trying to force them on the family.

The Mexican-American nurse who identifies with the two previous statements may become defensive, and, in so doing, may only deny further that the Mexican culture has any specific factors that can and do influence her role with a Mexican-American family. The emphasis here is not that the nurse should not be defensive, but rather that she should examine her working relationships with Mexican-American families, and her real feelings toward them.

These situations are not without stress and anxiety. The author, too, is a product of two cultures. Where does one end and the other begin? Have they mixed so that one is more dominant than the other? No doubt, there are people who will reject this chapter because the word Mexican-American is being used. Factually, it is incorrect because we are not speaking of Mexican citizens but rather of American citizens, people who are second- and third-generation Americans. But because this group of people are referred to as a distinct group, the word Mexican-American will be used. The reasoning for selecting this word has also come from identification—a more positive and comfortable feeling of using the word Mexican-American and associating with it.

Even though the Mexican-American family has taken on American ways and customs, it still is influenced by many beliefs and practices of its ances-tors. Mexican-Americans have individual differences, just like any other group. One will find that they have delinquents and gang leaders as well as college graduates and professional people. There will be some Mexican-Americans who will have a firm commitment to their Mexican culture and others who have adopted the Anglo way of life in the United States. But circumstances and situations commonly experienced by Mexican-Americans have sometimes placed great stress on the individual. In order to cope with the stress or to be accepted, he may have chosen to play down the part of his culture that has been criticized and labeled as being "Mexican" with all the negative connotations that have gone with it.

Since the role of the nurse demands knowledge of a situation and the factors within the situation, the first step is to know who is the Mexican-American family and what is important to this family. What are their values? What is it that must be considered if the Mexican-American nurse or any other nurse is to be effective while working with these families?

CULTURAL FACTORS THAT INFLUENCE NURSING

The specific cultural factors considered to have a direct bearing on the nurse's relationship with the Mexican-American are: family life, Spanish language, respect for authority (both inside and outside the family), politeness and graciousness, a sense of modesty, the amount of pride, and the attitudes and beliefs regarding health and health care. The beliefs and practices regarding health and health care will be mentioned only briefly here since Section A of this chapter speaks specifically of this topic.

To elaborate with the many references and statements that are available on the role of the nurse and nursing functions would be superfluous. It would also be inappropriate to dwell on the past role of the nurse and to lament over what nursing was not. Time is too short, society is too precious, and the quality of life is too valuable to dwell on the past. Therefore, it is fitting that we look to today and to the future.

For the purpose of this chapter, the nurse is one who has been prepared for vocational, technical, or professional nursing. The nurse, it is assumed, has knowledge of the social sciences and related disciplines. She has knowledge and a beginning understanding of the behavior of people, the forces in society that affect the family, and the fact that the family affects society.

When working with the family, the nurse should have the family and their needs as the focal point. In nursing practice and nursing education we are taught how things should be done; but when we do not follow through in practice, we refer to it as idealistic. Or as can be seen in some settings, our practice is very archaic. If we in nursing and the health services intend to accomplish our purpose for being, then the questions posed in this chapter are important, and an attempt must be made to answer them. Evidence is available that nursing for society is vital and more so with the present discussion of health care systems today (Lysaught, 1971).

Ida Jean Orlando, in her book *The Dynamic Nurse-Patient Relationship* (1961), gives nursing excellent guidelines that can continue to assist us in effectively providing nursing service to people. Her nursing process explains that the nurse must perceive the situation and the patient's behavior, respond to it, and then carry out necessary actions for effective nursing care. An attempt will be made to apply her process to the role of the nurse with the Mexican-American family.

Among the Mexican-American people, the family is the central focus for social identification. Seldom does the concern for the individual family member become more forceful than concern for the family as a whole (Samora, 1971). This is demonstrated by the gathering of the family members in various situations. Some of these situations are festive occasions, and others are times of illness or hospitalization. When a Mexican-American is hospitalized, it is not uncommon for the patient to be visited by his immediate family, aunts, uncles, and good friends. The visitors usually come together. This becomes a difficult situation for the family and the nurse. It is difficult for the family because they know that not all the visitors will be allowed to visit. It becomes difficult for the nurse because she is the one who usually must inform visitors that they may not all enter to see the patient. It will also become difficult for the nurse if she does not understand the closeness of the Mexican-American family. If the nurse is Mexican-American, she may be embarrassed by all the visitors, and there may be a tendency for her to be rude since she may not wish to identify with them.

The Mexican-American nurse may be embarrassed by cultural traits that differ from those the nurse perceives to be typically American or by behavior of the Mexican-American family that is often criticized by the Anglo culture. This embarrassment causes stress, and the nurse's reactions to the embarrassment will have an effect on the family and on the effectiveness of the nursing service provided.

The place of the elderly Mexican-American within the family structure is an important family characteristic. The elderly Mexican-American family member accepts assistance from his children, but this assistance will not be readily asked for. The nurse's perception of situations as they arise when working with the elderly can prove to be very useful when discussing the situation and alternatives with the elderly family members and with the children who are concerned. It is not uncommon to find a great desire for independence among all people who are elderly. They do not want to be dependent on people, especially their children. But with economic costs as they are today, it is found in all cultures in America that often elderly couples or individuals do without the necessary food, medicines, and health care because they cannot afford it and will not ask for it unless absolutely necessary. But if assistance is suggested or offered in a respectable manner, they will gladly avail themselves of the offer. The nurse, knowing this, can then intervene by suggesting various alternatives, and exploring means and methods with the family members. This can be in relation to more adequate or suitable living conditions, necessary medication, and adequate health care.

Authority in the Mexican-American family is paternalistic. It belongs to the father or, as is often seen, to the eldest son in the family. This authority deals with permission to do such things as wear lipstick, cut one's hair, date, seek medical assistance, and follow through on health care recommendations.

Nursing contacts with the family are usually made at a time of day when the father and husband is at work. In attempting to meet the health needs, nurses identify situations and needs and then plan for necessary nursing intervention and health care. At the same time, nurses add to the stress of the health situation by demanding that the mother make an immediate decision that, according to their culture, may have to wait until the father is home to discuss the situation and make the decision. What is our goal in nursing? What are the specific goals when working with families? If individual family situations are truly being assessed, and the nursing service provided is being evaluated, then it should be evident that the mother of the family may make a decision; but it may not be carried through. When this happens, nurses usually continue to reemphasize "how important it is to follow through," to make more home visits, to send postcards and reminders. When it is seen that this has not brought results, there is a tendency to conclude that the mother is not interested or that she is "uncooperative." An expression often heard in nursing settings is, "They just don't understand." After proper assessment and validation of the assessment, it is the nurse who usually did not understand or did not realize that other factors were contributing to the situation. Some questions that may prove to be most helpful in such situations are: "What does your husband think of this situation?" "What does your husband think is wrong?" "What do the two of you do when such a situation arises?" "Where does your husband prefer you take the children for medical treatment?" "What does your husband think about your taking the children to the doctor?"

The following is an example that demonstrates the cultural factor of authority within the Mexican-American family:

During a Head Start immunization program, the children were vaccinated against smallpox. Permission had been obtained from the parents by signing an immunization card. In 3 days a father and his five-year-old son came looking for the nurse who had given his son the vaccination. The father was very upset because there was a reddened and swollen area where the vaccine had been administered. He said that he did not give permission for something like this to happen. To his way of thinking this was an infection, and he felt that his child would become ill.

Realizing that the man was upset for two obvious reasons, the nurse took him and his son aside and explained the normal "take," or reaction, of a smallpox vaccination. She told him that this was evidence of his child's immunity against smallpox, and that he was correct. This was an infection, but not the type that we usually associate with illness. The nurse, although frightened, did not become defensive. She sincerely told the man that she and other nurses wished that more fathers would get concerned about the type of care and service that their children received. At later meetings regarding health teaching, he and his wife were present and always ready and confident in expressing their doubts regarding certain health care teaching.

Orlando's nursing process can be readily identified in the above illustration.

The Mexican-American knows that he is different from the Anglo. He knows that he is not fully accepted. His language is often different. Does the Mexican-American nurse feel the same way? Is this one of the reasons why she sometimes refuses to speak Spanish with a family that has difficulty understanding English, assuming that the nurse knows how to speak Spanish? Frequently the family will be watching for the nurse's response or reaction to the family situation. Two questions Mexican-American families ask themselves while waiting for this response are: "Is she like one of us?" Or, "Is she one of those who thinks that she is better than we are?" If the family gets an affirmative answer to the last question, they will not hesitate to ask for a nurse who is not Mexican-American.

Working with families would be most effective if, in the nursing situation, the family would be approached as a unique group of people with qualities that are important and vital to them. The nurse must work with them to identify needs and then to establish mutual goals. If the family were approached in this manner, then it might not be necessary for the family to set up defenses, attempt to deny some of their own values and beliefs, or accept those that the nurse is trying to force on it.

Recently it was explained by a young person interested in becoming a nurse that her reason for doing this is so she can be helpful, "not like some of the nurses from my own people" who treat poor Mexican-American families without any respect. The young person related that she has thought of this ever since she was five years old and had to receive medical and health services from a county institution. There her family encountered Mexican-American nurses who treated them "very badly," and she felt that this was because the nurses were ashamed of them because they were Mexican-American and they were poor. "We didn't speak very good English and we couldn't pay for care."

The Mexican-American family is a polite and gracious family. This is especially evident when the family sees that the nurse is also Mexican-American, by either name, language, or appearance. One does not have to know or work with a Mexican-American family for any great length of time for this to be evidenced. This may be in the form of a hug, a firm handshake, a very flattering statement, or a material gift. If the contact is in the home, this may be shown by offering a cup of coffee, a glass of water, or something to eat. How does the nurse respond to this? Is she embarrassed that this has been offered to her? Should she accept or refuse? Should she accept so that the family's feelings are not hurt? Should she not accept because this is not part of her professional role? Is it what is said and done that communicates more, or is it *the way it is said and how it is done that communicates more?*

Answers to such situations will depend on the nurse-family relationship. If the nurse believes that this family is inferior and that accepting this gesture would not be professional, then her response will be very different from the nurse who sees this as a sharing with the family and understands professionalism in a different context.

For some reason, when nurses have difficulty in such situations, there is a tendency to act or not act and to refer to this as being professional or not being professional. What is demonstrated and referred to as professional is often dehumanization. The literature has well defined what professionalism is and how this can be attained in nursing. So where do we get our own individual ideas of professionalism that demonstrate a firm, stiff, keep-at-a-distance, and do-not-get-too-involved manner? This too comes from our education and practice in nursing. But now is the time to rectify this, to take a second look, and to change where we see that change is indicated.

There is a great sense of modesty within the Mexican-American family. This cultural factor will also be related to beliefs and practices for health care. This sense of modesty is in relation to keeping personal things personal, especially in terms of the body. The nurse has many occasions to work with the family during pregnancy. Oftentimes, individual nurse's values are forced on these families. These are illustrated in the following statements: "You must go to the doctor." "You must go to the clinic." "It is very important that the doctor check you." "You must make plans early for delivering the baby in the hospital." The emphasis in these comments seem to be on the physician, the clinic, and the hospital. It seems that they are the important factors in such statements. Nurses must reexamine the reasons for stressing such issues. Is the family told why these things are so important? How is all of this going to benefit the mother, child, and family?

The institutional way of life and the hospital way of life are American. When we assume that the Mexican-American family will avail themselves of this we are in error. An example of how specific cultural and family clues are missed, and how nurses force their values on families—that all women should be delivered in hospitals by physicians and that this will be best for them— is illustrated in the following:

> A Mexican-American family was being visited by a Mexican-American nurse for prenatal care. This was the tenth pregnancy for this family. All previous babies had been delivered by midwives. No complications or difficulties had been encountered.
>
> When the nurse learned that the midwife delivery was planned, she attempted to talk with the mother so that arrangements could be made for a hospital delivery. The husband and wife chose a hospital that was noted for good care. The nurse felt this an accomplishment. She had accomplished her purpose, getting the patient to deliver in the hospital.
>
> Time for delivery came, and the patient was taken to the hospital by her husband. She was properly admitted and made comfortable in the labor room. In the hour that she had been there, the nurse had checked her frequently. When the nurse went in to check her again, the mother had her baby lying on her abdomen, but had not yet put it to breast. The woman did not complain, but she did admit that it was more difficult here in the hospital than when she had her babies at home. When she delivered at home, she did not have to do it all by herself. Her husband and the midwife were always there to help her. Here she had to do it all alone. She was very tired.

Do we in nursing credit ourselves with effective nursing intervention in this particular situation? What criteria are used in nursing to determine effectiveness? Is our criterion a count of hospital deliveries versus midwife deliveries? Is our criteria in reference to the family and how the family, mother, and child benefit from nursing intervention and the hospitals available for such care? Some comments from nurses when this situation was discussed were: "She was comfortable." "She had a clean bed." "She didn't have to worry about washing all the bed linen." What rationale do we have for assuming that she was not comfortable at home, that she did not have a clean bed, and that she worried about washing her linens?

If the mother-to-be tells the nurse she is going to have a midwife delivery, does the nurse respond in awe and insist that she go to a hospital? The midwife is an accepted practitioner in the Mexican-American culture. She is usually knowledgeable and skillful. Is the nurse aware of this? Even if the nurse is not familiar with this aspect of the Mexican-American culture, she has a responsibility to learn about it. Does the nurse attempt to find out who the midwife is and if she is a safe practitioner? Does she attempt to work with the family and the midwife?

One of the cultural factors of the Mexican-American family is pride. One does not expect something for nothing. They want to contribute, to help, and to understand. This desire and willingness to share home, ideas, advice, and food with people whom they trust and respect or who have done them a favor are considered to be a basic Mexican-American cultural characteristic. It is a custom among Mexican-American families to share different dishes that are prepared for eating. When the food is taken to the next family, the container (plate, bowl, saucer, or pot) is never returned empty. They return it only when they too can send it back with some type of prepared food or gift. To share with one another is basic to the Mexican-American culture. The Mexican-American family has a need to reciprocate and to show the nurse its gratitude. Perhaps this is the reason why Mexican-American families in the lower-economic levels do not always participate in various health services that are advertised as *free*.

In connection with immunization programs, it is often heard, "After all they are free, what more do these people want?" All people feel, or would like to feel, that they too have something to offer. The dignity of man is destroyed when he is not allowed to share, and to share is to be allowed to give and to receive. Possibly this is part of the problem of lack of participation in immunization programs. Another reason is lack of understanding or information as to what is meant by immunization. In health care practice this is accepted as a part of healthy living. The Mexican-American family accepts this concept partially, but in a different manner. He sees it as an agent that also causes the disease and feels that the person, usually a child, who received the immunization becomes ill. This too is correct. But nurses must help clarify this a little further so that it can be understood in a manner that is acceptable to the family. The same is true regarding the cost of immunizations. The immunizations are not free. They are usually provided by some level of government if the family is not required to pay cash. This family is living in the United States and also contributes to the taxes that support our health care governmental agencies.

It was mentioned earlier that language is a factor that distinguishes the Mexican-American family from the American and Anglo culture. What is the role of the nurse in this regard? Her foremost role is to determine whether the family identifies with the Mexican-American culture in this respect. As there are Mexican-American nurses who tend to deny any cultural traits with the Mexican-American culture, so are there families who do this. How can this be determined? This will depend upon the nurse, the family, and the situation. Is the nurse working in a community where it is the belief of many people that English should be spoken at all cost? If this is so, then the nurse must reexamine her own thinking and practice. If she too believes this, there will be difficulty in delivering nursing service to a population that speaks and understands Spanish better than English. If the nurse comes from a background that is more Anglo, and Spanish was not spoken in the home, she may not know how to speak it, or at least not well enough to assist her in her service. In order to improve her communications and her nursing service, she should then do whatever is necessary to learn how to communicate with the Mexican-American family. It has been reported by Mexican-American families that they prefer an Anglo nurse who knows a few words in Spanish or makes an effort at it to a Mexican-American nurse who denies that she knows Spanish and makes no attempt to speak it or understand it.

There is a large population of Mexican-American families throughout the Southwest. Depending on the specific states and regions, some people have continued to speak Spanish, and others do not use it at all. It is the nurse's responsibility to determine the practice of the individuals with whom she is working. One part of the Mexican-American culture deals with health beliefs and practices. Although the health practices of these families have already been covered, they will be mentioned briefly because of their impact on and importance to the effectiveness of nursing service. Even today there are practices with evidence of results that imply better health or at least a relief from the symptoms of illness. One will find these health practices believed and practiced by economically poor, middle-class, and professional Mexican-American families who identify with this cultural trait. The family will not admit to these practices if the nurse working with the family is going to ridicule and downgrade them. In an effort to keep the nurse from knowing of these practices, they will hold back information important in the assessment of the family health situation.

There is one isolated characteristic that has been observed while working with the elderly Mexican-American. This is in relation to the regularity with which medications are taken. They do not take medications for hypertension and cardiac conditions that must be taken daily as prescribed by the physician because, if the pills are taken this often, the patient will then "get used to them and will have to take them the rest of my life." This is a most difficult barrier; even after explanations regarding addiction and the taking of these medications are discussed, experience has not shown any great change in relation to this particular problem. One other reason for not taking the medications regularly is that they are very expensive and will be used up too soon.

SUMMARY

This chapter has concerned itself with the Mexican-American nurse's role in working with the Mexican-American family and has considered cultural characteristics that influence the nursing care provided. We in nursing can achieve our purpose for being if we continue to assess individual situations *with* the family concerned, and then mutually plan for the necessary health care desired and needed.

BIBLIOGRAPHY

Aranda, J.: "The Mexican-American Syndrome," *American Journal of Public Health,* **61**:104–109, 1971.

Burma, J. H. (ed.): *Mexican-Americans in the United States,* Cambridge, Mass.: Schenkman Publishing Company, Inc., 1970.

Lewis, O.: *The Children of Sanchez,* New York: Random House, Inc., 1961.

Lysaught, J. P.: *An Abstract for Action,* New York: McGraw-Hill Book Company, 1971.

Madsen, W.: *The Mexican-Americans of South Texas,* New York: Holt, Rinehart and Winston, Inc., 1964.

McWilliams, C.: *North from Mexico,* New York: Greenwood Press Publishers, 1968 (First Greenwood reprinting: copyright, 1948).

Orlando, I. J.: *The Dynamic Nurse-Patient Relationship,* New York: G. P. Putnam's Sons, 1961.

Samora, J.: *Los Mojados: The Wetback Story,* Notre Dame, Ind.: University of Notre Dame Press, 1971.

Sanchez, G. I.: "History, Culture, and Education," in J. Samora (ed.), *La Raza: Forgotten Americans,* Notre Dame, Ind.: University of Notre Dame Press, 1966.

Chapter 11

Working with Low-Income Families

Jean L. Sparber

What a pity this chapter should have to be written at all! If health care were, indeed, the right of everyone, then we should not have to separate our thinking about assistance to low-income families from help to those more economically endowed.

Indeed, there is a tragic gap between what should be and what is. This requires straight talk, not pretty talk.

PUTTING IT BLUNTLY

Working with low-income families is a professional field for people capable of growth, personal warmth, and maturity. It is hoped that those who cannot measure up to these standards will have the common decency to get out. The poor have troubles enough without having to cope with square professionals working in a round hole.

Generally, the person who works in the world of the poor goes home at night to a vermin-free bed. Close contact with poverty and deprivation is often shocking to the new student—especially to those brought up in protected wealthy and middle-class homes. At first, the deluge of negative impressions tends to disturb him to the point of taking the situation personally. His first impulses might be to organize a neighborhood brigade to mop, replace smashed window panes, or plan an overkill assault on the rat and roach population.

Unfortunately, the new health worker's enthusiasms are often chilled before getting his knuckles around a mop handle. He may feel a cool response from both community and professional people. His righteous indignation can sputter out into a sheepish feeling of foolishness. After all, indicates the community, how can this arrogant stranger eradicate problems which have defied so many experts before him? Unless the new health worker can retain some of his initial indignation, he will soon make an adjustment or truce with his job environment. He will gradually learn to forget the day's problems when he goes home at night. His submerged frustrations might take the form of occasional nightmares about injustice and wasted human lives. Unfortunately, the "poor" health consumer wakes each morning to find *his* bad dreams are *true*.

Warm, sensitive supervision and understanding are essential to the young worker. In the beginning, it is easy to become cynical and bitter about inequalities which appear to defy correction. A student from a protected background with limited life experience can be emotionally traumatized by exposure to writhing misery. These devastating feelings must be worked through if this person is to become an effective health care helper.

Nastiness exists. Those who study to ameliorate health conditions of the poor must be trained to "take it" while retaining their warm humane concern. This is no small order!

GIVE ME YOUR TIRED AND POOR

The United States may have got herself into some of this trouble through generosity. Historically, the country advertised itself as a haven for the world's underdogs. Millions of destitute immigrant families rose out of poverty by climbing Horatio Alger's ladder.

But the fabled land of opportunity did best for strong, clever, lucky, and racially acceptable families. Some people never got to the first rung of the ladder. And those who failed to meet the tests of success and status were somehow considered unfit for first-class citizenship. What a paradox that we have permitted generations of elementary school children to pledge their allegiance daily to a flag promising liberty and justice for *all* (Hurley, 1971, p. 6)!

Eventually, middle-income people began to wake up to some frightful truths. Social infections originating in neglected, rejected areas were spreading to "nice people's" children. Then, *horrors,* the costs of inhibiting the disease began to hit middle-income wallets!

Emotionally and socially crippled families not only tended to perpetuate themselves, they also resisted suggestions about cutting down their birthrate! Welfare costs, prisons, and police protection cut into funds which might have been used to promote preventive measures. To be sure, there were always humanitarian programs which sought to maintain dignity and snatch families from the jaws of pathology. Slowly, social reforms were legislated. Private and government agencies and church organizations launched pilot projects. Some steered straight courses. Others hit the rocks.

At this moment, remedial action remains fragmented. Misery exists on a massive scale. And some of that misery is that of sincere, thoughtful, intelligent professionals who are frustrated by their inability to deliver quality health services to low-income families.

Today, one can not work with low-income families without becoming aware of gigantic forces for change. The Constitution and Bill of Rights are taking on new meaning to the disadvantaged. Reactions range from nonviolent legal efforts to revolutionary resistance using desperate tactics. Families are changing, too, along with divorce and abortion laws, communal living experiments, and women's liberation (Wheeler, 1971, p. 19).

The nurse working in a hospital, making a home visit, or working in a storefront clinic must become involved with these larger socioeconomic problems if he is to understand those he serves. At this time in history there can be nothing routine and stereotyped about working with low-income families. In fact, it comprises a new interdisciplinary frontier—as wild and challenging as steering a covered wagon across a rampaging stream.

WHO ARE THE POOR?

One chilly evening after Thanksgiving, a dozen sorority sisters on an urban college campus called a traditional meeting. The agenda was simple and seasonal: What good work shall we perform this Christmas?

Being a sociable, sentimental group, easily touched by the plight of needy children, the decision was an easy one.

"We'll have a Christmas party for poor children!"

"Great! I can't wait to get started."

Plans thrust ahead rapidly. Animated committee heads urged their followers into enthusiasm. Soon, a storage room bulged with new and reconditioned toys, games, and dolls. A gigantic Christmas tree dominated the sorority house living room. Cheery notices went up all around town, proudly announcing the free event—the untold treats and surprises and the treasures available for needy children. What a welcome! What warmth and goodwill!

At 2:30 P.M. on that sunny pre-Christmas Saturday, the sorority sisters had every cookie and goodie in place. A costumed and very perspiring Santa fanned herself, especially around the pillowed stomach.

By 3 P.M., the truth had dawned. No one was coming. What redblooded American child wanted to be considered "needy"?

DEMOLISHING THE STEREOTYPES

We have plenty of low-income families, and the public has created an over-abundance of stereotypes to describe them.

The Deserving Poor

The most acceptable of all, epitomized by the characters in Charles Dickens' *Christmas Carol,* are the deserving, uncomplaining, and grateful poor. They reward their benefactors with blessings and cause us pangs of the deepest guilt that the "Little Match Girl" should have frozen to death unnoticed in the midst of plenty.

The Lazy, Shiftless Poor

These are a supposedly clever lot. They are unmotivated people who have made a career of leaning against shovels and avoiding work. The *Congressional Record* speaks of them on many occasions, especially when liberal health and welfare bills are ready for the vote.

The Loud, Complaining Poor

These people are never satisfied with the taxpayers' contributions. They grumble at low-quality goods and services as though they had a right to consumer protection.

The Unexplainably Wealthy Poor

Some of the shiftless poor acquire color television sets, drive luxury cars, and own products which most certainly could not be purchased on a welfare budget. Poverty seems to agree with them. They have a lot of fun, make noise, dance with joyous abandon, and let others take care of their rainy days.

The Lying Poor

These are the professional poor. They have every angle figured and know who to approach when grant money is being handed around.

The Scary Poor

This is a new kind. Oh dear, the anxiety they are causing! This is the "political-legal" poor. They can quote the Bill of Rights and the Constitution with no effort. Some can spout ordinance numbers and have been in personal contact with elected officials and the Civil Liberties Union. There are some members of the public who fear what would happen if these people really got the equality to which they are entitled.

The Nouveau Poor

You've heard of the "nouveau riche," now learn about the "nouveau poor." Here is a brand new stereotype we are creating with every rise in inflation. The elderly with what they considered to be secure pensions are joining this group. Educated men with obsolete jobs are edging in. These people simply will not permit you to put them in their "low-income" place! They will resist even the most temporary labels and make a big fuss about how they always had private doctors and never had to stand in line for foodstamps. This is a growing group. Watch out, *you* might even qualify for it yourself someday!

The Hereditary Poor

This is a lot of hogwash. Exciting new research is being done on the deteriorating effect of poverty on health, IQ, culture, family structure, emotional illness, and character formation. The temptation used to be to lump the families who tended to stay poor from one generation to another as a sort of Juke-Kallikak syndrome. This granddaddy of stereotypes is one of the hardest to break. Evidence is emerging which indicates our gross undervaluation of these families for too long. Unfortunately, the families with visible racial characteristics appeared to have got the worst of the deal (Hurley, 1971, p. 8).

The Criminal Poor

Facts are beginning to come out, especially through the Fortune Society, that we have been manufacturing criminals in our so-called reformatory system. We took fathers out of their homes and finally returned them to their families without a shred of dignity and no way of making a decent living or changing the factors which got them into prison in the first place.

There are also the unfortunates who never made it at all as criminals. Not only were they unsuccessful thieves, but they could not even learn criminal techniques from the skilled conmen they met while serving their prison terms.

The Voluntary Poor

An emerging low-income group, now coming up strong on the poverty scene, and just as stereotyped as the rest, are the people who are simply antimoney.

They do not value materialistic goods. Motivations differ, and very little is known about how the voluntary poor will develop. They might figure out some solutions we can use.

The above-mentioned categories of poor are stereotypes because they do not take into account the individual circumstances of the family being described. It is not our purpose to size up families and assign them with tags reading "poor risk," "fun to work with," "uncooperative," etc. It *is* our function to assemble as objective and fair a social history as possible. We should try to understand how the family feels about itself, what problems it thinks it has, and how it perceives the health care worker.

If the health care worker is to be of any positive assistance whatsoever in working with low-income families, the crucial test will be in his attitude. It is for this reason that this chapter concentrates on challenging the feelings and preconceived notions of those of us who are currently working or planning to work with low-income families. You may be assigned to a family with a "bad" reputation. It is your job to observe, record, evaluate, and to try to see them as human beings deserving dignity and the chance for rehabilitation.

In other words, we professionals are not entitled to preconceived, judgmental opinions. This does not mean we approve, but it does separate us into a clinical group capable of maintaining fairness as one of our major tools.

MAJOR PITFALLS AMONG HEALTH CARE WORKERS

We hereby list five of the most obvious and commonly found "characters" who perhaps, without realizing it, fall into habits not in the best interest of our clients.

The Defrocking of Lady Bountiful

In the long-gone years of garden parties, demure lawn frocks, and flowery picture hats, there was once a lovely Lady Bountiful whose serene reputation rested on her good deeds to the deserving and grateful poor.

We hereby rip off her many-buttoned, floor-length dress and strip her down to a Godiva nude.

You see, Lady Bountiful gave her gifts in a capricious yet charming manner. She might donate a basket of luscious pears to a child with a desperate need for eyeglasses, or distribute flower seeds to the villagers in need of basic tools for the cultivation of vegetables.

Do not think for a moment that Lady Bountiful has not been reincarnated among us. She exists among both experienced and uninitiated health care workers. She lives on, providing sturdy, unglamorous, prep-school-type sweaters and skirts to young girls desperately yearning for bellbottoms, hot pants, or whatever the current styles demand. All of us have the capacity to give unwanted services to families while enjoying the illusion of having done a good deed.

The Lady Bountifuls who occasionally remain backbones of our institutions and agencies carry the infection into higher echelon decision making. This can be exceedingly dangerous.

The victims of her gifts, on the other hand, can be caught in a treacherously embarrassing bind. Should they be grateful or speak out for their real needs?

Take the case of a Lady Bountiful who pounces on a federally subsidized plan to retrain low-income mothers on welfare for semiskilled jobs. All the lucky applicant must do is pass a small battery of tests and be evaluated for a variety of jobs. The proposed new careers hold the promise of a fast elevator ride from the lower- to middle-income living. This is an ingenious scheme for free education and a subsidy to the student's family will be covered at its previous level of poverty while mother studies.

"How could anyone in her right mind refuse?" thinks Lady Bountiful.

But the old girl is astounded to discover that Mrs. J., a most intelligent woman with a cooperative record, vetoes the plan at first hearing. She will not listen. Lady Bountiful becomes annoyed, surly, almost rude. Her negative attitude is not lost on Mrs. J., who now has a big conflict on her hands. She really does want to advance, but the J. family is so constituted that Mr. J. prides himself on supporting his family whenever possible. Now, if Mrs. J. is trained and advances to a higher-paying job, Mr. J. will lose confidence in himself. Mrs. J. is ashamed to admit this. Lady Bountiful is not sensitive to this, nor does she bother to explore it further with Mrs. J. If Lady Bountiful were a bit more concerned about the family, she might be able to dig up a similar training opportunity for *Mr.* J. Then, perhaps they both could be advanced, and the story might have a happy ending.

Lone Rangers

These are a breed unto themselves but also pop up occasionally in the best of us. We try, singlehandedly, and preferably without consulting with others, to solve a problem by ourselves. The results are occasionally gratifying but ordinarily stir up more trouble than they are worth.

The Eager Beaver: A Close Relative of the Lone Ranger

He goes around slapping his tail vigorously over minor issues. These give him a fine sense of importance and give everyone else a gnawing sensation that he is out for his own glory rather than that of the client. He can never see the forest for the trees.

The Establishment Preservers

These dear people are dedicated to the preservation of triplicates and interminable meetings to discuss grammatical trivialities. They also enjoy propounding policy statements destined for rehashing at annual delegate assemblies. They look very important.

The Sob Sister (or Brother)

Each of us has a soft spot. Some low-income families become experts at discovering these areas and learn to play one agency against another. Flattery can get them somewhere. Beware.

Undoubtedly one will find even more of these prototypes as one piles up years of service. Just be careful that *you* do not turn out to be one.

HONEST SERVICES POSSIBLE

Real, bona fide service can be and is being performed everyday. You must be open to the opportunity to get in and do your bit. This is only possible if you become increasingly sensitive to what people really want you to help them do.

FIRST STEPS IN OPENING ONE'S EYES TO REALITY

Millie and Mollie, experienced, long-term welfare recipients, leaned their gritty elbows out of the peeling lead-paint window sill and smirked at the student social worker retreating from their house four flights below. The interview had been a short one. Miss Watchamacallit had been nervous. She asked the same tired old questions, and Millie answered them mechanically. Miss Watchamacallit tried to smile with sympathy, but the general effect was self-consciousness.

Mollie thought the interview had been rather entertaining. Mollie did a hilarious and fairly accurate imitation of Miss Watchamacallit's unsuccessful attempt to ignore a cockroach crawling out of the sugarbowl.

"She'll be an easy one to twist around our little finger," observed Millie.

Meanwhile, several blocks away, Miss Watchamacallit, professionally known as Miss H. R. Watchung, collapsed onto a coffee shop counter stool. While waiting for the murky beverage to cool, she envisioned grand and glorious social changes in store for Millie and Mollie. She would personally lead these crumpled, unmotivated women toward better lives.

"By George," thought Miss Watchung, "I'm the one to do it!"

The preceding paragraphs are typical fantasy fragments in our current health care collection of illusions. Millie and Mollie have become cynical and "wise" to the young, idealistic, and inexperienced workers. The clients are tired of the solutions promised by fervent predecessors. They reject both excuses and panaceas. In some areas, because of high agency turnover, some families are lucky to get the same health care worker two times in a row.

On the other hand, the young, inexperienced worker may be in danger of promising too much, and permitting himself to indulge in overoptimistic fantasies. He can be "used" by the experienced low-income client. The result can be a mighty disillusioned young professional. It can drive good people out of the field, challenge them to become really good workers—or turn them into cynical, red-tape-loving health care robots.

ALL IS NOT LOST

The low-income family was not born yesterday. It has become adept at pulling heartstrings. There are both passive and active resistant methods of foiling the best worker's attempts to be of assistance.

While the low-income family is sizing up the professional, however, it might be in for a few surprises. For one thing, even a green health care worker may be a talented and trustworthy listener. He might not know the answers or make promises, but the consumer might find him to be exactly the right person to hear problems. If the health care listener is nonjudgmental and supportive, the relationship could easily take a positive turn.

What we are trying to achieve, then, is a nonstereotyped, sensitive give-and-take relationship between two or more human beings. This is true in working with families in *all* income brackets and also when working with individuals. However, the poor tend to have low self-images. This complicates the formation of the simple dignified relationship. The health care worker must, therefore, be especially scrupulous in respecting the family and avoiding every trace of condescension.

Words alone cannot communicate these qualities. The nonverbal undertones and overtones take courage to control. For instance, the aforementioned Miss Watchamacallit might have broken through to Mollie and Millie if she could have openly admitted her discomfort about the cockroach. By simulating an "I don't see the roach" approach, the trio never grappled with what was really happening around that table.

Most people appreciate honesty, even if they are sometimes suspicious about it. Part of honesty may be the frank admission by a health care worker that the environmental conditions are making him squirm. This gives the client or consumer the opportunity of verbalizing the problem. By allowing the "underdog" health consumer to be the expert in explaining hardships, there is a subtle switch of roles. The professional is no longer the "giver." He can receive advice and counsel. The disadvantaged consumer can teach him how to work in disagreeable neighborhoods. The low-income family can give tips to the inexperienced worker on how to walk a street or climb dark tenement stairs with greater safety. Why can't the professional relinquish his authority to the point of establishing a true working partnership with the family?

REALLY LOOKING AT A FAMILY

Each family is different. We see families changing in structure and wonder whether the institution will survive in the future. There are migrant families, rural families, and woman-dominated families. Then there are ethnic and racial differences. These factors are important if we do not permit these labels to become stereotypes.

Working with a family is different from caring for one individual. One must size up that family's power structure. Who proposes decisions? Who appears to make the problems? Who blocks their solutions? Is some family member being protected at the expense of all the others? Is one member unconsciously terrorizing the family by using illness, martyrdom, or control of money?

Why have these people been classified as low-income? Were their parents poor? Do they have areas of untapped strengths? Perhaps there are longings and hopes just waiting for some skillful, kind, and sensitive worker to explore. Are there undiagnosed emotional or physical problems?

Most important, and this can not be emphasized too strongly, what are the family aims? Some homes show interests in several directions simultaneously. The mother wants material goods. The father wants simplicity and solitude. Be careful. Siding with one member of the family might upset the balance among the other relatives.

Then, one must think very hard about how the family fits into the social structure. It is possible that a family is an antisocial one. Think hard. Are they harmful to others? Should the family be evaluated by experts to determine if they are unfit to exist freely within our society? A dangerous family can harm other families trying to live decent lives. These are extreme examples, but nonetheless real. They will require help from wise and experienced supervisors and many social agencies.

On the other hand, what if a health care worker discovers a treasure— a family member of such positive potential or talent that it would feel like a crime to waste it? Again, one must return to the true aims and motivations of the family. The parents might not wish the child's gifts to be developed. It is their right to refuse.

Getting to know a family's real interests and motivations may not be impossible. There are ethnic, racial, class, language, and intelligence barriers, to name a few. We are not always able to achieve communication. It is a bitter pill to swallow, but we can fail.

Nevertheless, a loving health care worker can often get across complex ideas by exercising the simple human force of caring. Trust can grow in the most unlikely places. Did you ever see a fragile, beautiful flower growing from a rock crevice hardly wide enough to contain a fragment of soil?

AVAILABLE RESOURCES

Health care workers meet the recipients of our services in many settings: hospitals, streets, migrant labor camps, furnished rooms, social agencies . . . anywhere.

There is a continuing controversy. Should we reach out to families or wait to be asked in to help? There is some virtue in crisis intervention. On the other hand, many families are much more apt to accept service when they state their wish for it. Let this controversy be resolved for the present in a simple, basic way. It would not hurt to at least start to establish a friendly, nonthreatening relationship with a family. It could be the basis for a genuinely needed relationship at some future date.

Referrals to existing social agencies is a usual way of handling problems. There are many available community resources. In this day and age, it is difficult to keep up with the new ones springing up in low-income areas. Older agencies are reevaluating their purposes and sometimes abandoning long-term policies. Referrals can be valuable. But again, they cannot be done in a stereotyped or thoughtless way. For example, one might suggest that the Jones family solve an after-school problem by enrolling ten-year-old Benny in an afternoon play group in a local schoolyard. Mrs. Jones goes there and finds there is a waiting list. Or maybe Benny is too young. The fee may be more than they can afford. Maybe the play group has a reputation for starting kids off on drug experimentation. Look harder. A mechanical referral may make the worker feel good, but it may be no solution. Also consider that Mrs. Jones might only be trying to please the worker, and might actually prefer Benny to stay home where she can keep an eye on him.

A referral looks good on paper. It can enhance an agency record. If there is enough volume, perhaps the agency will have its funds renewed. But be honest—nothing replaces the family's complete participation in the plan and the health care worker's sensitive follow-through. If the plan turns out to be a poor one, get rid of it with the family's consent and look for something better.

This boils down to something simple and basic. Be friends with your families. This should not be confused with unprofessionalism. Just be real friends. The families and you will know the difference and everyone can benefit.

WHERE MATURITY AND COMMON SENSE COUNT

Standing on One's Own Principles

Principle #1: You are the tool for serving others. Be as clean, sharp, and true as possible.

Principle #2: Be tremendously concerned. Listen very hard to what the family is trying to tell you. Try to understand it from their point of view whether you agree with them or not.

The health care worker will grow in the job if he permits himself to do so. Agencies, hospitals, and institutions at this point in history appear to be in a state of flux. One can no longer rely on the mimeographed policy book for the answers. Some agencies are in decay and do not know it. You might find yourself working in an organization, doing a job, and suddenly be hit by a thunderbolt of insight! The agency may be perpetuating more wrongs than righting injustices!

What is the next step for you? Do you quit in a huff? Is it more courageous to stay and try to work out positive change from within? This can sometimes be the wisest course.

Now here is another touchy one. Can you trust your supervisors? Are they unalterably aligned with the old established policy? Have they forgotten the needs of the people? Can you discretely work with an authority figure and reawaken some of his former sensitivities?

Everyday one is bound to hit a problem that is not in the rule book. You will bump into unspeakable, embarrassing situations that are not supposed to happen, or that workers in the past have chosen to ignore because there was no ready answer for handling them.

Here are some examples and a sprinkling of comments to stimulate your thinking about how to find some sort of solution of your own.

1 "Your family" on welfare seems to have plenty of cash for toys. The kids have the latest gadgets advertised on television. You do not want to be suspicious, but it is strange. You see evidence of numbers slips. You think the oldest brother is involved in illegal gambling. *Comment: First of all, do you know anything about the numbers rackets, how they are set up, why low-income people seem to enjoy playing the numbers? Shouldn't you learn more about the legal side of the situation? What is considered proof? If you decided to bring this to the attention of the legal authorities, would you have to appear in court? How does your suspicion about this illegal process affect your feelings about the family? Do you think all of them sanction dishonesty? Might not the parents be concerned about having the numbers in their home? Would you rather forget the whole thing*

than "rat" on the family? Would you go off and say, "I'm only here to be a health care worker, the numbers aren't my business."

2 The mother listens carefully to your detailed explanation of how she should administer medication to a child recuperating from surgery. You check her records. Everything seems in order on paper. Something tells you to look at the medication bottles. There seem to be many more pills than there should be. Is she lying? *Comment: The medication is very important, and it would be an excellent idea to straighten this out for the patient's sake. What are the facts? If the mother is not giving the medication properly, why not? Is she afraid it is habit forming? Is she suspicious of side effects? Is she using this as a way of showing unconscious hostility to you? Does the medication taste bad and the child have trouble swallowing it?*

3 You accompany your "family" on a visit to the out-patient clinic of a hospital. You have waited for almost 2 hours on the hard benches. Little Jackie needs a change of dressing and a treatment. The mother spots the physician who customarily treats little Jackie. As he passes, she gently reminds him that her son is becoming exhausted from the long wait. Dr. X. is furious. He snaps back that he is overworked. Besides, he says loudly, clinic patients cannot expect the same service as private patients. *Comment: It is usually not good policy to sock a physician on the nose in front of a lot of witnesses. Can the entire problem of long waits, discourtesies, etc., be opened for discussion with medical students? Can a coalition of students and sensitive workers challenge this outrageous, undignified kind of treatment? Can any of us afford to let it stand as a tradition?*

4 You are sending a report to a social agency asking them for additional services for a member of your "family." The forms are complex. One of the questions, if you answered it honestly, would indicate that the child is ineligible for service. In confidence, the mother has indicated that while she was married she had an extramarital affair, and the boy is not legitimate, in the strictest sense. Meanwhile, you hear rumors that the social agency in question has a reputation for carelessness with handling confidential material. Do you manipulate your report to disguise the facts? *Comment: This is an "elegant" compounding of establishment errors. One must consider why legitimacy has any bearing on the child's current needs. More urgently, how can our society permit erosion in the area of confidentiality? The health care worker is thus put into the position of stretching the truth or perpetuating outmoded values. As for confidentiality, is there no longer a reliable check and balance system within our institutions? Or is this only reserved for middle- and upper-income families?*

5 An unmarried woman, supported by the state, had produced six children out of wedlock and has become pregnant again. You broach the subject of family planning. The woman becomes furious, claims you are suggesting genocide. She feels strongly that you and your kind are trying to eradicate her group from the world. *Comment: If you find a way of answering this one, let us know.*

6 Your "family" makes grammatical errors to the point of murdering the King's English. They also use a colorful lingo, liberally sprinkled with terms related to waste elimination and sexual activity. Do you attempt to make them feel more at ease by falling in with their method of speaking? Or do you maintain your ordinary high school English syntax and refrain from adding "in-trend" phrases? *Comment: It depends upon how comfortable you are in the dramatic arts. Ordinarily, one makes fewer errors if one stays in one's own character.*

7 Would you sincerely congratulate a fourteen-year-old girl on the birth of her second illegitimate baby? *Comment: How does the girl feel about the blessed event? If you think a new baby entering the world is cause for joy, then why not say so? If you are adversely affected, then no one says you have to be a hypocrite.*

8 If a teen-aged boy in your "family" confided to you that he was "splitting" and moving out of the state as soon as he got his high school diploma, would you feel it important enough to tip off his family? What if the family was depending on his presence in order to survive? *Comment: This is a much more complex problem than meets the eye. For instance, it indicates an awesome lack of communication within the family. There are depth-charged feelings behind his decision to leave without giving his folks a chance to prepare for an alternative solution. One could try to find out why the young man felt the way he did, but offhand, this is a matter to be handled by an experienced and very sensitive professional. Try to find one to help you out.*

9 A ten-year-old has an odd look in his eyes, and you wonder whether he has been experimenting with drugs. In numerous casual discussions with the family, the parents openly pride themselves on their kids being strong enough to resist temptations of the neighborhood. *Comment: You will need more than a hunch to go on. There are other knowledgeable people who may have contact with the boy. Maybe you can piece the facts together. Who knows, you might be wrong.*

10 Your "family" is sheltering a son who has broken parole. Do you feel obligated to report him to the police? *Comment: Try to contact a member of the Fortune Society, a fast-growing group of former convicts with a firm grasp of the heres and nows of the parolee situations. You need not reveal the name of the parolee to them, but the society might be able to track down the man's parole officer and give you a line on whether the man is going to get a fair shake. It might be that by careful handling, the young man could get into some worthwhile rehabilitation situation. Also consider what you discuss with your "family." After all, it's their son, and there is a trust relationship involved.*

11 Do you accept a cup of coffee from the lady of the house when you visit a low-income home? What if you preferred tea? Would you ask for it instead? Would you offer her one of your cigarettes if she were out of them? *Comment: Some of this has to do with agency policy, but it is pleasant when one can do what comes naturally.*

12 Should you accept or buy underground newspapers, handouts, and giveaways on the streets near where your "families" live? Might not people think you are some sort of radical or maybe even belong to a bunch of bombmakers? *Comment: How can you ever know what is going on if you never try to find out? Perhaps you and your close friends will want to go a few steps further and speak with the people distributing the ideas? You might be surprised to learn that your families may have either positive or negative feelings about these ideas. Your interest may also lay the groundwork for further talks.*

YOU ARE THE EXPERT; YOU ARE THE TOOL

Skim through professional journals, résumés of seminars, or conference critiques. Can you sense the fear about our crumbling institutions and agencies?

There is no longer a confident clear-cut way to "solve problems." Consumers do not always trust agencies enough to use their services.

You will find plenty of speakers and writers with exciting new theories on how to eliminate poverty and the misery it causes. Some of the ideas undoubtedly have merit. Each of these solutions is subject to interminable debate. The discussions appear to be as savage among the friends as the enemies of the ideas. There is so much vested interest. There is so much status to protect. It is very easy to become confused. And what if everyone agreed, then there would still be laws to be passed and funds to be appropriated. Who would get the cash, and how much of it would get into greedy hands instead of into the pockets of hungry people?

THINGS ARE CHANGING

Well, maybe something new is happening and changes will be forced upon us. Poverty exists on a worldwide basis. Our mammoth agencies and traditional institutions may not exist in a few decades.

This may sound hopelessly overwhelming. Perhaps it is a new opportunity if we use the situation in the best interests of all people of all races and nationalities.

HOW CAN WE SALVAGE THE SITUATION?

Perhaps we must simply return to ourselves. To be sure, there are many frightening aspects of change going on. Yet that is the most important time to become even more sensitive than before.

We must find small groups of people willing to open themselves up to trust.

WHO ARE YOU?

We all have a lot to learn about ourselves. Working with low-income families, especially those with troubles, can be personally difficult to tolerate. Partially submerged fears and anxieties begin to surface. This is another good reason to become allied with sensitive and mature people with aims similar to your own. You will need emotional support.

LOOK AT YOUR MOTIVES

Are you in the "helping game" because you want power over others? Are you essentially a gullible kind of person who wants exposure to "real life"? Will encountering harsh realities tend to change you into a cynic? Will it make you hard? Or, with the help of others, can you grow in sensitivity and compassion?

How will you handle frustration or discouragement? Would working in difficult areas give you a ready-made excuse for tantrums and other regressive behavior?

After a day of meeting people living in squalor, would you go home feeling guilty, almost wishing you could ease your conscience by desecrating your own comfortable home? And then, there are the daydreams of glory— how you personally will salvage an entire neighborhood and earn the praise of all!

WHAT IS PROFESSIONALISM?

Whether you are being trained for nursing, medicine, social work, physical therapy, rehabilitation, etc., you will get certain basic skills and knowledge. Let us hope it is useful. Being professional, to some extent, encompasses much more than having the right training and the right degree or license. Professionalism is not too different from good manners.

For instance, a professional would approach a $1,000-a-year family with the same attitude as one with a $20,000-a-year income. You would hesitate to invade the privacy of either. One would certainly not betray confidences. It is only right to give equal respect to rich and poor alike.

This may seem simple. It is not. How many times have you been softened up by a high-status, well-to-do person? So watch it.

WHAT TO WATCH FOR IN YOURSELF

Try for a "here and now" realistic view of the family. Your sight will often be clouded by past experiences. You will not immediately recognize submerged prejudices. Don't be alarmed. All of us have these. We must have the patience and courage to root them out. Our sensitive friends can often point them up. You need not change your prejudice or point of view if you are aware of it and take it into account when making a decision.

For instance, if you come from a home where the bathtub is usually clean and the garbage pail routinely emptied, will it make your skin crawl on entering a smelly, infested house? If so, face it. How will your personal disgust affect the way you relate to the family? Will gamey socks and a stained undershirt on a man admitted to the emergency room alter your attitude toward him as the patient? Will you find it more difficult to give him his due as a first-class, full-quality patient?

Watch yourself and ask trusted coworkers to help you spot these personal reactions. Many observations will become obvious to you as you continue watching for them. For example, will you accept a reply to your questions from a neatly aproned housewife in the same way as from a slipshod one with a hint of beer on her breath?

How about judgmentalism? Are you turned off by a loud shrill voice? Does a person who uses a four-letter, sex-oriented vocabulary seem less credible to you? Do you learn how to cut through the language and hear what he may be desperately trying to communicate to you?

As if this were not enough, are you aware of your own stake in the situation? Do you expect some sort of thanks or reward in a spiritual, if not a concrete, form? If a family deteriorates while under your care, do you tend to repudiate it—to look for ways of blaming them or yourself? Are you working to help the family, or to get praise and a good rating from your supervisor?

This is why only a person capable of growth, warmth, and maturity should attempt to work with low-income families. It is not that you could not hold down the job, pass the tests, fill out the forms, etc. We owe these people superquality service until we can get them up to equal par with the rest of our citizens.

REWARDS

We should speak of humility. It is not taught and some people never learn it. Warm human contact with those who survive and occasionally thrive under awful conditions can start you on a path to humility. Observe those with so much less than you, who make so much more of what they have. You can learn from a family and let them know about it. How wonderful for all of you to share an experience of coping with life.

Maybe you will be a creative health worker and find a better way to give assistance. There is a psychiatric hospital somewhere in New York State which offers vacations to the families of chronically emotionally ill patients. They simply take the patients back as short-term guests. This gives the ill person's relatives a chance to stretch, enjoy, and prepare for the continued battle against mental illness.

So many new ideas are needed: more free clinics, new kinds of halfway houses, day care, night care, etc. Could you be the one to develop something original, simple, and inexpensive?

NEVER FORGET YOU ARE ONLY A TOOL

A capable carpenter keeps his tools in good shape and stores them in a proper place. Should not the health care worker take the same care to keep his skills, knowledge, and attitude in fine working order? We can all get stale or fall in with the easy routine established ways of working. This is very easy to do while working with low-income families because a "who cares" attitude so often prevails among the professionals.

Find others like yourself among all the health care disciplines. Groups of mixed peoples can check on each other in a spirit of maturing relationships.

THE ULTIMATE AIM

Would it not be best if each family could decide its own aims and work out its own problems, financial or otherwise? Is not our job to help and then get out?

There are ideas under discussion about ombudsmen—neighbors of families who are friendly, trained visitors. These should be thoroughly acceptable to the family and used as resources as needed. Could not such a trained neighbor refer a sick child to a specialized agency as well as prepare the family for what it can expect? We are not sure that people prefer to receive assistance from racially or ethnically similar professionals, but we could learn to be more sensitive to what they do feel and do more about establishing a more realistic basis of trust.

Working with families in low-income areas is so huge a subject that it can not be covered in a chapter of this size. But it can be explored as one human being to another and as one increasingly aware person learning to live with himself.

BIBLIOGRAPHY

Fromm, E.: *The Art of Loving,* New York: Bantam Books, Inc., 1967.
Hurley, R.: *Poverty and Mental Retardation,* New York: Random House, 1971.
Jonas, G.: *On Doing Good, The Quaker Experiment,* New York: Charles Scribner's Sons, 1971.
O'Gorman, N.: *The Storefront,* New York: Harper & Row Publishers, Incorporated, 1970.
————: "Storefront," *Columbia Forum,* **13**:3, 1970.
Wheeler, G. R.: "America's New Street People: Implications for the Human Services," *Social Work,* **16**:19-24, 1971.

The Expanding and Contracting Family

This section discusses the expanding and contracting family. It is time for all health team members to be aware of the normal needs of families at different stages of their development. Only when the normal is known and understood can delivery of care be directed toward health maintenance and health promotion.

Part Two discusses general considerations of family planning, as well as those of the expectant family, the adopting family, and the guidance of families with infants, young children, adolescents, and elderly family members.

Chapter 12

Family Planning

Miriam T. Manisoff

The modern term for the measures taken to achieve family size aspirations is *family planning*. For many, the earlier and better-known phrase *birth control* (although the two terms are synonymous) became associated only with preventing pregnancies. As now used, both in scientific and popular context, family planning includes measures to delay and prevent pregnancies, to overcome infertility, to permit adequate intervals between births, and to assure that only wanted births take place.

After centuries during which birth limitation was shackled by legal, social, and religious taboos, family planning gained recognition in the United States, and in most countries of the world, as an integral part of comprehensive health care. Medical specialties without exception associate adequate family planning directly with maternal and infant health and as a precondition for the health and stability of the family. The American Medical Association, the American Public Health Association, and the American Nurses' Association are among the many professional organizations to identify with these health needs. To the nurse, for whom health education is a traditional basic responsibility, family planning in family-centered care is a logical concern.

HISTORY

Viewed historically, the emergence of a nurse as the founder of America's birth control movement appears less as a chance development than as the inevitable consequence of professional responsibility in the person of a dynamic, dedicated missionary of health. Margaret Sanger, of course, combined the talents of a brilliant organizer and a pioneering fighter for women's rights and the resolution of the world's great "movers and shakers" with her practical career in nursing. Working in the teeming slums of New York City's East Side early in this century, she witnessed lives destroyed by butchered, illegal abortion; young mothers prematurely aged by repeated unwanted birth; poverty intensified and compounded by births in families already too poor to maintain themselves. Mrs. Sanger's first birth control clinic, established in the Brownsville section of Brooklyn, New York, in 1916, found lines of women extending for blocks when the doors were opened. The word spread. Women came from many cities and from across state lines for professional assistance in spacing and limiting pregnancies. Within a week, authorities closed the clinic doors and sent Mrs. Sanger to jail for 30 days.

But this frontier-smashing nurse lived to see her vision of a society in which women could determine their own reproductive destiny become fact. She saw taboos smashed; laws against birth control struck down; national acceptance gained in government and law, in professions and in religions, and in all popular groupings. Universities conferred honorary degrees upon her. Her books, papers, and other memorabilia found an honored place in a repository at Smith College. In the fall of 1971, the United States government issued its first family planning stamp.

Although family planning—as currently offered and practiced in the United States—is something new, there is nothing new about the concept of birth limitation. It is specifically referred to in an ancient Egyptian papyrus dating back nearly 4,000 years. Greek philosophers were debating suitable measures at least 2,400 years ago. In India, documented methods go back 1,600 years. China's first literary medical reference appears in a text nearly 1,300 years old. Birth control historians are convinced that the urge to space and limit pregnancies and to make independent decisions about family size is as old as mankind itself.

Philosophically, Thomas Robert Malthus, the nineteenth century clergyman, is identified as the developer of the rationale for modern birth control. Although regularly refuted by generation after generation, his "Essay on the

Principle of Population," written in 1798, refuses to become obsolete. His contention that population, when unchecked, increases in geometric ratio while food increases in arithmetic ratio was proved wrong when plagues curbed the growth of human numbers and improvements in agriculture vastly extended food resources. But when modern sanitary and medical science began to protect life and lengthen man's longevity, death control became a fact; and Malthus and his theories remain as timely as this morning's newspaper.

Where Margaret Sanger and her contemporaries stressed the relationship between voluntary family planning and health, Malthus stressed the relationship of family planning to population growth, food, land and prime resources, and the economics of societies and individuals.

THE LEGISLATIVE SETTING

In the name of crusading against vice, Anthony Comstock sponsored the laws which for decades banned birth control education and service in the United States. In 1873, Congress passed the Comstock Law, making it a crime to import, mail, or transport in interstate commerce obscene literature or "every article or thing designed, adapted, or intended for preventing conception or producing abortion." Little Comstock laws were enacted in the states. While these restrictive statutes remained on the books, the United States' voluntary birth control movement, founded first as the Birth Control League, in 1942 became the Planned Parenthood Federation of America, and developed and struggled for legality.

Not until 1965 did a United States Supreme Court decision strike down Connecticut's law which stated that birth control was unconstitutional. This verdict, which enunciated the right to privacy in decisions about spacing and limiting pregnancies, marked the beginning of the end of the Comstock era. While remnants of restrictive laws continued to hamper some aspects of family planning in the United States, a new legal climate had come into existence—one in which legislative action now became a means of expanding, rather than curbing, information and service.

In 1966, the U.S. Department of Health, Education, and Welfare promulgated the first official positive family planning policy. By Congressional action, not less than 6 percent of HEW funds allocated for maternal and infant health were earmarked for family planning. The 1967 amendments to the Social Security Law mandated public welfare bureaus to provide family planning information and service to appropriate persons. In 1970 and 1971, states began to liberalize and repeal abortion laws, facilitating access to abortion where it might protect the health of the mother. Attitudes towards sterilization were relaxed, and voluntary sterilization is now legal in all fifty states. In 1969, in an unprecedented message to Congress on population problems, President Nixon said:

> It is my view that no American woman should be denied access to family planning assistance because of her economic condition. I believe, therefore, that we should establish as a national goal the provision of adequate family planning services within the next five years to all those who want them but cannot afford them. This we have the capacity to do.

In December 1970, President Nixon signed into law the Family Planning Services and Population Research Act. Its purpose is to:

> Make comprehensive voluntary family planning service available to all persons in the United States.
> Coordinate domestic population and family planning research with the present and future needs of population and family planning programs.
> Provide the trained manpower needed to effectively carry out programs of population research and family planning services.
> Develop and make available information (including educational materials) on family planning and population growth.

Congress authorized expenditures in this area of nearly $73 million for 1971. This could increase to $129 million in 1972 and over $180 million in 1973. In fiscal 1970, federal funds above $50 million were allocated for these family planning purposes.

RELIGIOUS ATTITUDES

Such sweeping changes in contraceptive law and practice could take place only within the framework of transformed religious doctrine. Churches, which at one time found birth limitation outside moral sanction, reexamined their policies and found family planning to be an obligation of responsible parenthood in today's world. All the major faiths approve in principle the right of couples to limit the size of their families, although there is continuing disagreement over acceptable methods.

A significant sector of the Catholic world seeks liberalization of the Roman Catholic papal edict, issued by Pope Paul VI, giving sanction only to the rhythm or abstinence method. Catholic nurses, serving in nonsectarian institutions offering family planning, are usually authorized to stand apart from delivering the service, if they consider it in violation of their conscience and their faith. However, in practice, no significant issues of staff opposition have emerged.

Sister Mary Helen of the University of San Francisco School of Nursing, in the March 1967 *Nursing Outlook*, stated that nurses should "recognize that the goal of family planning is the strengthening of the family." Since then, Catholic physicians, priests, nurses, lawyers, and parents in great numbers have expressed positive attitudes about family planning in general. Statistics about birth limitation practices indicate Catholic acceptance is approaching that of other groups nationally.

HEALTH INDICATORS

When family planning services are made an important component of overall health care, individual health is improved and family life strengthened. Drs. Wallace, Gold, and Dooley (1970), in an article in *Advances in Planned Parenthood*, noted that successful family planning enables mothers to regain full physical and mental strength between pregnancies, reducing the "syndrome of depletion." Family planning also helps to improve the quality of family life and to raise the standard of living by decreasing the numbers of dependent children requiring intensive personal care, education, food, shelter and clothing, and other necessities.

High-risk obstetrical patients, particularly those in the lower-socioeconomic groups and the minority groups, have significantly higher birthrates; maternal mortality and morbidity rates; fetal, neonatal, perinatal, and infant mortality rates; and low birth weight incidence. Low birth weight was shown to be directly related to birth spacing, in a study by Bishop (1964). He found that with birth intervals of 2 years, there was a 7.8 percent incidence of such low birth weight, but the incidence rose to 10.3 percent when the interval was 1 to 2 years and to 18 percent when the interval was less than a year.

Perinatal and neonatal mortality is higher among births to those under seventeen or over forty years of age, and there is increased perinatal mortality beyond the third birth. The recourse to illegal abortion for unwanted pregnancies has been held accountable for about 20 percent of maternal deaths in the United States.

When medical or nutritional problems are identified, it is important to be able to delay pregnancy until they can be treated or corrected. Family planning is also indicated in patients who have a history of previous pregnancy difficulties or failures, in diabetes, toxemia, heart disease, repeated abortion, stillbirth, premature labor, repeated caesarean sections, and certain genetic diseases.

Unwanted pregnancies among the lower-socioeconomic groups may carry increased dangers, because they not only intensify family poverty but compound the risks to mother and child. The avoidance of out-of-wedlock pregnancy among teenagers with its high costs in terms of health dangers and limitation of opportunities is of much importance. The preventive role of family planning in the maintenance of emotional health has been recognized by psychiatrists. The abused child syndrome, frequently the result of an unwanted pregnancy, is an increasing phenomenon, for which contraception or abortion can provide a partial solution.

From the public health point of view, the family planning center serves as an ideal setting for a wide array of preventive medicine. Such clinics can and often do screen for hypertension; breast masses; cancer of the cervix; venereal disease; anemia; nutritional problems including obesity; diabetes; urinary tract infections; susceptibility to tuberculosis; cardiac and pulmonary diseases. Sickle-cell anemia screening and counsel are increasingly becoming a general part of family planning clinic service.

A BROADER ASPECT

Helping Americans realize their own family size aspirations may hold the answer to United States population growth problems.

Every day in the United States an average of almost 10,000 babies are born, about 5,000 persons die, and over 1,000 more persons enter the country than leave. This adds about 6,000 a day to the population, or over 2 million a year. If this growth rate were to continue, it would increase the United States population from a little over 200 million to more than 300 million by the year 2008.

The Census Bureau estimates that if families were to average three children over the next few decades, and immigration were to continue as at present, we would reach 300 million in 1996. But, if we average two children, we would delay reaching that mark until 2021. The present family size averages about 2.5 children.

Our population would continue to grow until the year 2037 when it would be a third larger than now, even if immigration from abroad ceased and families began to average two children each. This is because of the relationship between the greatly widened base of people in their childbearing years and the extension of the life span. More people are being born and live longer.

The greatest United States population today is concentrated in cities and towns outside metropolitan areas, where more than three-fourths of the growth of the 1960s occurred. Suburbanites now outnumber those in cities. The farm population declined from 15 to 10 million, and about half of the nation's 3,000 counties lost population. Another one-fourth of all counties had low growth rates because more people moved out than moved in. But in-migration is not responsible for population growth. Seventy percent of the growth of metropolitan population occurred as a result of natural increase, not as a result of floods of people from rural areas. The in-migration from farm to urban dwelling does appear to favor a smaller family since agriculture has traditionally fostered larger patterns of family life than does the urban environment.

Perhaps more significant as a factor in voluntary reduction of family size is the extent to which women enter the work force. More than 30 million women in the United States, over 12 million of them mothers of children under eighteen, are now earning a living. This represents a steadily increasing sector of the working population. The desire for a two-salary family and its significance in improving the standard of living heighten individual desire to limit family size and greatly strengthen interest in measures to prevent unexpected pregnancies. The growth of women's liberation organizations—greatly varying in their approach to militance—reflects a contemporary trend toward more work outside the home and for greater personal control over reproduction.

There is impressive evidence that a substantial percentage of the 3.5 to 3.7 million babies being born annually in the United States were unwanted at the time of conception. The Westoff-Ryder National Fertility Study, based on married women's own reports of their childbearing experience, indicated that one-third of the married couples had already at least one child more than they had intended. In the period 1960-1965, nearly 20 percent of all live births were reported as unwanted by their parents. Three-fourths of all parents reported they had not been completely successful in preventing unwanted and unplanned pregnancies.

Unwanted births not only intensify the population problem; they also often represent serious cost to the family. For families living close to the poverty line or those in which the mother's earnings represent the difference between an adequate or an inadequate income, an unwanted birth can mean sudden alteration of life plans. Family stress is intensified; the stability of the family itself is endangered when the wage earner finds the home too crowded and the burden too great for his capacities. Among the very young, unwanted pregnancies lead to barriers to higher education and the acquisition of working skills, school dropouts, hasty marriages, and out-of-wedlock births.

Voluntary family planning, already demonstrated to be an integral part of preventive health programs, may offer a major method of helping couples, rich and poor, in the United States realize their own aspirations, protect their health and welfare, and contribute toward the nation's solution of the population problem, without employing coercive measures.

Studies of patterns of United States fertility have repeatedly shown that:

1 Virtually all United States couples at some time during marriage use a method to limit family size.

2 Both the well-to-do and the medically indigent want about the same number of children, but the poor are less successful in achieving the family size they desire.

3 At any given time, approximately 5.4 million low-income fertile United States women between the age of fifteen and forty-four desire access to free or low-cost family planning service. But in 1969, only 1.1 million were receiving service.

4 Ninety-nine percent of United States women deliver their babies in hospitals; but in 1969, 509 hospitals, or less than 15 percent of the 4,305 nonprofit general hospitals reporting births, offered family planning guidance. Public health departments were reported to be providing some family planning in 1,436 of 3,072 counties. No program could be identified in 1,636 counties, 53 percent of the United States total.

5 Wherever free and low-cost medically supervised family planning service is offered on terms of dignity, respect, and convenience, substantial enrollment is reported.

A study of estimated need for subsidized family planning services, made for the Office of Economic Opportunity by Planned Parenthood's Center for Family Planning Program Development, found this distribution of the national case:

Type of agency	Number of agencies reporting	Number of patients	Percentage of total
Hospitals	505	311,583	28
Health departments	1,177	418,104	38
Planned Parenthood	146	271,537	25
Others	155	92,823	9
Total	1,983	1,094,047	100

More than half of the women in need of subsidized family planning live in the 445 metropolitan counties of the United States standard metropolitan statistical areas. The remaining 45 percent live in the 2,627 nonmetropolitan counties. More than four-fifths of all patients reported in the study lived in the urbanized counties.

The Office of Economic Opportunity, with forty-five comprehensive neighborhood health centers and 115 family planning projects in 1969, was serving more family planning users than any other single public or private agency.

BASIC NURSING ROLE

In the light of widespread public acceptance and government and medical approval of family planning as a factor contributing to individual and family health, it is no longer necessary to justify the active participation of nurses in family planning. It may, however, be useful to postulate some dimensions of their role. Briefly stated, this can be seen as a three-pronged concept—case-finding, parent education and counseling, and case-holding; or simply stated—reaching, teaching, and keeping families. Utilizing such a concept, all nurses, regardless of their field of practice, have a role in family planning. Effective communication is, of course, essential to functioning in these areas. So is understanding of possible barriers to and facilitators of proper utilization of services. Among the barriers are those relating to lack of adequate services, offered without due regard for patient sensibilities and needs with regard to costs, transportation, hours, and eligibility. There are obstacles which relate to attitudes, feelings, and values regarding family planning that are operational both within patients and within the staff providing services. When these are negative—moralistic or racially prejudiced—they can be serious hurdles to achievement of patient acceptance, hurdles which are insurmountable for some. The methods of family planning themselves can be a barrier, since none of those currently available are ideal, and the most effective require access to a physician and entail a pelvic examination which may cause fear and embarrassment for many women.

Negative attitudes among patients may stem from lack of understanding, fears or dislike of available family planning methods, religious beliefs which consider their use immoral, and misconceptions that family planning will interfere with sexual enjoyment or cause sterility. Among minority groups there may be suspicion that family planning programs are intended simply to reduce their numbers, and impoverished people may be concerned with the costs of obtaining the service or may have had previous experiences with poorly administered clinics which deter them from returning to seek additional medical care. The facilitating effect of nurse intervention can be a decisive factor. Through careful, sympathetic, and open discussion with patients, nurses can attempt to ascertain the existence of the possible barriers as seen by the patient and to offer assurance and correct information coupled with empathetic understanding and acceptance.

The goals of communication in family planning are to offer information in such a way that the woman will know what her options are, to help patients translate a knowledge of family planning into regular and effective use, and to create an atmosphere of mutual respect and understanding and response to patients' needs.

All women within the childbearing years, regardless of age, income, parity, or marital status, can be considered potential patients. Family planning should be considered the rule, rather than the exception. Low-income families in particular should be given special attention because, lacking access to private medical care, they are less likely to have had information and help in family planning offered to them by a physician. Family planning is particularly appropriate during the obstetrical experience—prenatally, postnatally, and during the hospital stay itself. It should also be considered before discharge of all patients, male or female, and after hospitalization for physical or mental illness. Child health conferences are also an appropriate possibility for case-finding.

The provision of information, counseling, and referrals to a source of service is a second important area of nurse functioning in family planning. The nurse can explore the woman's interest and level of understanding, and selectively offer accurate knowledge, reassurance, and encouragement. In counseling families it is useful to use a problem-solving approach by helping them to define the problem, helping them to identify possible solutions and testing their assessment of the results of such solutions, and finally, helping them to make their own decision.

While case-holding is mainly the responsibility of nurses and staff within family planning clinics, nurses who have referred patients to such services can follow through to see if the woman has acted on the referral, whether she is satisfied with the services or needs additional guidance in using her prescribed method or has other problems or questions. Where the problem is service-connected, nurses can act as family advocates to see that they are provided with needed assistance or to bring about improvement in service that may be called for.

A TOTAL APPROACH

In order to make family planning universally accessible and acceptable to all who need and want to plan the number, spacing, and timing of their children, a total approach is indicated. There needs to be equality of opportunity to obtain quality services; research into the development of new and improved methods of fertility control; improved basic and continuing education for professional groups such as physicians, nurses, social workers, teachers, and pharmacists; wider community education and dissemination of knowledge on parental responsibilities, human reproduction, and contraception to all Americans through all means and mass media, including the schools. Every hospital and out-patient department and health department should provide high-grade dignified family planning services and education at convenient times, at low or no cost. All welfare departments and other social service agencies should see that their workers are prepared to offer and guide clients to suitable family planning services. Industries and unions should include education and services to their employees and members. In view of the inherent importance to the individual and society, the financial and manpower investment required by such a program is well justified.

FAMILY PLANNING METHODS

Methods of fertility control include both the temporary, readily reversible techniques involving continuous use by one or the other partner, and those which are achieved through surgical sterilization of the male or female. The latter are considered permanent and irreversible, although some limited success has been achieved in reanastomosing the fallopian tubes or vasa deferentia.

Contraception can be achieved through intervening in or changing the usual chain of reproductive events in either the male or the female so as to prevent pregnancy from occurring. Current methods are based on preventing the meeting of the sperm and egg cell, either through interposing a barrier, mechanical or chemical; inhibiting ovulation; or altering some of the uterine conditions needed for implantation.

Experimental methods under research are utilizing or exploring the possibilities of other changes in the reproductive process which are vulnerable to controlled interference. In the male these include effects on sperm production, maturation, and motility or transport. In the female, vulnerable areas are passage of the sperm through the cervical mucus, changes in the activity of the myometrium or musculature of the fallopian tubes, preparation of the endometrium for nidation, function of the corpus luteum, tubal patency, and embryonic development.

While not a method of contraception, the use of abortion to remove the product of conception is widely used to prevent unwanted births. It is now legal on request in four states—New York, Alaska, Hawaii, and Washington, and thirteen additional states have liberalized their restrictive abortion laws. A number of organizations, including the American Public Health Association and Planned Parenthood-World Population have recommended that abortion be considered a matter of medical and personal judgment to be decided between doctor and patient, without legal interference.

The most effective methods of birth control available today are those which require a doctor's care, examination, and prescription. These are the oral contraceptives, intrauterine devices, diaphragms, and voluntary sterilization. Although a detailed discussion of these methods is beyond the scope of this text, it is clear that all health workers have a responsibility to know this information and to share it freely if effective family planning is to be a reality for all who wish it.

BIBLIOGRAPHY

Bishop, E.: "Prematurity, Etiology and Management," *Post-Graduate Medicine,* **35**: 185-188, 1964.

Bumpass, L., and F. Westoff: "Unwanted Births and United States Population Growth," *Family Planning Perspectives,* **2**:9-11, 1970.

Commission on Population Growth and the American Future: Interim Report, Washington, D.C.: U.S. Government Printing Office, March 16, 1971.

Douglas, E. T.: *Margaret Sanger: Pioneer of the Future,* New York: Holt, Rinehart and Winston, Inc., 1970.

Dryfoos, J. G., et al.: "Eighteen Months Later: Family Planning Services in the United States, 1969," *Family Planning Perspectives,* **3**:29-44, 1971.

Helen, Sister M.: "Family Planning within the Curriculum," *Nursing Outlook,* **15**:42-45, 1967.

Himes, N. E.: *Medical History of Contraception,* New York: Gamut Press, 1963.

Kessler, A., and S. Kessler: "Health Aspects of Family Planning," in E. Diczfalusy and U. Borrell (eds.), *Control of Human Fertility,* New York: John Wiley & Sons, Inc., 1971.

Lieberman, E.: "Preventive Psychiatry and Family Planning," *Journal of Marriage and the Family,* **26**:471-477, 1964.

Manisoff, M.: *Family Planning—A Teaching Guide for Nurses,* New York: Planned Parenthood-World Population, 1971.

————: *Family Planning Training for Social Service,* New York: Planned Parenthood-World Population, 1970.

————: "Counseling for Family Planning," *American Journal of Nursing,* **66**:2671-2675, 1966.

Schwartz, R. A.: "The Role of Family Planning in the Primary Prevention of Mental Illness," *American Journal of Psychiatry,* **125**:1711-1718, 1969.

Wallace, H., E. Gold, and S. Dooley: "Relationships between Family Planning and Maternal and Child Health," in *Advances in Planned Parenthood,* Amsterdam: Excerpta Medica Foundation, vol. 5, 1970.

Westoff, L., and C. F. Westoff: *From Now to Zero,* Boston: Little, Brown and Company, 1971.

Chapter 13

Anticipatory Guidance
of the Expectant
Family

Rosemary Kilker and Betty L. Wilkerson

We look at the family into whose circle a child is to be born as going through three periods of normal crises. Within these periods, we have found there are levels, or phases, of crisis. It is in one of these phases that the expectant family and the nurse first meet. At this meeting, the nurse and the family conduct a mutual assessment. The family begins by raising the basic question, "To whom should we turn to aid us in having our baby successfully?" This occurs whether it is the first or subsequent expectant experience. The assessment begins upon verbal telephone contact with the proposed maternity service. Is this verbal communication warm, reassuring, welcoming—or is it cold, curt, too impersonally businesslike? This exchange of words sets the tone for the family's first confrontation with the health services engaged for this pregnancy.

When the expectant mother arrives in the maternity clinic, she reviews and evaluates in her mind that which she has heard about the clinic and, now, the environment in which she finds herself. With these assessments in mind, she meets the medical team, anticipating the answers to all her questions, besieged by undefined apprehension.

The first member of the medical team who meets and assesses the patient is usually the nurse. From this assessment the nurse begins to develop the guidelines she will use to take this mother and her family through the ante-partal, intrapartal, and postpartal crises.

While obtaining the usual medical statistics, the nurse assesses this mother and her life style, so that the health team can view this mother as an individual, as a member of her family, and as a member of the community. The assessment is built on evidence noted in the verbal and nonverbal com-munication. The nonverbal assessment includes general appearance—the mother's concept of self in regards to cleanliness, tidiness, her method of walking and talking, her wearing apparel, her facial expressions, and how she uses her hands and feet. The inflections of the voice, and the tone of delivery, are also noted. She notes whether the patient seems to be listening, is she hearing, taking in?

The communication includes determining the expectant mother's vo-cabulary, then translating medical jargon into *her* language. This is a "must" if the nurse hopes to give proper practical guidance and to draw a baseline for the principles of learning.

Activities of the patient's daily living are discussed—sleep patterns, rec-reation, work, elimination, and sexual drives. Nutritional health needs for mother and her family are to be evaluated very critically, such as when the big meal is eaten each day, what foods are eaten on a "typical" day, how the foods are prepared, and how the family's culture influences their eating habits.

To help the mother plan for this child and to help her plan for her own health, it is necessary to inquire about living facilities. Are there laundry facilities? Is the residence on one or two floors? Where is the bathroom located? How many families share the home?

If the expectant father has not been present at this first visit, he should be encouraged to come at a later visit to meet the health team, and to tour the maternity unit. This is a way to make him feel more comfortable at the time his wife is admitted, to answer his questions, and also to help him be of more assistance to his wife and more a part of the total experience.

Following this initial contact, the nurse needs to "sift out" her impres-sions of the expectant family at this stage of crisis, and to make tentative plans for nursing intervention. The nurse must consider the mother's desires, and what she can do to assist her in attaining them.

For this assessment to be useful, the same nurse and the same health team should be with this family throughout the maternity experience. The nurse becomes the "cue taker." By making each patient a special person, she picks up innuendos from the patient in regard to her well-being, her family's well-being, and their interaction. Old wives tales and "coffee klatch" fears, such as the belief that it is harmful to paint, must be dissipated with logical answers. It must be explained to the mother that the harmful part of the painting is climbing on ladders, and on and off chairs. Another myth is that putting the hands above the head causes the umbilical cord to wrap itself around the baby's neck. It must be explained to the mother that her movements will not displace the cord.

We must continually involve the husband in the mother's care and plans. Husbandhood and fatherhood develop from the knowledge the husband gains and the amount his involvement is increased. The mates learn from their own experience (Schaefer and Zisourtz, 1964). This means the nurse must establish communication with the father-to-be. Besides preparing him for his wife's labor and delivery and for their new baby, the nurse must prepare him for his wife's emotional swings and the changes of mood of which he and the family will be a part. Most important is his understanding of the change in his wife's sexual desire, such as there being little difference in the woman's sexual appetite during the first trimester. However, during the second trimester, the wife usually has an increase in sexual desires. According to Masters and Johnson, this increase is sometimes beyond that of the prepregnant state. During the last trimester, sexual interest is again decreased, which is perhaps due to the protuberance of the female abdomen and generalized physical discomforts. Restrictions by some physicians during this period are also imposed (Masters and Johnson, 1966).

As pregnancy continues, the nurse reassesses the woman at each visit. This reassessment is made to determine her health, her understanding of her progress and to meet new needs as they rise. It may be necessary to expand the health team to include a social worker, a dietitian, or other community agency personnel. In these situations, the nurse intervenes as a coordinator, or liaison person. At no time should the nurse be the "decision maker" for this family. She must continually encourage their independence in planning both before and after the baby's arrival.

As the antepartal period continues, the nurse progressively builds the theme that childbearing and childrearing are a family affair. There are developmental roles for both mother and father during this period. The developmental roles are greatest for those in the first pregnancy. The woman must remain a wife, become a mother, and yet maintain her individual personality. The man, while retaining his identity as a man, is now both a husband and a father.

Though the wife may have come from a very "close" family, where ties were strong and secure, she may secretly feel very anxious that she will now have to step into "mother's" role. All the marriage and family sociological classes with which she was involved are now far removed as pregnancy progresses.

The expectant father enters the antepartal period often unknowing about what will evolve. The type of family environment in which he was reared may well determine his feelings during his wife's pregnancy. Was it a "not talked of" subject? Was sex considered wholesome and included in family discussion? What did his mother tell him concerning her pregnancy and deliveries? He needs to feel wanted and needed by his wife, and he also needs to feel a part of the events occurring inside his wife's body. The physician and nurse must include him. They must guide the wife's "dependency" needs of pregnancy toward the mate. Otherwise, the physician may encroach upon the expectant father's role, if the wife turns to him to meet these needs (Wonnell, 1971).

The family should be encouraged to attend parent classes. Anticipatory guidance needs to be given to prepare them for the final phase of this first crisis—the beginning of labor. The expectant father's role in supporting and sharing this experience cannot be underestimated or overemphasized. Both parents should understand the nature of labor; how to cope with it; how to make decisions, when feasible (i.e., the type of anesthesia to be requested). The parents should, finally, be instructed in the care and feeding of the new baby. This is the "ideal" situation; however, the cultural and ethnic backgrounds of people influence the degree of involvement of the father.

If the expectant family has had a "peak" experience during the antepartal crisis, it is much easier for them to make the transition to the labor and delivery room health team during the second crisis of the maternity cycle.

The amount of involvement of the husband in his wife's antepartal experience is easily detected by their verbal and nonverbal behavior during this crisis. The anticipatory role of the nurse will greatly help to alleviate the tension and nervousness present in labor. The nurse in the labor unit must be able to speak with conviction. She should convey confidence to establish the emotional "climate" conducive to providing a meaningful labor experience for this couple. Hopefully, more expectant parents will be able to meet the labor and delivery room personnel on an antepartal hospital tour. This was emphasized by a patient, Mrs. T., who stated how comforting it was to have the nurse she met on her antepartal tour with her during the course of labor and delivery. Mrs. T. said, "When you arrived, I wasn't afraid anymore." Another value of antepartal tours was verbalized by Mrs. A., gravida one, who with her husband, was taken on a tour of the labor and delivery rooms antepartally. Both labor and delivery rooms were viewed, and the nurse explained the items of equipment. The fetal monitoring room was also included and reasons given for its use. During Mrs. A.'s labor, the fetal heart tones became irregular, necessitating the use of the fetal monitor. During the puerperium, Mr. and Mrs. A. both verbalized how beneficial the earlier explanation of fetal monitoring was in decreasing their apprehension.

The husband can be the source of comfort and support to his wife during this experience if the nurses and health team so guide their interrelationship at this time. After all, he, too, is having this baby! Father can be mother's best relaxant and pain reliever. The nurse should instruct and support the husband in such actions as sacral pressure, wiping the brow, and moistening her lips. An example is Mrs. S., para one, who expressed her gratitude to the nurse for showing her husband how to massage her back and relieve her back pain. Her comment was, "I couldn't have gone through labor without him."

He should feel his wife's contractions with his finger tips; he, too, can be able to anticipate the contractions and help his wife with the various breathing techniques. He and his wife should be able to listen to the baby's heart tones, if they desire. This brings the reality to both the mother and the father that this baby is real and soon to be born as an individual personality. Truly compassionate nurses remember that this soon-to-be-born infant started as a seed from father and an egg from mother in a physiological and psychological experience. The embryo was the result of cooperative effort. Since then the mates have shared together the 9 months of pregnancy. It is fitting that the nurse's role be that of a catalyst. She acts as the thoroughly concerned person protecting and promoting the health and safety of mother, father, and child.

In the meeting of the needs of the laboring couple, it is paramount that the nurse keep ahead of the labor process and, with anticipated planning, assure a smooth transition from the labor bed to the delivery table.

It has taken decades, but many nurses and physicians have come to the realization that the delivery room is not sacrosanct. With adequate preparation, and at the discretion of the couple, the husband can be there with his wife. Who else, indeed, belongs there, if not the father? If for a personal or medical reason the father is not present for the actual delivery, he should be involved in the event by continual communication. He should be kept appraised of his wife's progress; he should be promptly notified of the arrival of the baby, and he should be allowed to visit with his wife as soon as possible. When the father is not in the delivery room, the mother and baby should be transferred together, and together greet the father.

The new family is now engaged in surviving the third crisis of the maternity cycle. The first phase of this third crisis is the realization of the parents that the baby is here and that new or added responsibilities have arrived. Nine months of anticipation are over. Wife and husband are now mother and father. The "to be" has become an "is." "Blessed event" is now "baby in reality." A *family* has been completed: father, mother, and child.

Father and mother must go through an adjustment phase. Both have mood swings. Following the elation mood of "The baby is here!" and becoming aware of the consuming need of "spreading the word," the father perceives how the arrival will change his role and responsibilities. These untried roles and new responsibilities involve finances, self-image of maleness, and the duties of parent and husband. At times, in this crisis period, the father is moody, withdrawn, and distracted. It is easy for him to develop a "poor me" attitude as he now falls into the background, and the baby becomes the new center of the family universe.

The beginning of this crisis is fraught with tremendous mood swings of the mother. She initially is euphoric; she has completed her work; she has brought new life into the world. Slowly, she begins to realize her responsibilities to this new baby and to her husband who is now a father. At times, these new concerns seem overwhelming, and she becomes depressed. She, too, feels dispossessed as the baby takes center stage. These feelings begin in the hospital and may carry over to the first days at home. She vacillates between periods of dependence and independence, and to help her gain a stable independence, the nurse must assume the duties of listener, teacher, and supporter. The nurse is unable to give specific anticipatory guidance. The guidance and support is an "on the spot" situation. The nurse must have an instinct for the time that is appropriate for the mother to relive her labor experience. She must sense the time that is appropriate; when feasible she must reeducate wife and husband to the role of mother and father. This instruction includes baby's care and health, mother's care and health, and the family's care and health. This health is all encompassing, it is both physical and mental. The nurse must orient the couple to team effort: the best decisions that parents make are made jointly in common discernment and resolution.

The second phase of the third crisis is preparing the family for leaving the hospital, to take up the old and adjust to a new pattern of family life. If there are other children, plans need to be made concerning sibling rivalry and sibling acceptance. Discussions should be held in regard to ways of harmonizing the care, love, and safety of the new baby with adequate concern for siblings. Feelings also need to be explored concerning the "significant others"—the grandparents, aunts, uncles, and close friends. The inescapable question must be faced of setting limits to unsolicited help from relatives and friends.

Before leaving the hospital, the opportunity should be given for the parents to discuss their sexual needs and family planning. This must be done by an initiated member of the health team very closely associated with this couple throughout the maternity cycle.

The last phase of the third crisis is "homecoming." Anticipatory guidance on this "homecoming" is a *must*. The excitement and the tensions of dressing the baby in all his finery; packing the suitcase for home; gathering up of the flowers, letters, and gifts; and bidding goodbye to the hospital personnel explode 5 minutes after the family arrives home. The baby reacts to the strange environment; he becomes cross and irritable. The mother sees all that needs to be done; the father, after unpacking the car, feels helpless and useless. The baby has to be settled. The first feeding has to be faced. She quickly becomes exhausted, while he usually returns to work. This phase simply has to work itself out, as each couple is different. Things usually become easier as practical wisdom of adjustment and know-how grows with time and experience.

The anticipatory guidance, such as that of the nurse, can steer the new family to survive the perils of this crisis. The postpartal nurse and health team contribute to the nurturing of the family while still in the hospital and to the future in the family home.

Through all three crises, the nurse and maternity service team have helped the husband and wife to grow in love and appreciation; they have mutually guided the first steps of the new mother and father in their evermore closely knit union by sharing in the incorporation of the living link—the child—that completes the family circle.

BIBLIOGRAPHY

Caplan, G.: *Concepts of Mental Health and Consultation,* Washington, D.C.: Children's Bureau, U.S. Department of Health, Education, and Welfare, Welfare Administration, 1959.

———: "Psychological Aspects of Maternity Care," *American Journal of Public Health,* **47**(1):25-31, 1957.

Jessner, L.: "Pregnancy as a Stress in Marriage," in E. Nash, L. Jessner, and D. W. Abse (eds.), *Marriage Counseling in Medical Practice,* Chapel Hill, N.C.: The University of North Carolina Press, 1964.

Masters, W. H., and V. E. Johnson: *Human Sexual Response,* Boston: Little, Brown and Company, 1966.

Rubin, R.: "Basic Maternal Behavior," *Nursing Outlook,* **9**:683-686, 1961.

———: "Maternal Touch," *Nursing Outlook,* **11**:828-831, 1963.

———: "Puerperal Change," *Nursing Outlook,* **9**:753-755, 1961.

Schaefer, G., and M. Zisourtz: *The Expectant Father,* New York: Simon and Schuster, Inc., 1964.

Scott, D. U.: "Crisis Intervention," in B. Bergerson, E. N. Anderson, M. Duffey, M. Lohr, and M. H. Rose (eds.), *Current Concepts in Clinical Nursing,* St. Louis: The C. V. Mosby Company, 1967.

Selye, H.: "The Stress Syndrome," in J. Folta and E. S. Deck (eds.), *A Sociological Framework for Patient Care,* New York: John Wiley & Sons, Inc., 1966.

Weidenbach, E.: *Family-centered Maternity Nursing,* New York: G. P. Putnam's Sons, 1967.

Wonnell, E.: "The Education of the Expectant Father for Childbirth," *The Nursing Clinics of North America,* **6**:591-603, 1971.

Chapter 14

The Adopting Family

Katherine Gustin

Adoption is the legal process devised by society and assumed to be the best solution in providing care for children who, for some reason, cannot live with their own parents. To adoptive parents go all the privileges and obligations which are removed from or relinquished by natural parents. The one exception is the situation in which the natural parent is also the adoptive parent, as in the case of a father adopting his illegitimate child.

When we speak of the adoptive process, it becomes apparent that not only the adoptive family and the child, but also his natural parent or parents, are integral parts of the process. This chapter will be addressed to a discussion of all three components in adoption.

Many children are placed through social agencies to whom either the parents have relinquished the child voluntarily or to whom the courts have assigned those removed from their homes. A greater number are placed independently either by parents or by a third person who may be a relative, friend, or professional person such as physician or lawyer. Another group of children is sold on the "black market" by a third person for profit. In all but the case of children removed from their home by court action, parents sever legal ties with the child by signing relinquishment papers which provide temporary custody to the agency or person designated. Adoption is not final until the appropriate court so designates.

AGENCY PLACEMENT

Placement through a social agency seems desirable for protection, not only of the child, but also of the natural and adoptive parents. Most children become candidates for placement because they are born out of wedlock.There are also those whose parents are, or were, married and unable to rear their children because of some existing difficulty, such as mental illness, broken homes, or financial problems. Organizations which work with adoption may be welfare offices, juvenile courts, or religious and private agencies.

Social agencies are able to assist unmarried mothers in several ways. Sometimes they provide living arrangements such as a maternity home or financial help and temporary care of the child until placement is accomplished. Agencies offer counseling in several areas. For example, reality factors regarding the feasibility of either keeping or relinquishing the child, or whether to marry the child's father are discussed while the mother is given sufficient time to decide which course she wishes to follow. Sometimes the client is quite ambivalent about relinquishment, and casework treatment can be an asset. For the most part, an effort is made to enable the mother to come to her own solution, but, at times, protection of the child may indicate a need for the worker to support relinquishment if planning for the child seems impossible in the mother's circumstances.

Casework treatment during this period should have as one of its goals a helping process which will aid the mother in establishing healthier methods of handling needs and problems so that, hopefully, the illegitimacy will not be repeated. Social workers have long operated from the hypothesis that pregnancy out of wedlock does not usually happen by chance, but is embedded in parent-child relationships which produce unconscious motivation toward unmarried motherhood and do not provide a basis for the healthiest functioning of the individual. This probably applies to the father of the child as well as to the mother.

Young (1954) has discussed the apparently purposeful, though unconscious, behavior of the unmarried mother. The family or life situation has not been one in which relationships enable her to achieve a normal psychosocial development, and the child becomes a means of meeting neurotic needs. The child, consequently, is usually of little concern to her as a person, although the degree of health in the personalities of unmarried mothers varies, and some are able to love the child. Young also finds the degree of illness in unmarried mothers is greater when their cultural background contains strict moral codes. Thus, it is possible for a greater degree of health to exist in the personality of those mothers whose cultural milieu is more permissive in its moral standards. The author points out that although little social work has been done with the unmarried father, evidence tends to indicate he has also experienced a background which interferes with a mature psychosocial adjustment.

Social agencies assist the mother in obtaining proper health care throughout pregnancy and delivery. She may also be helped in planning for her future after delivery in such matters as schooling or employment. Emotional support, as well as other casework treatment, is given as long as needed.

Since some unmarried mothers do not seek agency help or even prenatal medical attention, a public health nurse may be the only professional person she might see prior to delivery. Nurses can be helpful by suggesting referral to an adoptive agency and explaining the many services which can be offered. A nurse can be a supportive person throughout pregnancy, delivery, and in subsequent contacts. They are especially helpful to unmarried mothers who decide to keep the baby and in educating the mother in childrearing practices.

If adjustment problems are developing in the child as he becomes older, a nurse following a family is in a good position, because of her relationship with the mother, to discuss referral to a social agency such as child psychiatry or family service for treatment in parent-child relationships. She may also refer the family to some other social worker in the community, such as a medical social worker, who will assess the situation and make appropriate disposition.

A nurse, in assessing a child's adjustment, may gather the information from observation of his behavior and interaction with other persons or through communication with the mother or others in the child's environment who may be aware of problems he or the family may be having. How the child relates to family members and to other children is an important area. Adjustment to school, in terms of behavior and grade achievement, can be explored. The child's and his family's interests and recreational activities should be noted. In general the illegitimate child has the same needs for good physical care, warmth without overprotection, and consistent, reasonable limit setting, as any other child.

Couples usually decide to adopt only after a period of years in which they are unable to have their own child. The route which offers the safest course is application to a social service agency which handles adoptions. These agencies discuss the reason for an inability to produce children and usually refer the family to a physician, if they have not already sought medical advice. Some of these adoptive applicants are then able to have their own children. A nurse seeing a family who wishes to adopt but does not wish to contact a social agency and has not sought medical help has the opportunity to explore the situation. Educating the family about the adoption process could help lower anxiety and enable them to approach an adoptive agency or physician.

In agency placements the prospective adoptive parents are assured that proper legal procedures are observed. The identities of the two families will be unknown to each other. Unfortunate circumstances can result when this is not observed. For example, visitation by a natural parent may be disruptive to the child and adoptive family and even result in natural parents regaining custody after the child and adoptive parents have become emotionally attached to each other.

The methods and also the competence of adoption agencies vary greatly, but the aims and process have similarities. The goals are to serve a protective role, primarily for the child, who must be the main concern, but also for the natural and adoptive parents. Agencies, in general, try to place a child in a stable home which will best meet his individual needs.

When prospective adoptive parents approach an agency, they probably feel a sense of failure because most have not conceived their own child. They are probably fearful, too, of not being accepted as adoptive parents, as most people are aware there are not enough babies to place with every family wishing to adopt. The supportive approach of social workers should be beneficial to all applicants, particularly those who are not accepted as adoptive parents.

Social agencies explore areas such as financial security, duration of the marriage, absence of gross emotional instability, physical fitness, the number of adopted or natural children already in the home, marital status, and age of the couple. There is variation in standards on these various aspects, but all are given consideration. For example, adoption by a single person has occurred, but social agencies have generally believed that a child needs both a father and a mother.

The more intangible aspects, such as personality factors of the applicants, their interaction, and their ability to provide such things as warmth and reasonable limit setting in a parent-child relationship, are more difficult to determine and should be evaluated by the most highly skilled social workers. Since adoptive applicants know there are more people seeking adoption than there are children available, they wish to present a good picture of their home and are not likely to discuss problems openly. Because most applicants are childless, there is no opportunity to assess the adjustment of a child in the home or to discuss differences the couples might be having regarding child-rearing methods. Another difficulty is that people cannot readily verbalize unconscious material in which conflict in the matter of parenthood may be buried, and are aware only of the conscious wish to have a child.

Many of us in the behavioral field have questioned, formally or informally, why the large group of prospective parents who have no diagnosed physical reason preventing conception are unable to achieve this. We know of instances in which couples do have their own children after initiating or completing adoption. It is not known, of course, whether they would have conceived regardless of adoption, but one wonders if taking the step to apply for a child represents a readiness to accept parenthood which for some reason was not previously present.

Agencies vary in the amount and type of background information required from prospective adoptive parents. In the area of relationships with parents and siblings it would seem helpful to explore parent-child relationships rather carefully. Experience in the area of problematic parent-child relationships indicates that parents' method of relating to their children arises rather directly in discernible ways out of experiences with their own parents. Consequently, this exploration should be somewhat predictive concerning how prospective applicants will relate to a child in their home.

Prospective adoptive parents are asked the reason they wish to adopt a child. This is necessary as agencies must try to eliminate homes in which the motivation arises out of purely narcissistic reasons or ulterior motives. In the writer's experience, most families have said they wish to adopt because they love children and have been unable to have their own. Sometimes applicants wish to adopt in an attempt to save an unstable marriage, but casework experience indicates that a child added to a situation of this type only increases tensions and problems and creates a poor environment in which to rear children. Other applicants are motivated by the desire to replace a child who has died; and, in these cases, it must be questioned how much of the concern is motivated by the applicants' own needs rather than by awareness of the child's. Others may wish to adopt in order to provide companionship for an only child.

In general, agencies prefer that prospective adoptive parents be mature enough to focus upon the child's needs rather than exclusively upon their own. Sometimes applicants never move from the wish to have a child simply because their lives are incomplete. Applicants who are too rigid in the type of child they will accept and will not consider any other also fall into this category. Prospective adoptive parents who accept an agency's evaluation and answer questions willingly in a direct manner are probably more mature persons who realize the agency must be careful into whose hands the life of a child is committed. Those who are resentful of the process may tend to be motivated only by their own interests.

After a social worker has talked several times with applicants at the agency and in the home, and the family is considered one in which a child would thrive, they are placed on a waiting list which may involve a few weeks to several months. The list is studied in order to select the home which is thought to be best suited to the individual child who needs adoption.

Agencies have attempted to match children with their adoptive parents to some extent. It has generally been considered advisable that the child is not too different in appearance from the adoptive parents. It formerly was a policy to select a home in which the religion is the same as the child's although there are exceptions to this, and the emphasis being placed upon matching is diminishing.

CHANGING POLICIES

Agencies policies regarding age of infants at time of placement have changed in recent years. The infant used to remain for 6 months or longer in a temporary foster home in order to ensure that his development would be normal. Since most defects can be detected shortly after birth, we know now of babies being placed within 3 weeks after birth or even directly from a hospital. The baby's family history, together with a pediatrician's evaluation, is probably the most reliable estimate of his intelligence at this early age. This change in agency thinking arises partly from the recognition that adoptive parents can give much more freely of themselves to a child than can foster parents who realize the relationship will be temporary. The importance of maternal care in the early stages of life is widely recognized and is an important reason for early placement.

Agencies are also changing policies regarding the criteria for determining if a child is adoptable. Emphasis is beginning to be based upon the child's social and emotional capacities for relationships rather than concentrating upon a particular handicap. Franklin and Massarik (1969), in a study of methods and results in placing medically handicapped children, found more failures in placement existing in middle-class families than in those such as business and professional groups on the one hand and in "blue collar" families on the other. These authors believe this is possibly associated with middle-class families being absorbed in a desire to achieve economically and socially. Previous experience in rearing children also seemed to be advantageous in adoption of a handicapped child.

Prospective parents are made aware of any handicap prior to placement. If they are interested in the child and the agency believes they can cope with the problems, handicapped children are now placed in adoptive homes.

Jane, born out of wedlock, was found to have cerebral palsy shortly after birth. At that time, children with this diagnosis were not considered adoptable, and the child was placed in foster care. She was a bright, personable child and eventually, with medical care, was sufficiently ambulatory to take care of personal needs. The foster parents were older people who were quite fond of the child and gave her a secure early childhood. Years later, this child, then a young teenager, was seen by the worker at a child psychiatric clinic when she came in for evaluation prior to placement. The foster mother had become unable to care for Jane, and she had been placed in another home. Consequently, the child went from foster home to foster home and had no family ties. It now seems certain that an adoptive family could have been found early in her life, and that the experience could have been a rewarding one for both child and parents. With the change which has taken place in adoption policies, a child such as this would probably receive an adoptive placement.

Many children are held in foster or institutional care because for some reason their parents will not relinquish custody, even though they cannot provide a home themselves. It does seem a change in law should be considered so these children could become adoptable by court action. Then adoptive parents, subsequently selected, could feel free to become more emotionally involved with the child as it would be a permanent relationship.

After a child is placed in his adoptive home, there is usually a waiting period of 6 months to a year before adoption is considered permanent by the court. In an agency placement, adoptive parents are protected in that the natural parents do not know where the child is placed. The natural parents are also protected in that their identity remains unknown except to the agency.

Social agencies vary regarding how much information about the child is given to adoptive parents, but it is considered necessary to relate details of the child's and his family's medical history. Adoptive parents vary also in how much information they desire from the agency. Children do have a right to know something of the circumstances of their birth and why they were placed for adoption. The way in which a social worker tells adoptive parents about the natural parent or parents is important. If adoptive parents can understand and accept natural parents as persons even though they may not approve of their actions, then they are in a better position to transmit this feeling to the child. Jolowicz (1946) has discussed the effect on a child's well-being if he cannot think of his natural parents as acceptable as persons, even though some of their behavior cannot be condoned. There is always some identification with natural parents, and a child may feel he is bad in some way if those with whom his past and present are linked are undesirable as persons.

HOME SUPERVISION

During the 6- to 12-month period of supervision after an agency placement, the social worker visits the home several times, providing an opportunity for adoptive parents to discuss any problems which may emerge and guidance in parent-child relationships. Study of growth and development is a part of social work training; and, if problems in care develop, the family is encouraged to seek the services of a pediatrician. The major focus needed in following an adoptive placement is in the area of relationships. The period of supervision can be a smoother one in the case of an infant than that of an older child, who may misbehave in testing the strength of the adoptive parents' acceptance of him. Sometimes, too, older children have had a series of previous placements and do not feel secure with another change of homes. Older children also have a stronger identification with natural parents as many have lived part of their lives in their own home.

When the adoptive home being supervised has an infant in placement, the social worker must discuss fully the problem of telling the child, as he matures, of his adoption. While most parents readily agree to this intellectually, the actual experience of talking about this to the child over the years is difficult. This is not a matter of one session with him, but a continuing situation which must be handled according to the maturational status of the child. Adoptive parents, out of fear of the child's feelings about adoption, sometimes handle this poorly, if at all. Experience has indicated it is much better for the child to hear it from people who love him than in an unforeseen way from someone else in the community. The writer has known several persons whose adoptive parents failed to tell them they were not their own child, and then they heard it from someone else in the community. These people spoke of their anger over the fact that the adoptive parents had not been honest with them. The news was not catastrophic in any of these situations, so we assume good parenting otherwise was more important; but the fact remains that any person has a right to know something of his heritage. Since the adoptive family is usually not followed by an agency after adoption becomes permanent, a public health nurse who might be following a family for some reason could be helpful if a situation of this type is encountered.

The general goal involved in the supervisory period is to enable family members to adjust under the new circumstances and become a healthy, integrated unit. Throughout the adoption process the main concern must be protective service to the child in the continuing task of selecting and supervising a suitable home for him. The following case illustrates some of the problems which can develop in an independent adoptive placement:

Baby boy S., age 2 weeks, came to a large medical center with a severe, congenital cardiac defect. He was the second illegitimate child born to the mother and was to have been placed for adoption by the referring physician who was working with a lawyer on the case. The first problem confronting the medical center was to obtain written permission for surgery, and it was not clear who had custody. Through the local juvenile court, permission was obtained from the natural mother to perform necessary treatment. Open heart surgery was done, and the baby was restored to good health. The next problem was a financial one as it was also not clear who would be responsible for payment. This was eventually assumed by the prospective adoptive parents who applied for assistance through the state agency for crippled children. It was not possible to learn very much about this couple or to work with them as the local physician did not want them to talk with anyone at the medical center.

When the infant was ready for discharge from the hospital, the local physician was assured of his good health. He had some difficulty in locating the prospective parents as they had gone for a vacation in another state, and the physician did not know their exact location. They were located by him after some difficulty; and, after several days' delay because of this and the couple's need to apply for financial help, the baby was discharged to the adoptive father, who came to the hospital and asked for the S. baby, indicating the child's name was known to him.

This case is representative of several aspects which are better handled by an adoption agency. There would have been no problem in regard to obtaining permission for surgery as an agency would have temporary custody through relinquishment papers and would have assumed responsibility for any necessary papers giving consent for medical care. There would have been no problem regarding the hospital bill as an agency would have arranged for this. Of even greater importance is the fact that the baby's name would have been kept secret, offering protection to the natural mother and to the adoptive parents. In connection with screening prospective adoptive parents, we would have to question the strength of the motivation to adopt in view of this couple's taking a vacation trip, whereabouts unknown, when they realized placement could occur within a few days. In the writer's experience, this is not the usual behavior exhibited by prospective adoptive parents. Any ambivalence toward adoption should be carefully considered, and we do not know whether there had been any other evidence of the couple's doubts about adopting prior to this incident. Parenthood is a serious undertaking for anyone and in the case of adoptive parents there is added the fact of facing the inability to have their own children plus taking the child of another into their home. The isolated fact of going on the vacation trip would not necessarily preclude their being accepted as adoptive parents, but the behavior should have been evaluated. In addition, we have no assurance of follow-up supervision in which the family could be helped with the adoptive process, although judges do sometimes appoint a social worker to evaluate the home and supervise placement at the time the couple approaches the court for the adoption. However, both social workers and judges are more reluctant to reject a home when the child is already placed as they do not wish to disrupt family relationships unless home conditions are quite detrimental to the child's welfare.

At the present time, more children are placed independently by the mother or a third party than by agencies. It appears that placement of children should be done by agencies employing highly skilled social workers who could constantly examine and thus improve child-placing methods. The responsibility assumed in planning for a child's whole life is an awesome one and a process which should receive the best efforts of society.

SUMMARY

In this chapter, adoption has been defined as the legal method devised by society and assumed to be the best solution in providing for care of children who cannot live with their own parents. The child, his natural parents, and adoptive parents are integral parts of the adoptive process. Children may be assigned to adoptive agencies by parents or courts or they may be placed independently either by parents or by third persons. Acquiring the services of these social agencies would seem to offer the most desirable course of action because of the protective services which can be received by all parties involved. Some recent changes in policies of adoption agencies have been reviewed. These include placing the child at an earlier age than previously, shifting focus from a child's handicap to his social and educational capacities in determining whether he is adoptable, and placing less emphasis upon matching a child with adoptive parents. The nursing profession is seen as having a helping role to the child, natural parents, and to both adoptive and prospective adoptive parents.

BIBLIOGRAPHY

Benedek, T.: *Psychosexual Functions in Women: Studies in Psychosomatic Medicine,* New York: The Ronald Press Co., 1952.

Cominos, H.: "Minimizing the Risks of Adoption through Knowledge," *Social Work,* **16**:73–79, 1971.

Festinger, T.: "Unwed Mothers and Their Decisions to Keep or Surrender Children," *Child Welfare League of America, Inc,* **50**:253–262, 1971.

Franklin, D., and F. Massarik "The Adoption of Children with Medical Conditions," *Child Welfare League of America, Inc.,* **48**:595–601, 1969.

Jolowicz, R.: "The Hidden Parent," paper read at the New York State Conference on Social Welfare, November 1946. (Mimeographed)

Rohr, F.: "How Parents Tell Their Children They Are Adopted," *Child Welfare League of America, Inc.,* **50**:298–300, 1971.

Smith, I. E.: *Readings in Adoption,* New York: Philosophical Library, 1963.

Young, L.: *Out of Wedlock,* New York: McGraw-Hill Book Company, 1954.

Chapter 15

The Nurse and the Expanding Family: A Mother's Viewpoint

Nancy K. Maebius

The purpose of this chapter is to inform nurses of one mother's viewpoint of the importance of the nurse's consideration of the entire family unit at a time when the family constellation is being altered and enlarged. This expression of a mother's perception of the role of the nurse with the expanding family may allow the nurse to consider some new and effective methods of providing health care to the expanding family unit, based on the needs of individual family members. By recognizing the constantly changing needs and roles of each member of the expanding family, especially those of the mother, the nurse may be able to individualize health care and at the same time take care of the family as a unit.

The author has selected and commented on some wants and goals, beliefs, feelings, attitudes, and values of members of an expanding family, based on experience as a mother of three preschool age children. Considerations of family structure, motherhood, fatherhood, the role of the child, family interaction, and nursing intervention are presented from a mother's point of view.

The focus of this chapter is on the expanding family unit, on some of its dynamics and its efforts to cope with unaccustomed roles and responsibilities, and on the nurse who is working with the expanding family. Key functions of the nurse, seen from a mother's point of view, include observation, assessment, determination of family behavior patterns, deliberative interaction, anticipatory guidance, and health teaching. Aspects of the expanding family to be presented include the new mother, the crisis of parenthood, the new infant, maternal and infant health services, and family organization and integration.

THE EXPANDING FAMILY STRUCTURE

The birth of a child adds a new role to each member of the family. No two relationships within the family are identical. Each set of relationships is a unique relationship between two members. Biopsychosocial differences in children create uniquely individual relationship potentials. Sex, age, shared and unshared life experiences, and other factors are operative in making each mother-child and father-child relationship unique (Rubin, 1964).

What is observed at the time a new member is added to the family is not just an assimilation process into an established organization; in addition, there is diffusion and realignment of roles and relationships. Identification and reidentification of the nature and needs of the new member are prerequisites to be accomplished by each member in his own way, according to his own needs and wishes, and in his own role in a unique two-way relationship (Rubin, 1964). The family's equilibrium depends on the complementariness of the roles.

The birth of a baby is a crisis for the family; understanding the phenomena of family crisis requires an understanding of the role changes inherent in periods of transition from one life stage to another. Crisis situations change the role patterns of families, impede the functioning of the family, and may cause anxiety and insecurity. If the family members can perform their roles with some efficiency, strengthened by their unity as an integrated family with a successful experience with a previous crisis, they will be able to effectively adapt to the expanded family situation.

CHILDBIRTH

Childbirth is a process in the family's life that is governed by complex interactions (Chertok, 1969). The course of confinement during childbirth and the way in which it is experienced and felt have significant importance for the mother and the future mother-child relationship. The assessment of childbirth itself becomes critical, as childbirth represents a biopsychosocial event of particular significance for the family. The inception of early contacts between mother and child is a determining factor in their later lives.

The nurse needs to recognize the meaning of labor to each individual woman. Observation of the mother's behavior and recognition of its meaning guide the nurse's actions. An example of the nurse's lack of observational abilities and lack of recognition of meaning of labor to the mother may occur when the nurse sends a mother to the shower after a long and exhausting childbirth experience. She may be unaware of the mother's need to talk about the labor and delivery experience, or the mother's need for rest; and thus, she will not meet the mother's needs for expression of these feelings or for rest.

Toward the end of labor, nothing exists for the mother beyond herself. This self-reference necessarily limits perceptions. In the postpartum period, a reverse process occurs over a period of days. The mother needs help initially in grasping the idea that the baby has been born and that her labor and delivery have been successfully accomplished. Labor is a crisis situation; if it is not dealt with, the person will be less able to cope with and adjust to the demands of ongoing life. If the mother is given the opportunity to review her labor and delivery, to fill in the missing pieces, and to really understand what has happened, then she will be ready to move on and assume the role of motherhood (Rubin, 1961a).

At this time, immediately after childbirth, the mother needs to feel that she and her baby are the most important persons, and it is thus a very valuable experience for the mother to talk about and clarify her labor experience. She will do this more easily with someone who has shared that experience with her; this author felt very strongly this need to discuss her delivery with the obstetrician, and with the nurse who had been with her during labor and delivery, and with her husband. Supportive skills and communication skills are important qualities for the nurse who is working with the expanding family at this time. The mother, during the first 2 to 3 days postpartum, is apt to greatly treasure a gift brought to her as she is very concerned about and feels somewhat proud of herself and her role in the delivery of the child. A gift brought to her by her husband or a friend may give her added recognition.

In family-centered maternity care, the months of pregnancy, the actual labor and delivery, and the postpartum period are experiences to be shared by husband and wife. The birth of the baby and the subsequent hospital stay should be a culmination of, not a break in, an ongoing family relationship. The need to operate as a family unit from the day the infant arrives is paramount. The parents must be active participants in decisions that affect them and their new child.

The observation of early mothering behaviors, as well as the evaluation of the childbirth, can be accomplished by the nurse and discussed with the mother. The first look at the child, the first words, and the way in which the early mother-father-child relationships develop must be considered by the nurse as she works with the expanding family.

MOTHERHOOD

Maternal behavior is a learned behavior, evolving and changing, largely dependent on the nature and kinds of significant interpersonal experiences and on the individual mother's evolving self-concept. The mother's perception of herself as a mothering person in relation to her new child needs to be realized (Rubin, 1961a). The nurse has a wonderful opportunity to pick up cues that identify maternal attitudes and feelings and to observe the cyclic interaction between the mother and her infant (Clark, 1966a).

Mothering, the function of the mother role, involves skill and a certain understanding of the developmental process of the child. Motherliness is an emotional feeling that develops as the mother increases contact with her children. The maternal claiming process is evident in an initial or early mother-newborn contact. The need for reassurance that she is now, in fact, a mother is of paramount importance. Such initial events as an infant who sleeps through feedings when brought to the mother may create anxiety for the mother and, in turn, for the infant and possibly for a future mother-child relationship (Robischon and Scott, 1969).

Maternal Functioning

The mother's own concern for her ability to function in a mothering capacity is evident in the early postpartum period. Childbirth, the first time she feeds her child, the first time she changes her child, and the first time she dresses or bathes her child are extremely important events to her, as she begins to realize and evaluate her maternal functioning. If the first performance in a mothering act succeeds relatively well by the mother's own criteria, subsequent performance becomes increasingly less anxiety filled and more comfortable. If the first performance fails to be relatively satisfactory, she may approach subsequent experiences of the same mothering act with anxiety and increased tension (Rubin, 1961a).

As reported by Klaus (1970), mother-to-infant eye-to-eye contact appears to be an important exchange during the development of affectional ties. In observing the beginnings of a mother-child relationship, identification of the partner in the relationship is a universal prerequisite. A new mother who has not held her baby apparently does not feel that she has a baby. The holding of the baby is at first a passive interaction, a receiving of contact (Rubin, 1961a). Mothers usually begin feeling the babies with their fingers and later use their palms, moving from first feeling the child's extremities to later feeling his trunk (Rubin, 1963). Any frequent and intimate contact with the thriving infant, such as breast or bottle feeding, has a stimulating and integrating effect on motherliness (Benedek, 1970).

The role of the nurse includes acting as a sounding board, validator, supporter, and a reliable source of health information. The initial contact of the nurse during the early postpartum period can foster an openness which makes the mother more willing to talk; the mother usually welcomes the nurse as a helpful contributor in planning her care and the care of her infant.

Mothering Tasks

A crucial function of the nurse working with the expanding family is the observation and assessment of interaction patterns of the mother and infant. The nurse is able to observe childbirth, early mother-child relationships, and any difficulty experienced by mothers in carrying out mothering tasks.

The mother's tasks, as presented by Reva Rubin (1961b), are as follows: (1) identify the new child, (2) determine her relationship to him (this includes altering her patterns and style of living to accommodate this new relationship), and (3) guide and reconstruct her family constellation to include a new member. An important point for the nurse to recognize is that the tasks of this period of adjustment are not easier after the first child. The mother may be more self-confident in her abilities but she also has a more complex family situation to reintegrate.

As pointed out by Spaulding (1969), the nurse considers the following variables as she collects and orders data which will assist her in facilitation of the mother's achievement of the mothering tasks: ethnic background, length of hospital stay, type of delivery, condition of mother and baby, socioeconomic level, and the number of other children. Other variables include age, education, previous experience with babies, help at home, occupation, and the hospital where delivery occurred.

Three important developmental mothering tasks enumerated by Spaulding (1969) are: (1) assuming responsibility for care of the baby; (2) learning how to anticipate and to recognize needs of the baby; and (3) regulating demands of the infant, self, and environment. These were three of the author's most crucial needs as a mother following the births of each of three children.

A frequent need of new mothers assuming responsibility for care of the baby that is often overlooked by the nurse is instruction in feeding techniques designed to keep the baby awake until he has taken enough to sleep until the next feeding. Problems identified by mothers, such as getting the baby to complete a feeding at one sitting, certainly have implications for the nurse working with the expanding family.

The mother's tasks of recognition seem to depend on establishing communication with the infant and are apt to reflect the mother's attitude toward her baby, her empathy, and her own observation abilities (Spaulding, 1969). The nurse is a key figure in helping the mother accomplish these tasks.

The new mother is preoccupied with her own learning of mothering actions 2 to 3 days postpartum. The nurse can approach health problems by helping the mother to recognize her infant and his condition and focus on what to look for in his behavior. Suggesting an action which is not in keeping with the mother's experience is not helpful. It is interesting to note that in a study done by Spaulding (1969) a total of seventy-three mothers out of a total of ninety-nine reported deviations from health, such as skin rashes, frequent regurgitation, and stuffy noses in their babies at 10 days of age. This author also observed minor health deviations in each of her three children and felt the need for anticipatory guidance.

Some common conflicts of motherhood include idealized motherhood versus lack of confidence in ability to function as a mother, need for dependence versus independence and responsibility, feelings for baby versus feelings for other family members, and self-realization versus motherliness. Personal expectations and reality need to be coordinated. The role of the mother is individualized according to her own personality structure.

A mother needs reinforcement and support in her mothering efforts. She needs the opportunity to validate her observations and approaches. Her coping abilities can be observed as she attempts to master mothering tasks. Coping can be judged by what the mother had to cope with—kinds and numbers of problems—or in terms of how well the mother had handled situations to either prevent or minimize problems (Spaulding, 1969). It is helpful if the nurse places emphasis on how the mother handled the situation or coped with a problem and not on what happened to the baby. It is important to note that mothers who have taken care of children rely on previous experiences in caring for their baby rather than on instructions given by the nurse (Spaulding, 1969). In teaching or in providing anticipatory guidance to the mother as a family member, the nurse considers previous experiences as well as the structure of the family, in order to learn what the mother's needs for help are and how they can be met.

FATHERHOOD

As described by Josselyn (1956), fatherhood involves feelings of tenderness, the ability to empathize with others, the valuing of a love object more than self, and the finding of a living experience in the experiences of others. These qualities and feelings are quite different from a father's pride in his child as a symbol of his virility. The role of the father has definite implications for family life. The nurse may be able to observe and assist him in developing his own optimal level of fatherliness. A woman often is unable to express motherliness until her husband can adjust to fatherhood (Robischon and Scott, 1969). In viewing a family approach to maternity care, the father should have unlimited visiting privileges, be included in the health teaching and anticipatory guidance given, and have assistance in adjusting to his new role of father. Fathers also need to be made aware of the infant's development, such as changes in feeding techniques as new growth levels are reached and sudden normal changes in the newborn's breathing patterns.

THE CHILD

A whole chain of new relationships is started with the birth of a new child. The baby may become a brother or sister to other children. Each baby is unique. Each has his own ways. The pace of life around him affects each baby differently. From the outset the mother experiments with her baby to find how to apply what she knows in the way that suits him best.

The identification of the child by the mother as a separate and real being goes on as a parallel activity to that of assessing her ability to function as a mother. Association and differentiation occur as a part of this identification process. The sex of the child is identified by the mother as she associates her views of maleness and femaleness with expectations of the child. Before the infant is seen for his own characteristics, his features are fixed by association; he is said to look "like" someone else (Rubin, 1961a). Mothers need to know that the baby is whole and intact. It is difficult for mothers to touch the child before they have seen him, and to care for the child until they have touched him (Rubin, 1961a). During the first week, each of the infant's normal bodily functions is checked on by the mother.

Until the infant responds, meaningfully and personally, to father and to siblings, he may not be viewed as a valued family member. It takes about 3 months for the infant to contribute to the mother-child relationship, another 6 months for him to contribute to the father-child relationship, and still another year before he can acquire the appropriate responses for a sibling relationship (Rubin, 1964).

THE NEW FAMILY

The nurse needs to consider the forces of personality, family interaction, the social system, and nursing intervention as a unit. In caring for families, nurses observe and analyze role behaviors. Nurses are often called upon as respected and reliable sources of information for a particular situation in which a member of the family finds himself. Nurses can assist and share concerns and goals of the family with the individual family members. The nurse should encourage each family member to express his feelings and concerns, and she can plan with the family the discharge from the hospital. In doing this, she is continuously assessing family behavior patterns, coping mechanisms, and needs. By being alert to parents' comments, or lack of comments, the nurse recognizes needs, present or future, and plans to meet them.

The ability to listen carefully, to understand the needs of the family, to be a supporting person, to utilize communication skills selectively, and to ensure that follow-up care is available and that the family is aware of this after they leave the hospital are important functions of the nurse as she works with the expanding family.

Principles of family-centered care in the hospital and at home include not separating the mother from the framework of the family, recognizing that each person is an individual, knowing growth and development patterns, meeting learning needs of parents, and involving parents in the planning of health care (Hogan, 1968).

The nurse, utilizing the nursing process, can assist the expanding family and plan nursing intervention by determining (1) the critical times or incidents in the family life cycle in which positive health interventions will yield the most promising results and (2) the comparative outcomes in changes in family health behavior when the nurse works with the family group and when the nurse does not work with the family unit (Spaulding, 1969).

The family is the initial setting in which an adjustment to a crisis occurs or does not occur. The nurse must consider how the family and the infant adjust. Factors affecting adjustment are: ability to perform roles as family members, family adaptability, family integration, relationships among family members, and previous experiences with crises (Johnson, 1969).

When this author returned home, 5 days after the delivery of her third child, she found the need to reestablish bonds with her two other preschool children. Family members were redefining roles at this time. Some time was needed to reintegrate before taking in a new family member. In 2 weeks, this reintegration was accomplished; evidence of this was seen as the other children played with each other as the baby was fed and as they helped with certain aspects of infant care, such as the baby's bath and changing of diapers.

The first month, the neonatal period, is surely a new parent and new family time as well as a new baby time, with its own special stresses for the mother and father and for other family members. As the family is reintegrated, sharing patterns, responsibilities, budget, space at home, family routines, and communication systems are altered. New stresses of parenthood involve balancing the needs of the mother and the father with those of the infant. Social pressures occur as family, friends, and neighbors call and visit. A valuable social contact at this time was talking with other new parents, and this author relied trustingly on advice given by them. The other children in the family face new developmental tasks. As stated by Benedek (1970), motherliness is probably tested each day with each child during the phasic development of the newborn. Because of the special family stresses which occur during the first month, health care provided by the nurse should be based on an understanding of family developmental tasks.

At home, the mother is very concerned about taking care of her infant adequately. With this author's third child, she felt she did not need advice as much as she needed help in evaluating her performance as a mother; she would have appreciated help from a nurse in identifying what she was doing and the reasons for her performance. Assistance from a nurse in developing a deliberative and problem-solving dimension to her coping mechanisms would have been very helpful at this time. The mother needs to acquire and refine maternal skills; to develop increasing self-confidence; and to know about such things as expected behavior of infants, the sounds babies make, and their breathing patterns. With the first baby, she spent a great deal of time checking him frequently to see if he was all right. Even when he was asleep, she observed him over and over because she was afraid he might not cry or somehow indicate his possible distress. Other concerns centered on feeding techniques and feeding schedules. Rubin (1967a) points out that the infant's sphere of action and interaction is enlarged around the experience of being fed. Maternal giving can be accomplished in a variety of creative ways; the way the mother responds to the infant in carrying out mothering tasks will influence the baby's social responses and learning.

As has been pointed out, the interpersonal relationships within a family are changing as the new member is added. Parents need to recognize and accept the fact that older children may be jealous, and then respond to the demands of other children for extra attention needed initially. Children may experience feelings of loss, and they need to reestablish trust in their mother at the same time she is paying so much attention to a new baby. It was very helpful to this author to take several walks a day with all three children; this was one activity they all enjoyed equally. It was also important to spend a few minutes at least with each child individually, hoping to preserve the personal autonomy of each family member. Those persons who brought presents for the older children at the same time they brought presents for the baby helped meet the needs of the other children for added attention during the first few days at home. A key thought presented by Rubin (1964) with respect to relationships within the expanding family is that the parents' capacity for a variety of individualized relationships with their children may well be a strong basis for the development of family creativity.

NURSING INTERVENTION

The primary role of the nurse with the expanding family is to understand the mother's perception of the childbearing experience and to facilitate the family's effort to respond to and cope with family expansion (Wiedenbach, 1965). Nurses may also be called upon to initiate action planned to promote normal movement through the childbearing process and to foster normal growth and development of the baby (Wiedenbach, 1965).

In planning nursing intervention, nurses need to establish meaningful communication patterns between labor-room nurses and nurses who care for the mother and infant. Family-centered nursing implies decreased separation of the mother from the family and decreased compartmentalization within the hospital. New babies and mothers need each other; rooming-in arrangements may encourage early mother-infant interaction. First-time mothers often want their babies close by to learn the principles of infant care with help from the nurses. Multiparous mothers may want to get to know this baby and plan how best to reintegrate the family when they return home. The nurse needs to be able to individualize the care of the infant and the mother and to help the baby establish his own unique feeding schedule and his other unique patterns of living. The nurse needs to spend time assisting the new family to become acquainted with and become confident about the care of the new baby. Nursing intervention focused on helping the mother express her feelings, acknowledging and encouraging maternal feelings, and seeing that the relationships between the mother's behavior and that of her baby expand, may lead to the mother's feeling a sense of security in her new role. Nurses may play an important role in the development of a healthy mother-child and, later, a family-child relationship (Warrich, 1969). The nurse is able to assess and observe interaction patterns of the mother, father, and infant, and to set criteria for referrals based on these interaction patterns as well as on the more traditional criterion of the physical condition.

The nurse, by listening to the mother, is able to develop a supporting, sustaining relationship with the family. The nurse can establish needs and needs for help by listening to the mother exclaim such feelings as how hungry she is, especially during the first 2 days postpartum, and how flat her abdomen is. Only by listening and observing can the nurse know needs of the mother and the family. Not only must she know how to listen, but she must plan time to listen (Hogan, 1968).

The taking-in of the maternal role is a quiet, self-active, continuous process based on the motivation of the mother to really *become* a mother (Rubin, 1967a, p. 240).

Two to three days postpartum, the mother is very anxious to talk, is concerned about the baby's feedings, and is concerned about her own sleep and food needs. She initiates little herself during this taking-in phase (Rubin, 1961b). Nursing intervention consists of allowing the mother to express her feelings about her childbearing experiences, about changes in her bodily functions, and about the new mother-infant relationship.

Rubin (1961*b*) then describes the third day, at which time the mother is ready to meet the present. Maternal concern is developing. After the mother has coped with the functions of her own body, she is ready to face the mothering tasks. As she copes successfully with the mothering tasks, her perception increases, and she then becomes concerned about her home and family. This latter phase lasts 10 days (Rubin, 1961*b*).

The nurse, having evaluated the progress of the childbirth experiences, observes the infant's growth and development. Observing the early mother-infant interaction and "maternal touch" (Rubin, 1963*b*), the nurse can judge whether the mother is satisfied that the baby is whole and intact, or whether the mother is anxious to examine the baby from head to foot. The parents' first total inspection of the infant can be a learning experience and may relieve anxiety. It is meaningful to involve the parents in this assessment, after the nurse has completed an initial assessment of the newborn. The nurse can allow the parent to look, and she can serve as a reliable source of information when questions are raised by them.

Anticipatory guidance related to the mother-child relationship may prepare the mother for future developments in her relationship with her child. It would be helpful for the mother to know that changes in her behavior from 3 weeks to 3 months following childbirth are largely related to the maturation of various characteristics of the infant. Because the increased confidence of the mother, her greater familiarity with the infant, and her developing attachment to the child at 3 months as compared to 3 weeks also account for changes that occur in the infant during this time period (Moss, 1970), the nurse should begin assisting in the development of these abilities as soon as the mother is concerned about them and desires help.

As the infant increases his time spent in smiling, vocalizing, and looking at the mother's face, he becomes an interesting and responsive person. The mother's social reactions to him during this time parallel the infant's increasing social responses (Moss, 1970). Anticipatory guidance, utilizing information from studies such as the one by Moss (1970), along with knowledge about developmental growth of the infant and of the family should be shared by the nurse with family members at the time the mother becomes concerned about the family unit and her return home.

Nursing intervention involves assisting family members to assist themselves, and helping each individual family member develop to the fullest extent of his own unique capabilities.

CONCLUSION

The nurse can play a primary role in providing new parents with personal interest, an empathic nursing approach, emotional support, anticipatory guidance, communication about family behavior patterns, and health teaching needed to cope with the adaptation problems which occur as the family expands. Nursing services continued in the home during the postpartum period would be a valuable service (Clark, 1966b; Peckham 1969). There is a great need for the mother to focus attention on the family as a unit as well as on individual family members. The importance of nursing care for the expanding family is significant. If anxiety felt by parents is transmitted to the infant and other family members, the crisis of the childbearing experience may be left unresolved, and the family may be unable to move on to other developmental tasks. A process of negative feedback may be established leading to feelings of frustration (Clark, 1966b). The way in which the family masters assimilation, diffusion, and realignment when the family is enlarged will affect the way the family copes with future crises.

BIBLIOGRAPHY

Anthony, E. J., and T. Benedek (eds.): *Parenthood: Its Psychology and Psychopathology,* Boston: Little, Brown and Company, 1970.

Benedek, T.: "Motherhood and Nurturing," in E. J. Anthony and T. Benedek, *Parenthood, Its Psychology and Psychopathology,* Boston: Little, Brown, and Company, 1970.

Chertok, L.: *Motherhood and Personality,* Philadelphia: J. B. Lippincott Company, 1969.

Clark, A. L.: "The Adaptation Problems and Patterns of an Expanding Family: The Neonatal Period," *Nursing Forum,* **5**:92-104, 1966b.

————: "The Beginning Family," *American Journal of Nursing,* **66**:802, 1966a.

Duval, E. M.: *Family Development,* 3d ed., Philadelphia: J. B. Lippincott Company, 1971.

Hennel, M.: "Family Centered Maternity Nursing in Practice," *Nursing Clinics of North America,* **3**:289-298, 1968.

Hilliard, M. E.: "The Evaluation of a Maternity Nurse," *Nursing Forum,* **4**(2):6-29, 1965.

————: "New Horizons in Maternity Nursing," *Nursing Outlook,* **15**:33-36, 1967.

Hogan, A. L.: "The Role of the Nurse in Meeting the Needs of the New Mother," *Nursing Clinics of North America,* **3**:337-344, 1968.

Johnson, E.: "Utilization of Behavior Science Concepts for a Family in Crisis," in *American Nurses' Association Clinical Conferences,* New York: Appleton-Century-Crofts, 1969, pp. 164-169.

Josselyn, I. M.: "Cultural Forces: Motherliness and Fatherliness," *American Journal of Orthopsychiatry,* **26**:264-271, 1956.

Klaus, M. H., et al.: "Human Maternal Behavior at the First Contact with Her Young," *Pediatrics,* **46**:187-192, 1970.

Moss, H. A.: "Sex, Age and State as Determinants of Mother-Infant Interaction," in T. D. Spencer and N. Kass (eds.), *Perspectives in Child Psychology,* New York: McGraw-Hill Book Company, 1970, pp. 51-61.

Peckham, B. M.: "Optimal Maternal Care," *Obstetrics and Gynecology,* **33**(6):862–868, 1969.

Robischon, P., and D. Scott: "Role Theory and Its Application in Family Nursing," *Nursing Outlook,* **17**:52–57, 1969.

Rubin, R.: "Attainment of the Maternal Role: Part I," *Nursing Research,* **16**(3):237–245, 1967*b.*

———: "Attainment of the Maternal Role: Part II," *Nursing Research,* **16**(4):342–346, 1967*c.*

———: "Basic Maternal Behavior," *Nursing Outlook,* **9**:683–686, 1961*a.*

———: "The Family-Child Relationship and Nursing Care," *Nursing Outlook,* **12**:36–39, 1964.

———: "Food and Feeding," *Nursing Forum,* **6**:195–205, 1967*a.*

———: "Maternity Care in Our Society," *Nursing Outlook,* **11**:519–522, 1963.

———: "Puerperal Change," *Nursing Outlook,* **9**:753–755, 1961*b.*

Seacat, M., and L. Schlacter: "Expanded Nursing Role in Prenatal and Infant Care," *American Journal of Nursing,* **68**:822–824, 1968.

Spaulding, M. R.: "The Effectiveness of Tape Recordings with Primiparas of the Lower Socioeconomic Group in Coping with Mothering Tasks," in M. V. Batey (ed.), *Communicating Nursing Research,* Boulder, Colo.: Western Interstate Commission for Higher Education, 1969, pp. 107–118.

Spencer, T. D., and N. Kass (eds.): *Perspectives in Child Psychology,* New York, McGraw-Hill Book Company, 1970.

Warrich, L. H.: "Femininity, Sexuality, and Mothering," *Nursing Forum,* **8**(2):212–224, 1969.

Wiedenbach, E.: "Family Nurse Practitioner for Maternal and Child Care," *Nursing Outlook,* **13**:50–52, 1965.

Chapter 16

Anticipatory Guidance
of Families with Infants

Susan Nelson McCabe

Expectant parents are primarily interested in fulfilling their immediate needs: pregnancy, labor, and delivery. It is difficult to stimulate interest in infant care when the prospective parents have these concerns, but it is even more difficult to make the information available after the infant's arrival. Infant care information either has been ignored on the grounds that only that which is of primary concern will be heard and retained or has been introduced as feeding, holding, and bathing demonstrations, in the hope that this information will be remembered when needed.

Various techniques have been used to stimulate interest in child care. New parents can come to a class and bring their baby. This sometimes works very well if the parents are relaxed enough to tolerate a crying baby should he become fussy during the class. In addition, they must feel comfortable about the way they are doing things but be receptive to alternative suggestions discussed by the group. Movies showing characteristics of normal infants and some aspects of infant care are used to stimulate the expectant parents' interest.

In experiences with mothers of young children, this author has become convinced that they are not well prepared to care for their infant. Because they lack information, they frequently make comments such as, "The first 3 months were absolute hell, but now we really enjoy him," or, "If only you could throw the first one away and start over after you know something." Nursing has a responsibility to do something about this.

SLIDE PRESENTATION AND DISCUSSION

To provide anticipatory guidance for expectant parents, about 70 slides of my own child during her first year were shown. Some of the slides were taken with this teaching purpose in mind, but most were not. Many aspects of the infant's early development are not included; however, the slides serve as a take-off point for discussing family feelings about a new addition, concern about being a good parent, and specific information that parents of infants need to know.

Approximately five groups of expectant parents saw these slides. They were primarily middle-class, college students, and professional people. Both husbands and wives were invited, and the slides were shown at one class of a series of prenatal classes. The same teaching technique could be used with any cultural group, provided it was adapted to their particular needs.

Each group was encouraged to ask questions, make comments, or volunteer information both during and after the slide presentation. The focus differed somewhat depending upon the group; however, there were five general areas covered. These were: changing family life style, learning to pick up cues from the baby, providing sensory stimulation, providing physical care, and being a good consumer of child care literature. Obviously these areas cannot be separated from one another; and, when discussing one slide, points were covered that include three or four different areas. As the slides were shown, personal handling of situations and the ways in which they were handled in other homes were discussed. An attempt was made to provide balance to the discussion. For instance, if the conversation seemed to sound as if this baby were going to be nothing but fun, I might tell the story of the time I called a friend with two children in diapers to wish her a happy birthday; and when I asked how it felt to be thirty, she replied, "I haven't had my head out of the toilet long enough to know." What various authorities have written on certain issues was described, and it was pointed out that sometimes authorities agreed with each other while at other times they differed. For example, Dr. Spock says, "I don't think you need to worry much about spoiling in the first month or even the first two months" (1968, p. 191). He indicates that if the mother continues to give in to the infant's cries by picking him up after this time "he becomes increasingly disagreeable and tyrannical in demanding this service" (1968, p. 192). Dr. Dodson, however, says, "Cuddle your infant as much as you want, you won't spoil him. Feed him as often as you want, you won't spoil him. Sing and coo to him as much as you want, you won't spoil him. Pay attention to him as often as he cries, you won't spoil him" (1970, p. 70).

The following is a composite description of how the slides and group discussion were used to provide anticipatory guidance for parents expecting, in most cases, their first infant.

CHANGES IN FAMILY LIFE

As an illustration of changes in daily routines, a picture is included of myself with the new baby over my knee and my dinner plate beside me on the couch. My hair is uncombed, and I am wearing no makeup. The discussion (after everyone stops laughing) centers on alternative ways mealtime can be handled. For example, some families would prefer to put off meals or attempt to plan them for a time when the baby is sleeping or quiet. This, of course, sounds easier than it may turn out to be. Other families may be able to let the infant cry for awhile, in another room, while they finish dinner and can then feed the infant in a more relaxed fashion. Another frequently used solution may be to place the infant nearby in a seat where he is able to see and hear what is going on at mealtime. The family's usual meal patterns, the behavior of the individual infant, and the circumstances at a particular time may all influence the choice the family makes. Comments from the group about this particular slide have ranged from, "That's the way we always eat anyway," to, "I just couldn't stand that."

Grandparents

A picture of my child feeding birds with her grandfather frequently stimulates a discussion of grandparents (Figure 16-1). Usually some mothers express concern that grandmother will take over, or will impose some old-fashioned ideas. These same mothers, or others, may also recognize a real need for help from grandmothers. Various family situations may be discussed. How much help is available to the mother? Can the father take a vacation? Has the mother had experience caring for infants? How does the grandmother feel about helping, and what kinds of things does she expect to do? Can the couple comfortably discuss with the grandmother when they would like her to come and what they would like her to do? There is also some discussion about the idea that our parents did raise us and we turned out pretty well, so even if some methods are different than ours, we may be able to tolerate them as it is quite unlikely they will be really harmful to the baby. Some people are able

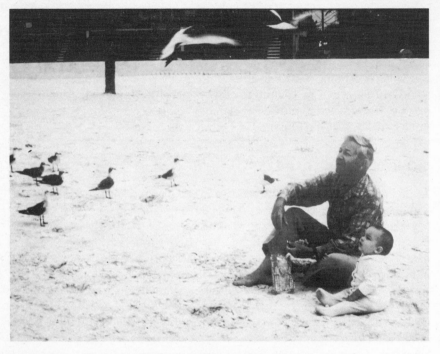

Figure 16-1 A baby and her grandfather feeding birds.

to say, "You can do it that way, but I prefer this way," or, "You can operate that way when you have him at your house, but here we're going to do it this way." Although there may be this type of discussion, this slide is used because it illustrates the special quality of relationships between infants (and children) and older people. A child cannot help but respond to the pleasure the grandparents feel in being with their grandchildren.

Dependence and Independence

The slides illustrate the total dependence of the infant at first and how much independence he gains in 1 year. There is discussion of the difficulty some parents have adjusting to someone so totally dependent on them, while it may be difficult for other parents to allow the infant the opportunity to gradually become more independent. Slides of the infant attempting to feed herself, pulling herself up, and getting into drawers stimulate discussion of what you can let them do when. Since there is no slide of the child in a playpen, if the question is not asked, the alternatives are pointed out. In some homes the parents have decided to use the old furniture until the children are older, and it is easy to put all dangerous items out of reach, or close off potentially dangerous areas. This family may have little use for a playpen. Other mothers could not possibly get the necessary tasks in the home done if they did not make use of a playpen. Some children do better in a playpen when they are able to see their mother as much of the time as possible, while others seem more content alone in a room with, of course, toys in the playpen and possibly some music.

Other topics discussed in the area of changes in family life include going out with the baby, traveling, babysitters, and the working mother. Again specific alternatives are suggested by the author and members of the group, but these suggestions are considered in light of the particular interests of the family, the amount of child care each parent is willing or able to be responsible for, and the economic situation of the family. The need to communicate what needs to be done and how both parents feel about the various tasks is discussed.

LEARNING TO PICK UP CUES FROM BABY

Individual Differences

It is usually mentioned that it is difficult to distinguish a hungry cry from other cries by the sound alone. Often it's easy to make a correct guess if it is about time for the baby to be hungry. Although most of the slides shown are of the same baby, the ways other babies react is also pointed out. If it is about time to eat, the mother assumes the infant is hungry, but she still needs to watch for cues. Does he relax and seem content the minute he is held and not too enthusiastic when offered food or does he remain tense and squirmy even when receiving food? Mothers need to learn with each baby the kind of cues he will give. Sometimes it is frustrating not to know what he means, but getting to know one's baby can be fun and, of course, it does not happen overnight. The book *Infants and Mothers: Differences in Development* (Brazelton, 1969) illustrates well the different ways three normal infants eat. Some of these examples may be used with the groups.

Similarities

While recognizing individual differences, the slides also may be used to point out commonalities. For instance, many infants show a fear of strangers at about 6 months. If grandparents are planning a visit, they can be reminded ahead of time that this may happen; and, even though it will still be upsetting, the family will know (at least intellectually) that the infant does not dislike his grandparents.

Most mothers of infants had books or had read books telling the usual sequence of infant development. This appeared to be of little interest to the group of expectant parents, but it is essential to give some anticipatory guidance in relation to these developmental milestones. Frankenburg and Dodds' explanation of the differences in developmental scales is helpful. They say, "These differences may be due in part to the use of different population groups. Another possible reason is that some of the investigators may have placed an item at an age when 50 percent of children could accomplish the task, while others may have placed it at an age when a larger or smaller percentage of children could perform the same item. The discrepancies may also be the result of differences either in the manner of administration or in criteria used for passing or failing an item" (1967, p. 182). It also needs to be pointed out that frequently perfectly normal, healthy children fall behind on one or two items in these scales, sometimes for no identifiable reason and at other times because the parents and/or children were simply not interested in this type of activity.

STIMULATION

Many of the slides show simple ways to vary stimulation for the infant. They show how simple it can be, and how early it can be done, as illustrated by the

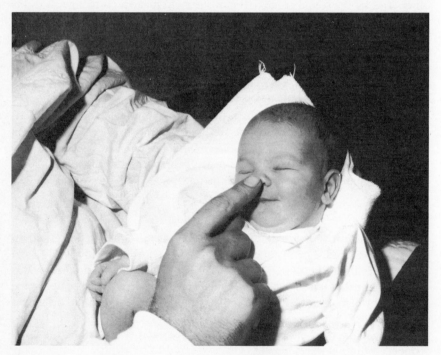

Figure 16-2 A new father touching his infant daughter's nose.

picture of the infant's nose being touched while her father talks about her "tiny little nose" even before she leaves the hospital (Figure 16-2). A number of the slides depict the activities or games suggested in *Baby Learning Through Baby Play* (Gordon, 1970). Recognition is made here that this kind of activity may come easily or more naturally to some parents while others have to work at it, particularly until the time the baby begins to respond.

Toys

There are usually questions about toys. What are the best toys? Is such and such a good kind of a toy to have? Again individual differences in terms of both the families and the particular child are discussed. There is some discussion of the merits of not providing toys for the child, because then he must

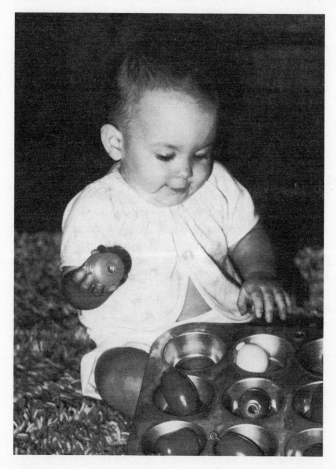

Figure 16-3 A baby playing with a muffin tin and pop-it beads.

learn to use his own inventiveness, versus the need to expose the child to the technology of today. There is also discussion about the proper age to give a child certain toys. One slide depicts an eight-month-old looking at a cloth book. This is used to show that, although she is interested in the bright colors and the action of turning the pages, she is not interested in a story. A book with paper pages is not appropriate unless it is all right for the child to rip out the pages; this would be a very good activity with an old magazine. This same illustration can be used with other toys. If the child is using the toy inappropriately but seems to enjoy it, that's what counts. Of course, if he is destroying an expensive toy or becoming frustrated because he cannot work something, then it would seem logical to put it away for a while. Also included are slides of a number of items commonly used around the house: bowls that stack and are different colors, tin cans which can be stacked inside each other and have been checked for sharp edges, and muffin tins with pop-it beads in the cups (Figure 16-3). There are illustrations of toys that may be used briefly and then thrown out, such as the boxes prepared foods come in. These are usually brightly colored and have pictures on the outside that the mother can talk about.

Safety

Some safety aspects of toys are pointed out, such as, the need for the parent to check the toy first and give various small parts a good hard tug rather than a gentle pull to see if they could come off in the infant's mouth. One slide shows the child playing with an old nylon stocking which fascinated her, probably because of the different texture, the noise you could make by rubbing two pieces together, and its elasticity. This is a good toy to use with supervision, but since it could become tangled and wrapped around her neck, she could not be alone while she was playing with this toy. Then some of the problems of providing a safe environment are discussed. The problem is often that parents do not want to restrict the infant so much that he does not have ample opportunity to explore his environment, but they do not want to take any risks with his health and safety. There are discussions of the importance of exploration together with the need to protect the child's safety by closely supervising his investigations. A slide is shown of an infant reaching out to touch a mushroom, but her mother's hand is right there, knowing that the infant's way of exploring is to get the object into her mouth. The slide of the infant investigating the toilet (Figure 16-4) usually stimulates a discussion that shows some families can tolerate types of exploration that others cannot.

Overstimulation

The last slide shows the child at Christmas with all sorts of toys, bows, and paper around her. Grandparents and parents are all focusing their attention

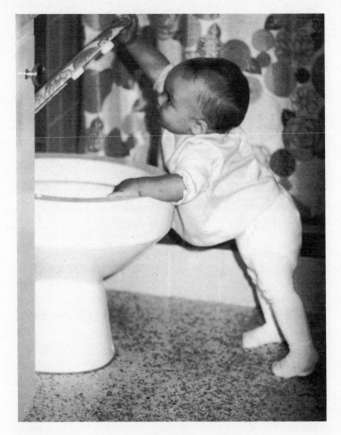

Figure 16-4 A baby investigating the toilet bowl.

on her. The situation is obviously one of overstimulation. While pointing out that this does happen occasionally without dire results, this slide also shows the possibility of too much stimulation. Since much time is spent discussing stimulation, it seems wise to also remember that both parents and children need quiet times when they are alone. Children need to learn to entertain themselves.

PHYSICAL CARE

Timing

There are some people who like to wake up and know fairly well what they will do for the day. Obviously, for these people to be able to put much of the physical care into some type of routine will make life more pleasant for both themselves and the baby. They will be happier when they can predict to some degree when the baby will eat, sleep, and be bathed. They may find they need to take some clues from the baby and devise a schedule that is relatively comfortable for everyone, recognizing that sometimes there will be interruptions. People who like to wake up and just let the day develop will probably have less of a schedule but may find that a little planning will make things easier. For example, if a mother discovers her baby is often fussy late in the afternoon, she will probably begin to plan her day so she can do the grocery shopping earlier if she takes the baby with her.

Bathing

There are numerous books such as *Baby and Child Care* (Spock, 1968) and *Infant Care* (Children's Bureau, 1963) which give the mother a detailed account of most aspects of the physical care. These are mentioned as good and helpful *guides,* but each person again will want to do things in the manner which suits them best. There do, however, seem to be some basics that apply generally. The bath slide shows the infant's head and neck being supported by an arm and the same hand holding her arm, leaving the other hand free to rinse the baby. It is mentioned that gathering equipment for the bath before starting makes a lot of sense. If they have the water, a basin, and a towel, they have the bare essentials, and the other things suggested may or may not be helpful; as long as they can get the baby in, rinse him off, let him feel and enjoy the water, and wrap him up before he gets cold, they have accomplished the major purposes of a bath. Then for next time they can consider what else they would like to gather for bathtime. There is further discussion of various types of soap, ways to prevent cradle cap, temperature of the water and the room, etc. The author usually mentions that her baby sometimes went 2 or 3 days without a bath and survived quite happily; but some mothers find a certain routine, especially a bath, comforting and calming to the baby, so they rarely miss the daily bath.

Feeding

There is some discussion of the many different feeding regimes. It usually becomes obvious that most of them work quite well for most infants. Basically, we probably do not need to get as concerned over what our infants eat as we seem to. We probably do this because our society values and praises large chubby babies, and, of course, one of the things we like to do for the people we love is feed them well. Some babies, consequently, end up being fatter than need be and sometimes uncomfortable because of the extra fat. It is important to know there is a wide range of normal weights. Parents are encouraged to ask the pediatrician to explain about the child's growth, such as whether he is following a normal growth pattern or curve. One slide shows the infant in her high chair holding a spoon. There is cereal all over her. This slide shows the growing independence of the infant and that her desire to attempt to feed herself was somewhat frustrating as things were so much neater and faster when fed. The knowledge that at some point she would have to make a mess in order to learn, and her pleasure at being able to do this, plus a large plastic apron-type bib made the experience more tolerable. Some groups asked specific questions about beginning solids, breast and bottle feeding, etc., but others did not.

Sleeping and Crying

There are times when one wants to sleep and the baby does not want to. No matter how much one reads about colic and babies crying for 3 to 4 hours straight and that there is very little that can be done about it and it will go away in about 3 months, after about the first 15 minutes of crying one begins to wonder what is wrong with the baby and what is wrong with oneself that you cannot handle it. Even if one decides it is nothing serious and there is nothing to do to help, it is almost impossible to ignore the child's cries. Probably the main reason is because a parent cannot really convince himself that everything is all right. A possible aid to getting through this is for parents to take turns just getting out of the house for an hour or two. It is probably not as hard as it may seem to find a babysitter who could tolerate the crying so you could go out together for a time. It seems to be more possible to cope with an unpleasant situation if you can get away for just a short time, but you really have to put some effort into dragging yourself away.

Some groups have questions about bedtimes and nap times and how many naps a day at what age. Again these questions need to be looked at by the group in relation to the family's habits. What time does the husband get home? Does he want time with his child then? Some men are too tired to enjoy a prolonged period with their child while others find it a pleasant change. Again the parents need to watch for cues indicating the child is tired, such as fussiness, blinking or rubbing eyes, less interest in family activities, or a sort of frantic hyperactivity. Individual differences in children need to be considered too; some need more sleep than others.

Clothing and Equipment

Clothing and equipment also need to be discussed in light of the family economics, the amount of space available, and how the family functions. The number of children they plan to have may determine the amount they are willing to spend. For instance, if they plan to have one or two children, they may get a less expensive playpen and stroller or carriage (if they decide they need these things) that they know will be less durable, but will probably last through two children. It is also suggested that as exciting as it is to buy these things while you are waiting for the baby there may be better ways to direct enthusiasm, because sometimes when the baby actually arrives one discovers that what he thought everyone needed just does not seem necessary. If purchases are made ahead of time, consider what they will be used for in your home instead of just assuming that it is necessary because friends have one. Some children use a high chair for only a period of months while others still use one, pushed up to the table, without the tray, when they are five years old.

The same principles apply to clothing. Many mothers find that during the first year to year and a half they need more tops than bottoms because the infant is drooling and messy when eating; but, when they begin toilet training, they need more pants than tops. Again, the individual situation must be considered; my child only ate at mealtime when she had a bib on and she did a minimum amount of drooling, therefore extra tops were not needed. Pants that can be worn with a variety of tops were helpful when toilet training, but extras were unnecessary because I had laundry facilities available in the home and could wash daily if necessary. If friends recommend certain brands, mothers are encouraged to ask why they are better than some other brands. This helps them to see if this brand will meet their expectations.

Calling the Doctor

Expectant parents indicate some concern about when to call the doctor, and mothers who already have infants indicate this is a real problem. They do not want to bother the doctor unnecessarily or appear stupid, but they also want to get the necessary care as soon as possible, and they are genuinely concerned about their child's welfare. A hurried pediatrician who intends to relieve a mother's concern may tell her it is nothing to worry about and leave her feeling that she has been stupid to call him.

It is suggested that parents discuss with the pediatrician what types of things he would like to be called about. They also need to go prepared with specific questions such as, during the first year, "If he runs a temperature of 101°, should I call you after office hours?" "If he vomits most of two consecutive feedings, should I call you after office hours?" These kinds of questions cannot, of course, cover every possible situation, but they show the doctor the kind of concerns the mother has and give him an opportunity to explain with examples how and when he believes the parent should communicate with him. In other words, this is a tool the parents can use to facilitate communication.

CONSUMERS OF CHILD CARE LITERATURE

Usually someone mentions an article they have read about some aspect of child care. Frequently it is controversial. Someone often asks who wrote the article. The discussion then revolves around who is really qualified to write on this topic. Just because the author is a nurse, doctor, or child psychologist does not necessarily mean the author is qualified to write about a specific topic, for example, pacifiers. If he makes definite statements either pro or con, his reasons for stating this need to be clear. As group members tell why they agree or disagree with the author, their comments can be used to show how the author's beliefs could apply in one family setting, but not in another. If for example, the author says that most young infants should have a pacifier in order to have sucking needs met, and some parents just cannot stand pacifiers, they need to look carefully at what evidence this author had to support his statement. They also need to look at what some other people have written about the sucking needs of young infants and how they can be met. After they have done more reading and/or talking to other people, they would then be able to decide if pacifiers are so important that they should attempt to overcome their negative feelings or if there are other ways of meeting sucking needs which would be more acceptable to the parents and therefore most desirable to their family.

The class is told about the infant care group they may join which has a well-stocked library on various aspects of childrearing. In other cities, child study groups have the same service. Some public libraries seem to have a better selection of these books than others, but many books are now available in paperback; and, if a few mothers would get together and buy different books, they could borrow from each other, thus not being limited to one person's opinion on a subject.

CONCLUSIONS

This description of a slide presentation with group discussion has been presented as a beginning attempt to provide anticipatory guidance to parents of infants. Obviously, it would be impossible to include here all the discussion included in the classes. Only selected examples have been used. No real attempt was made to evaluate this method of teaching. I became aware that people began making a special effort to tell me they had been in one of the classes and it had been very helpful. They rarely mentioned specific things that were helpful, but said the whole thing had made it easier when the baby arrived. One father stopped me before his baby arrived and said he just wanted to tell me that the night of the class he had realized for the first time that they would really be having a baby in their home. Obviously, it is much more likely that people with positive feelings would seek me out personally than those with negative feelings. Classes like this need to be evaluated by the participants (probably 3 months or so after delivery), anonymously and with some indication of those things which were helpful and those which were not. Some questions also need to be designed to determine how much of the information received during pregnancy was retained and used appropriately.

There is value in using slides in this manner. Certainly you can tailor the talk to the individual group, spending a longer time on some slides. It seems likely that the semidarkened room with people's attention focused on the screen may make it easier for some people to ask questions. One disadvantage to this more flexible approach is that it is much easier to forget content you believe is important.

Slides such as this could be used by any well-prepared nurse. If she does not have children or slides of her own children, she could plan those things which she would most like to illustrate and use the child or children of friends or patients. It is not easy to get the slides even with your own child and becomes more difficult as you plan times with other people. If you end up ready to take pictures and the baby starts crying, you may not get the planned pictures; but you may get some excellent pictures of a crying baby and frustrated parents!

This is not to suggest that this is the best way to educate expectant parents. It is one way, and some of the ideas could be used with other approaches. This is reaching a very small percentage of the population that needs help with child care. Adapting this and other methods for television and other larger audiences needs to be considered by nurses. Then more time can be spent on a one-to-one basis with those parents having special needs.

BIBLIOGRAPHY

Brazelton, T. B.: *Infants and Mothers: Differences in Development,* New York: Delacorte Press, 1969.

Children's Bureau: *Infant Care,* Washington, D.C.: U.S. Department of Health, Education, and Welfare, 1963.

Dodson, F.: *How to Parent,* New York: The New American Library of World Literature, Inc., 1970.

Frankenburg, W., and J. Dodds: "The Denver Developmental Screening Test," *Journal of Pediatrics,* 71:181-191, 1967.

Gordon, I.: *Baby Learning through Baby Play,* New York: St. Martin's Press, 1970.

Spock, B.: *Baby and Child Care,* New York: Pocket Books, Inc., 1968.

Chapter 17

The Family with a
Young Child

Debra P. Hymovich*

Have you ever had a telephone conversation with the mother of a toddler or
preschooler? Is it usually interspersed with interruptions—answers to the
youngster's questions, commands or cries, or checks on the sudden quietness
in the house? Mothers of these youngsters use such adjectives as "busy,"
"frustrating," "delightful," "trying," "demanding," "tiring," "fun," and "in-
credible" to describe their days.

It is little wonder that such a variety of terms are used to describe life
with young children. Gone are the days when a telephone conversation meant
a few minutes to sit down and chat. Gone are the days of a quick trip to the
store to pick up a needed item. Gone are the days of the leisurely bath or the
quiet cocktail before dinner. To some extent, the father is less apt to be
interrupted by the toddler who still clings more to his mother. But he certainly
finds changes in the routines the family had settled into before the toddler

* This paper was written while the author was a doctoral student at the University of Maryland, Institute
for Child Study, supported in part by fellowship number 1 F04 NU27445-01 from the National Institutes of
Health, United States Public Health Service.

days arrived. Of course, there was some hint of what was to come when the baby was awake and crying just when dinner was on the table or when he developed a fever just as the parents were preparing for one of their few evenings on the town. And what about the parents with an older child whose games are constantly interrupted by the toddler? And who, by the way, often instigates the trouble the toddler gets into? Or the parents with an infant of whom the young child is jealous?

Here are the days of a child's first step, first sentence, and soon the first of many questions. Here are the days of teaching skills such as self-feeding, toileting, dressing, and communicating. Here are the days of pleasant and not-so-pleasant excursions, of increasing autonomy, and of shifts between dependence and independence and between tantrums and charming behavior.

DEVELOPMENTAL TASKS

Why are the terms used by parents to describe life with their youngsters so varied? Perhaps a partial answer may be found in the differing developmental tasks facing parent, child, and family unit. There are tasks for each member of the family as well as some which are shared by the parents and the entire family unit. There are specific tasks of the toddler and preschooler; of the mother in her roles as wife, mother, and woman; and of the father in his roles as husband, father, and man.

Developmental tasks arise at certain critical times in an individual's life, "successful achievement of which leads to his happiness and to success with later tasks, while failure leads to unhappiness in the individual, disapproval by the society, and difficulty with later tasks" (Havighurst, 1952, p. 2). These tasks may be biological, psychological, and/or cultural in nature. In addition to their individual tasks, the family as a social unit also has developmental tasks which it must master. Duvall defines a family developmental task as a "growth responsibility that arises at a certain stage in the life of a family, successful achievement of which leads to satisfaction and success with later tasks, while failure leads to unhappiness in the family, disapproval by society, and difficulty with later developmental tasks" (1971, pp. 149-150). The interaction of tasks of members within a family may be in conflict with or complementary to each other, or they may have both conflicting and complementary components. If, for example, the parents of a toddler are adolescents with the tasks of the adolescent, such as establishing identity, they may well have difficulty coping with their toddler's attempts to assert his independence and autonomy.

Tasks of the family are related to the physical maintenance; labor division; resource allocation; communication; relationship to the larger society;

morale and motivation maintenance; and reproduction, recruitment, and release of members (Duvall, 1971). Among the tasks shared by parents of toddlers and preschoolers are those of adapting the home environment to the changing needs of their expanding family and maintaining effective communication within the family.

When a parent, usually the mother, brings a young child for well child care, the focus of guidance is usually on the child's behavior and needs. It is suggested that, although it is imperative for the parents to understand this, perhaps their adjustment could better be enhanced if the focus of attention is concerned with the interacting developmental tasks of all family members.

The literature abounds with statements concerning the growth and development of toddlers and preschoolers. The needs and developmental patterns of these children are stressed. Increasing attention is also being given to the needs of parents of these youngsters. The purpose of this chapter is to show how, through the nursing process, the concept of developmental tasks can be applied by nurses and other personnel working with parents, toddlers, and preschoolers. Focus needs to be on meshing the tasks of each family member as well as those tasks of the entire family unit, so that the rights and responsibilities of all individuals will be considered.

NURSING PROCESS

A process of developing and carrying out a plan of care based on family developmental tasks is comprised of six steps. The actual performance of an assessment is necessitated by three of these steps; the utilization of data obtained by assessment is included in the other three steps. This process includes:

1 Obtaining the data pertinent to the developmental tasks of each family member and to the family unit. This assessment will involve both observation and communication. There are a variety of assessment tools available or modifiable to provide this information.

2 Organizing the data into a meaningful framework related to developmental tasks so that tentative diagnoses can be inferred.

3 Planning care based upon the diagnoses inferred from the organized data and validated by the family.

4 Implementing the plan of care. This implementation may involve gathering additional data so that more definitive plans can be made.

5 Evaluating, or reassessing, the care in relation to the developmental tasks.

6 Revising goals and activities as determined by the reassessment (Hymovich, 1970).

The Weiss Family

Consideration of some of the Weiss family's developmental tasks will serve as an example of how this framework can be used by nurses and others working with families with young children.

> The Weiss family consists of a mother, father and three children: Bryan, aged five and one-half years; Shelly, four years of age; and Tommy, fourteen months old. Mrs. Weiss brought Tommy to the pediatrician for his well-child evaluation. She stated to the nurse that she was still putting him to bed with his bottle and asked if this was wrong. With exploration, it was determined that this mother had read this was a poor practice, and although she did not think it was bad, she did want to check the nurse's opinion.

At this point, the nurse had assessed Mrs. Weiss's need to talk about the situation. Her plan was to listen and ask pertinent questions regarding Mrs. Weiss, Tommy and other members of the family as they seemed appropriate. It was not possible to determine at this point whether Mrs. Weiss needed any factual information regarding weaning. Thus, she would be gathering and organizing additional data as she implemented her initial plan to listen and question.

> Why was Mrs. Weiss putting Tommy to bed with his bottle? It started about 2 months prior to this discussion when the parents, who had weaned Tommy from the bottle, went on a vacation for a week. The baby sitter found that using the bottle was an effective method of putting Tommy to sleep. Several weeks after the parents returned, the family moved to a new home. At about the same time, it became necessary for the child to again wear a Denis-Browne splint at night and his mother felt that continuing the bottle would help him readjust to the bar. She also stated that when this youngster was up late, he awakened the older children, and the family received little sleep. Everyone's schedule was such that the family had to arise early in the morning, and it was difficult to get through the day without adequate sleep.
>
> Mrs. Weiss felt she had solved the problem so that it met the needs of her entire family. She and her husband were in complete agreement with this plan. Mrs. Weiss stated plans to eventually discontinue giving the bottle to her youngest child at night but saw no need to consider it at the present time. She believed it would be difficult at first, perhaps a few sleepless nights, but that it would work when the family was ready.

The nurse's tentative diagnosis was that Mrs. Weiss was confident in her decision and wanted reinforcement rather than additional information. This diagnosis was confirmed by Mrs. Weiss. The nurse's plan was to reinforce and support Mrs. Weiss.

Mrs. Weiss was supported by the nurse in her plan. The needs of each family member were discussed, and the nurse reinforced the parents' belief that the total family needs had to be considered in making a decision such as this. The needs of just one child or one parent could not be considered in isolation because they were so interrelated with each other.

It was noted that Tommy's developmental level had not been assessed in nearly 6 months. The nurse, therefore, planned to carry out the assessment at this visit in order to determine if he was functioning within the norms expected of a child his age. Tommy's developmental tasks were used as a basis for assessing his development.

Use of a developmental history and the Denver Developmental Screening Test to assess Tommy's developmental tasks at this time revealed that he was functioning within normal limits for a child of his age. That he was learning to use his body effectively could be seen in his manner of walking, stooping, and building a tower with blocks. He was learning to take food satisfactorily; he could use a spoon and a cup and was adept at using his fingers for this purpose! Evidence of his learning to adjust to others and of learning to love and be loved was seen in observations of his interactions with his mother and her descriptions of his interactions with others. Mrs. Weiss was not planning to teach him about bowel elimination until the family was once again settled into some organized routine. Their move took place less than 1 month ago.

She expressed some concern because Tommy did not go to sleep as well as her other children had at this age and because he sometimes woke up at night and disturbed the other children. She felt, however, that she was managing satisfactorily with this child and did not view his sleeping patterns as a serious problem. Rather, it was a phase which would pass. She was pleased to know the nurse supported her decisions and stated, "Each child seems to have his own problems but we manage to solve them as they come up and it's nice to know that others think we are on the right track."

The nurse assured Mrs. Weiss that "she was on the right track" and that her assessment of Tommy revealed he was developing normally. In reviewing her conversation with Mrs. Weiss, the nurse felt Mrs. Weiss needed continued reassurance and suggested that Mrs. Weiss could call her any time to discuss her decisions and that she need not wait for a visit. She suggested that if Tommy continues to have difficulty sleeping, Mrs. Weiss might like to discuss this. Following this discussion, the nurse evaluated the plans she had implemented and made the following plans: to review the developmental tasks of the other family members to determine if anything else needed to be discussed with Mrs. Weiss, to ask Mrs. Weiss how she was managing with the other children, to reassess Tommy's developmental abilities when he was eighteen months old, and to find out how Mrs. Weiss was managing Tommy's sleeping situation on her next visit to the office.

> Data about rest, sleep, and activity patterns; eating; elimination; communication; interpersonal relationships; temperament; and dependence-independence patterns revealed the following information related to the developmental tasks of five-and-one-half-year-old Bryan and four-year-old Shelly. They are mastering different tasks than their youngest brother and also, in some cases, different tasks or different aspects of the same task as each other. Both of these children have mastered the basics of good eating habits. Bryan has mastered some of his impulses and is able to conform to the expectations of others to a greater extent than Shelly. He has difficulty controlling his temper when Bryan knocks down his toys, but he does not hit Bryan at these times as much as he used to. Instead he screams at him. Shelly has an occasional temper tantrum, but these only occur when she is very tired. Both children are learning to handle potentially dangerous situations; however this is creating some difficulties for the family because Tommy now gets into everything, and activities which are safe for the older children are dangerous for Tommy. Bryan and Shelly are toilet trained during the day; Shelly remains dry at night but Bryan continues to wet his bed nearly every evening. Methods of handling this situation have been suggested to Mrs. Weiss by the pediatrician, and her feelings about the situation have been explored by the nurse.

Organization of this summary revealed that intervention had primarily been related to providing some suggestions concerning safety measures in the family necessitated by the different developmental levels of the children. In addition to this, guidance had been provided concerning Bryan's bedwetting and its meaning to Mr. and Mrs. Weiss. Some anticipatory guidance was also begun concerning the tasks Bryan will be facing when he reaches school. At this visit, the nurse inferred that Mrs. Weiss was coping with these problems satisfactorily. To confirm her diagnosis, she planned to ask Mrs. Weiss how she was managing with Bryan's bedwetting and if Tommy was still getting into everything of the older children. Further plans would be made and implemented depending upon the responses of Mrs. Weiss.

> During the toddler years of their oldest children, Mr. and Mrs. Weiss were able to master the developmental tasks arising during that period. They became competent and assured in caring for their children and were able to provide opportunities for each child's development within their resources at that time. They established healthful routines for their family which are altered as their needs change. When these routines are altered, such as Tommy's poor sleeping patterns at times or illness in the family, the Weiss's are able to make temporary adjustments.

Mrs. Weiss feels the need to keep alive some sense of personal autonomy and has decided to return to her high school teaching position in the fall when her oldest child enters first grade and her youngest has adjusted to all the recent changes in the family. Mr. Weiss, a university professor, has assumed major responsibility for earning the family income and views the income his wife will be making as a supplement but not a necessity. They will use it primarily for emergency situations which arise in the life of parents with youngsters and to perhaps purchase some luxuries they had not intended to buy.

The family had adapted housing arrangements for their young children but found it necessary to move to a larger home following the birth of their third child. They are finding additional adjustments necessary because their youngest son is more active and "gets into everything" much more than the older children did. The parents share some of the childrearing tasks, such as putting the children to bed and babysitting. They do not plan to have other children and have selected a contraceptive which is acceptable to both of them.

These parents are able to share and discuss their problems and solve them in ways which are mutually satisfactory.

The role of the nurse at this stage has been one of support, reassurance, and encouragement as they continue to master their developmental tasks. Questions are answered as they arise in relation to the youngsters and occasionally in relation to the parents. Anticipatory guidance is provided when indicated by assessment of the family's developmental needs. The day-to-day problems which arise are handled competently by this family and further intervention is unnecessary at this time.

TASKS AND PARENT DEVELOPMENT

Parents, as well as children, grow and develop in their roles as they are constantly adapting to changes in their family and in themselves. This continuous process is characterized by five successive stages (Friedman, 1957). During their child's infancy they are learning the cues their baby expresses in making his needs known. With each successive child, the parents will once again go through this stage as they adjust to the unique cues of each infant.

The second stage of parental development, learning to accept the growth and development of their child, occurs when the child is in his toddler years. It is just prior to and during this stage that parents, particularly parents with their first child, need guidance and support. They need to understand the tasks the child is attempting to master and his needs during this time for such things as safety, limits, and toilet training. They need to understand the concept of developmental readiness, or the teachable moment; they need assistance in recognizing when this time arises. At the same time, parents need guidance in understanding the tasks they are mastering during this stage of their development. They may need assistance in reevaluating their position within their expanding family, in providing and spending their income wisely, and in arranging their home to meet the expanding world of their youngster.

About the time their child becomes a preschooler, the parents enter their third developmental stage, which is one of learning to separate from their child. This stage continues during the child's preschool and early school years. Separation is often difficult for parents as well as for their children. Parents need guidance in understanding their feelings and in understanding how mastery of their preschooler's developmental tasks contributes to his increasing independence. Once again, setting limits needs to be discussed, for as the child's ability to handle his own body and potentially dangerous situations increases, his needs for limits will be altered. He needs limits for protection, but he also needs freedom within these limits to explore and satisfy his insatiable curiosity. The changes occurring in the child's emotional development need to be explored, and the parents need help in understanding their dynamics. Separation may occur in a variety of ways—daily separations when the child attends nursery school and/or the parents go to work; temporary separations, such as vacations, business trips, or hospitalizations; or permanent separation, such as the death of a family member or the child's pet. Each of these situations would necessitate guidance of parents and children. Preparation of the family for attendance at nursery school, day care centers, or head start programs, and later for school should occur during this stage.

Sometime during the child's school years, the parents enter the fourth stage of their development—learning to accept rejection without deserting the child. During the youngster's teen-age years the parents' developmental stage is that of learning to build a new life. The tasks of parents and their offspring during these stages are not within the scope of this chapter; however, the developmental task framework could be applied to these phases as well as to earlier phases.

DEVELOPMENTAL TASKS AND FAMILY INTERVENTION

The developmental task concept is suggested as a framework for organizing data and providing intervention when working with families with toddlers and preschoolers. Examples of the use of this framework in relation to a nursing process are presented through examples of intervention with the Weiss family. It is recommended that this framework be considered by personnel who are working with families with children of any age in any stage of development.

BIBLIOGRAPHY

Carrieri, V. K., and J. Sitzman: "Components of the Nursing Process," *Nursing Clinics of North America,* **6**:115-124, 1971.

Duvall, E. M.: *Family Development,* 4th ed., Philadelphia: J. B. Lippincott Company, 1971.

Friedman, D. B.: "Parent Development," *California Medicine,* **86**:25-28, 1957.

Havighurst, R. J.: *Developmental Tasks and Education,* 2d ed., New York: David McKay Company, Inc., 1952.

Hymovich, D. P.: "Assessing Patients Needs," speech given in San Angelo, Texas, to District 16 of the Texas Nurses' Association, May 16, 1970.

Chapter 18

The School-aged Child and His Family

Joan T. Large

The bittersweet nostalgic days of Tom Sawyer and Huck Finn are gone for one generation. The days of *Please Don't Eat the Daisies* and *Where Did You Go? Out. What Did You Do? Nothing.* are gone for still another generation. Should you not have realized the subtle changes taking place, just recall a few headlines, editorials, or magazine articles of recent vintage. For example, remember "Why Can't Johnny Read?" "Crime and Violence Increasing in the Urban Ghetto," "Gangs and Delinquency in Suburbia," or "Drugs and VD in the Elementary Schools"? The reference group is not adolescence but those "latent" years between six and twelve.

Heretofore middle childhood captured the attention of a few psychologists and educators. Parents were vaguely aware that learning theories were being tested, IQs were being measured, and heights were being graphed. Many believed children were marking time in school between weekends and vacations. Some parents during this period regretted losing "the baby" and anxiously awaited the dreaded teen-ager. There are some parents whose sanity is restored on the first day of school each year and some teachers who lose their sense of humor that very same day.

No one truly believes children mystically appear on the first day of school nor that they disappear at age thirteen. Nevertheless, the inexorable passage of time has meaning, if to no one else, than to children. Children alone, however, provide a limiting frame of reference as the following conversation with a five-year-old demonstrates.

Interviewer: What does Daddy like Mary to do?
Mary: Uh . . . to be pretty.
Interviewer: What does Mommy like Mary to do?
Mary: Uh . . . to help her and uh . . . to girl talk.
Interviewer: What does Mary like to do?
Mary: Uh . . . to wear jewelry and uh . . . to cook and uh . . . to sleep over. Can I sleep over with you?

Does this brief conversation provide sufficient clues to conclude that the five-year-old had resolved the sexual identification conflict and is ready to leave the protection of the family? If "sleeping over" is equated with readiness to start formal school, will the mandated school system provide space for five-year-olds? If parents are satisfied with the role-taking activities of five-year-olds, will they permit increased independent activities away from home? Are there sufficient clues to say this five-year-old has entered middle childhood?

If some five-year-olds are entering middle childhood, are some eleven-year-olds leaving this stage of the life cycle? It is somewhat a simple task to mark the end chronologically at thirteen years or physiologically at the onset of menarche. The complexity of the situation may be demonstrated in the following conversation.

Mother: Nurse, what am I going to do about Denise?
Nurse: Does Denise have a problem?
Mother: She don't think so. I'm the one with the problem. She's only going on twelve and already she acts like she's grown up. She don't have "the sign" you know but the girls she goes with does.
Nurse: What does Denise say about this?
Mother: Oh she don't pay me no mind. She says she can take care of herself and all the girls act that way. I'm afraid she'll get in real trouble.

If childhood had a beginning and if there is an ending, then what constitutes middle childhood? Surely the "helping" disciplines need to know. Advocates of children need to select the best of several approaches to make the intervention most meaningful. Advocates of parents need to select the best of several approaches to make assistance most supportive.

FRAME OF REFERENCE

The organization of available knowledge must provide a cohesive wholeness while recognizing the contribution of fragmented parts. Such a frame of reference should also provide sufficient data to imply alternative ways of utilizing the knowledge base. The model in Figure 18-1 proposes a frame of reference to answer, "What is middle childhood?"

The three phases noted in the model were not assumed to fit neatly between six and twelve years nor to outline the elementary school years. It was interesting, however, to note one teacher's exclamation, "That certainly fits children in the first three grades!" when she heard a description of a child in the phase of diffusion. And at another time, a school nurse said, "The description of disorganization surely says it all about the fourth, fifth, and sixth graders."

Diffusion is intended to represent a dissemination of discrete new elements into a relatively ordered life (early childhood), resulting for a time in a patchwork, mosaic design. For example, the child may perceive no inconsistency among what mother says, what teacher says, and what his friend says about the very same event. Disorganization assumes that disorder arises out of the complexity of these confusing expectations, often resulting in eruption of turbulent behavior. Lying, stealing, fighting, and bossiness are examples of behavior demonstrating this phase of development. Finally disposition becomes an arrangement of elements into ordered systems, appearing to offer harmony among adaptive behaviors. Willingness to do home chores, doggedness at completing projects, and enjoying the challenge of school work indicate for some time that all is right with the world.

It may or may not have been an easy task for parents to anticipate the next stages of development with younger children. Certainly there are less feelings attached to "soon your baby will walk," a physical motor experience, than to "soon your child will lie and cheat," a moral sanction. If independent

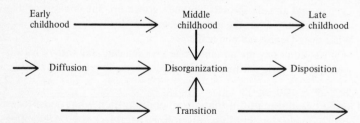

Figure 18-1 This model presents the passage of the child from early to late childhood. This conversion has been translated to represent three somewhat distinct phases of diffusion, disorganization, and disposition.

locomotion is to be anticipated, then is independent thinking any less desirable? Parents and other adults need to look at this stage of development with as much enthusiasm and excitement as "the first step." This model offers therefore, a way of looking at middle childhood.

SOME CURRENT THEORIES OF CHILD DEVELOPMENT

The outline of psychosocial and learning theories in Table 18-1 were selected as representative of current thinking. Areas of agreement and disagreement are to be expected. Admittedly, data were selected as best representative of the proposed frame of reference for middle childhood. Effort was made not to distort the basic theoretical framework of the authors. The reader may find it exciting to select his own favorite developmental theorist for analysis in such a frame of reference.

SELECTED DATA RELATED TO MIDDLE CHILDHOOD

With few exceptions all children begin formal schooling between the ages of five and seven. Surely parents, teachers, and children are reminded of the hide-and-seek game as each September approaches. "Here I come, ready or not," speaks for the ambivalence perceived by all those involved in such a momentous occasion. One child could be forcibly thrust out of the home into school. Another child could be released to embrace school. And still others are only reluctantly permitted to attend school. Given all the varied experiences these children possess, one experience which is held in common is a family which more or less controlled their world. The paradigm home and its possessions, family, and members admit to as many labels as United States society can contain. Home can be poverty or affluence, nuclear or extended, and stable or unstable. Whatever the label, it was indeed home and family. The child knew it and adapted to its parameters. Whether he starts out boldly as an explorer or reluctantly as a lost lamb, start out he must.

Diffusion

The school and its environs, the school group and its members establish parameters of the new world of the child. That it is not the futuristic adult society has not made it less real and full of personal meaning for this moment in time. Each child is capable of assimilating this new situation, however significant the new relationships will be. Some children will hear labels applied to them or their families for the first time. What does it mean to be poor, deprived, spoiled, bad, or dirty? What will it mean to have the family called

Table 18-1 Interpretations from *Theories of Child Development* for Understanding Middle Childhood

Frame of reference	Psychoanalytic (Freud) Period of sexual latency Development of superego		Cognitive schema (Piaget) Period of concrete operations Development of mental operations		Behavioristic (Watson-Skinner) Stimulus-Response Conditioned learning	
Diffusion	1	Sexual identity conflict resolved as it relates to parents	1	Limited to actual observation of real events	1	Generalized conditioning responses from previous adults and peers to new adults and peers
	2	Incorporates new thoughts and ideas about other adults and peers	2	Begins to perceive relationships between elements if pointed out	2	May begin new discriminating responses
			3	May not be able to use past judgment for present events		
Disorganization	1	Uncompromising superego	1	Conflict in understanding relationships among the concrete observations such as greater than, less than, higher than	1	New expectations for discriminatory behavior may lead to extinction or inhibition of previous learned responses
	2	Frustration, aggression, and delinquency may result from difficulty in maintaining own value system in face of others' value systems which differ	2	Inconsistent understanding of ordered events of time, space, and number	2	Intermediary responses may lead to learnable fears, avoidance learning, or inhibitory habits
Disposition	1	Development of conscience	1	Adapted to schema of concrete operations	1	Distinguishes between choices in sequence of events
	2	Value system more stable, flexible, and tolerant	2	Begins to perceive the universe of possibilities	2	Learns self-directed activities
			3	May begin to use hypothetical situations for solving problems	3	Can anticipate goal as a result of serial-learned events

Social-learning (Hull-Sears) People and environment as stimulus for learned responses	Organismic-Developmental (Werner) Orthogenetic timing for cognitive development	Family–Social system (Parsons-Bales) Period of moving away from coherent family structure
1 Has learned dependency behavior toward home environment 2 New social learning begins inhibition of dependency behavior	1 Fusion of qualities or characteristics leads child to perceive persons, emotions, colors as same meaning 2 Lacks differentiated, discrete thinking and behavior	1 Expectation to move to new social group 2 Family and child need support individually as units, reciprocally as an interacting unit
1 Inhibition of dependency behavior may result in hostility, anger, anxiety, and fear of retaliation behavior 2 Displacement of anger away from parent or authority figure toward dissimilar object seen in physical and verbal aggression such as fighting, teasing, and taunting	1 Rigidity in thinking and behavior 2 Strong concrete realism leads child to hold on to words and ideas even when it appears irrational—cannot sense the new idea is wrong	1 Conflicts arising from parents inability to "let go" may lead to maladaptive behavior 2 Conflicts arising from child's inability to transfer family interaction patterns to other adults and peers lead to low achievement, low status
1 Learns socially acceptable displacement activities 2 Learns to control impulsive behavior and resist temptations 3 Has feeling of guilt after transgressions 4 Learns variety of behavior patterns for making amends	1 Thinking behavior becomes discrete, articulated, flexible, and stable 2 Concrete realism significantly drops by age thirteen and leads to concrete symbolism 3 Particularly has acquired a symbolic language	1 Derives a sense of security from liking and accepting new status and performance 2 Derives a sense of adequacy from cooperating with team success and group achievements

Source: Adapted with permission from Alfred L. Baldwin, *Theories of Child Development,* New York: John Wiley & Sons, Inc., 1968.

unstable, broken, welfare, fatherless, or female-dominated? What will it be like to be called stupid, dumb, retarded, black, whitey, or kike? Some children may not be able to transfer the known behavior of parents to the unknown behavior of teachers with ease. Difficulties arise out of matching permissive parents with nonpermissive teachers. Reverse labeling of these authority figures can also result in a disrupted self-concept. "Look, Jimmy is a bad boy; he won't stay in his seat," will have meaning for Jimmy as well as his peers who have not equated "bad" with "staying in seat." Sharing the attention of teachers with so many others is likened to sharing the attention of parents with siblings. Similar patterns of responses to sibling rivalry have been noted in peer rivalry responses. Stamler and Palmer (1970) suspected that the loss of control perceived by the child in conforming to teacher authority and coping with peer rivalry may have resulted in repeated visits to the school nurse. While dependency needs of the repeaters was well-documented, the hypothesis that these children would be found in the younger age group in elementary school was not supported. One might suspect then that young children still use home as the focus for affectional support. Parents and teachers may not agree on authority and control of behavior, but they share a common expectation children will learn "something" in school. This something is most definitively associated with reading, writing, and other school subjects.

The propensity of starting school and enlarging the geographic and human neighborhood has not been perceived clearly except in popular comedians' jokes. The second new world of many children includes all those spatial and human relationships not labeled school and home. Crossing guards, bus drivers, policemen, and grocers know with certainty that the business of children would never be considered home or school curricula. Even in large city ghettos where mothers fear for the lives of their children, the smaller ones wander safely in and out of well-defined gang turfs. Suburban mothers realize with amazement how far their youngsters have traveled when another adult says, "So you're Johnny's mother." Children themselves report the frequency with which maternal interrogations begin with, "But who is he? And how did you ever meet him?" Finding a place for one's self in neighborhood peer groups is not an easy task. "Stop that or I'll tell my Mommy on you," indicates a strong need for adults to help control peer behavior. Speech as an extension of thinking aloud is not yet discriminatory in meaning. Being called "dumb" is tantamount to being dumb. Running home to mother or its symbolic intent, "I'll tell mommy on you," is tolerated in the very young. New ways of coping with peers demand very different patterns of behavior and must find expression in testing out only with peers. Early attempts to find a place in the community are observed in the imitative play of these early years. "Let's go wading," "Let's see how many lights we can knock out," "Let's go over to Mr. Bob's garage," usually have no relationship to adult rules, disobedience, or intent to do wrong. Being together and doing things together can be caused by the sheer pleasure of your company or an attempt to control immediate and present needs of the group.

Children in early middle childhood utilize home for bringing back to and testing out new ideas identified in school and in the neighborhood. Conversations and other behaviors demonstrate imitation of peers and comparision of other adults to parents. One father reported his delight in listening to the endless conversation of his six-year-old and the frustration of getting along with the nine-year-old. Many parents become polarized in their feelings about children exploring new ideas at home. Some parents may smile indulgently at the swearing, calling parents by given name, or beginning every sentence with "teacher says." Still others report with anger how very much they resent the influence of peers, "He eats, talks, and acts just like Tommy," and other adults, "I'll go crazy if he says, 'Mr. Bob says,' just once more." The ambivalence with which parents approach inhibition of dependency behavior during this period can be documented in the following serial comments of one parent.

"Why don't you grow up and stop acting like a baby?"
"Don't slam the door!"
"Wipe your feet!"
"Wash the back of your hands too!"

Disorganization

What happened to the mother's helper at five and the gay, talkative, and obedient six-year-old? "Mary teases all the time now." "Tommy taunts his younger brother." "Linda lies; I just know it." "I caught Sammy smoking, and he denied it to my face." "I am so ashamed to have other children at the house; Chuckie cheats and must win all the games." "Tim said he traded that truck at school; I don't know; it looks too new to me; I think he stole it." What did happen to the precious darlings of yesteryear? Why do parents report confusion and frustration about the child's behavior and loss of parental control? Is there an explanation for the number and frequency of runaways between nine and eleven? Why are so many teachers reporting behavior problems among fourth, fifth, and sixth graders? Schools blame parents in general and their childrearing practices in particular. Parents blame society in general and perhaps TV, films, and schools in particular. Children blame parents, siblings, friends, teachers, and whoever else may be near at hand. As children adapt to school life, various patterns become evident to teachers and peers alike. There are the good students and the bad, the popular students and the hangers-on, the bullies and the goody-goods, as well as the leaders and the followers. During this time, teachers are prone to say children have settled in to the school life style. There is, therefore, a certain freedom from extraneous factors which permits the child to concentrate on mental development. Family influence on mental development does tend to descrease as children move toward nonfamily members such as teachers and peers. Karen Morris (1968) was able to demonstrate the influence of the school system and teacher models on the development of self-concept in lower-class, black fifth graders. Self-concepts tended to be high when children were placed in traditional, segregated schools or with teachers who themselves evidenced high self-concepts. Some children, however, are unable to move from family influence to school influence.

> Denise, a nine-year-old, Negro girl, was a battered child. Continuous withdrawal from interaction with teachers and peers led to low achievement in school subjects and low status in her peer group. When placed in a class for slow learners, Denise became a happy, contented child. Yet I.Q. testing revealed above average test scores. How does one help Denise become willing to compete with her peers?

Sociometric procedures have indicated differences in perception between teachers and children. The child one chooses to work with in the classroom may not be the same as the one who is chosen to play with in the schoolyard or even the one who is invited home overnight. Similar discrepancies in individual behavior are reported by teachers who observe the busy, high achiever in the classroom as the aggressive bully in the schoolyard. Being human and responsible for large numbers of children, it may be impossible for the teacher to discern for each child the particular problem he is facing. How will he know that the same child who told her he forgot to take his homework from the kitchen table told his mother he forgot to take his homework book from school the night before? Most teachers are looking for persistent patterns of behavior which indicate a child is unable to cope with existing problems. Others may simply be interested in the child who disrupts group activity, interfering with the tasks of other children. Indeed, it is frequently impossible to identify which observable behavior is a problem to teacher or child.

The life of the child when not at home or at school is becoming more secretive. No longer does he take pleasure in recounting his activities to parents. It has become a matter of record that parents only learn of outside activities when other adults call to report misbehavior. The community at large begins to note with dismay the lack of regard for private property and the rigid, ofttimes cruel, regulations imposed on members of a group. Play is serious business. Children do not move easily from one group to another. Rules of conduct as well as the rules of games are not transferable. In the beginning, there may be much home contact, demonstrated in either crying or tattling behavior. Soon, however, there is "nothing to do" unless activity is originated and carried out within the group. As the child attempts to incorporate group values into his own behavior patterns, conflicts in parent-child relationships arise. Being punished for breaking a window when no other member of the group is punished for the same act is difficult to comprehend. His cry, "It's not fair," is echoed over and over in his handling of his own peer group. Being fair is the final criterion of judgment in group activity. Winning or being first appears to be unrelated to following exact rules of the game. Torg (1971), an orthopedist, clarifies the meaning of competition at this stage of development when he discusses the use of competitive sports in middle childhood. He believes Little League activities should be abolished in elementary school and competitive sports relegated to high school. Not only do children lack the physical coordination to be safe players, but they also lack the cognitive ability to comprehend adult rules and adult understanding of competition and teamwork. Playing together does not necessarily mean coordinated team effort but rather necessary processes leading to this ability. It may be heresy to suggest that organized group activities at this age are an invasion of privacy as well as an abortion of a necessary developmental stage.

Just as it would be a false assumption to believe that no teacher saw individual conflicts arising out of school behavior or that all adults perceived neighborhood activity to be secretive and deviant, so too one must avoid the generalization that all parents predict future thieves and juvenile delinquents arising out of the current behavior patterns of their children. Some parents view with alarm, and others with anger, their growing sense of impotence as they face loss of control of their children's behavior. The seeming compliance with peer group values is invariably in conflict with parental standards. Direct confrontation and challenge arise out of home- and family-centered activities. The teasing, taunting, and tattling which seem endless among siblings in the family are as much of a problem as challenging bedtime, eating patterns, bathing, and dressing activities. Some parents will react with more severe punishment, stricter rules, and limits so confining that child and parents are in constant opposition. At the other extreme are parents who are so permissive they offer no limits with which the child can test his new-found values; his socially unacceptable behavior may even go unnoticed. Somewhere in between are parents who seek comfort from like parents some days, pack the bags of potential runaways on some days, hide in the bedroom on other days, or just pray that this phase will not last too long.

Disposition

When it appears that neither families, schools, nor the children themselves can any longer tolerate the situation, calm begins to prevail. There is not only peace internally perceived but harmony with family, school, and community. The behavior of children indicates a sense of adequacy with which old and new situations are handled. Teachers report children approach schoolwork more responsibly. Parents are surprised when the child agrees with directions and limitations. Home chores are accepted more pleasantly and with less fussing. Activities around home and school, when permitted to be observed, are more organized. A sense of fair play exists. Unfortunately, even socially maladaptive behavior contains some of the same characteristics. Society may or may not sanction the adaptive behavior of these children. Expectations for this phase of development vary from one family, school, and community to another. For example, some communities may not become excited about the school dropout if he commits no vandalism. Some schools may not worry about low achievement as long as the child is not a disciplinary problem. And some parents may not be concerned about anything occurring outside the home as long as the child comes home "on time" or makes his bed everyday. Yes, even the life style of the ghetto child can be in harmony with his peer group's expectations.

Given the opportunity to experience success, children will begin to enjoy schoolwork. The fusion of work and play within the school setting allows for little distinction between the pleasure of learning and the business of schooling. Teachers report the intensity with which children approach the completion of each task. For most children, this sense of security about school occurs at the end of the elementary school years or the beginning of middle school (junior high school in some areas). Some parents are able to see this change reflected in the upswing of academic grades and improvement in conduct reports. The child, his teacher, and his school peers have reached a new high in their cooperative efforts.

The community is also reflective of the change in behavior patterns. Adults note with some surprise, "How nice Tommy is; why he puts my paper in a dry place when it rains." The peer group, now clearly circumscribed, will often be found cooperating with adults in community improvement efforts. While there is more evidence that individuals are accepting community responsibility, increasing effort is being placed on team activities leading to group success. The behavior of children who have not found success in school is also most evident in neighborhood activity. Children who have rejected parental control and who have failed in school are now reduced to only peer groups. While socioeconomic status presents no real barriers for considering deviant behavior, it is more observable in the low-socioeconomic level group, particularly in urban ghettos. These children must rely on each other for a sense of adequacy and purpose. The chronological age for deviant gang membership is becoming lower and lower.

Family living also demonstrates a welcome change of pace. Parents believe their persistent attention, sometimes constant nagging, is reaping its just rewards. Parents dramatically report the shock of hearing, "OK Mom, I'll do it right now." But the development of a sense of responsibility does not happen so suddenly. Conversations with children reveal the difficulty they have in understanding the importance of always hanging up clothes, taking out the trash, or raking leaves. These same children will report with pride their ability to babysit safely, stay by the house when parents are temporarily gone, and volunteer services to neighbors or to shut-ins. It becomes apparent that the task must inherently possess the need to prevent injury to others or to meet an overt human need. Whenever there is a failure to carry out their responsibilities, grief and guilt are subsequently followed by efforts to make amends. If one were to believe children in this age group, willingness to do home chores is simply a side effect of a new-found sense of self-worth. Parents become lulled into a false sense of security as they turn their attention to other, more pressing, family problems.

IMPLICATIONS FOR NURSING

In the normal course of events, it would be a natural summary to invite all nurses to participate in that delightful era called middle childhood. Yet nurses cling to the traditional activities of physical and dental examinations, sensorimotor screening, and supervision of the chronically ill child in school. Well-documented needs such as these are not to be negated. But is that all there is? Heretofore, nursing practice has directed its attention to stopgap, episodic measures almost exlusively related to physical or physiological needs of school children. In many instances the ability of parents or children to cope with this developmental period has been either overestimated or underestimated, but hardly ever seriously appraised. Just as nurses have been primarily concerned with physical health, so too teachers have culled out mental development as their special domain. If families are assessed at all, the frequency with which this leads to stereotyping is quite alarming. If the traditional perspective of the nurse has not been effective, and if there is a need to clarify the expected outcomes of middle childhood, what then become the essential competencies required of the nurse to assist families in middle childhood? The issue here is not how to do away with tradition, related to either physical health or mental development. The proposal assumes that professional practitioners want to support children and their families through a meaningful period of life.

Diffusion

The assumption during this phase is that relatively stable life styles are about to be mixed with new patterns. Basic understanding of where children are going demands concommitant knowledge of where they have been. Is it not possible to register children for school *and* interview mothers for a developmental history? In addition to the birthdate and place, the immunization record, and physical examination, ask if any of Johnny's friends are starting school with him. What does he talk about at home? What does he do when he is hurt? What does he do with his older and younger siblings? Who takes care of him most of the day? How can you tell when something is bothering him or when he is getting sick? Who will be bringing him to school? Taking him home? What do you think schools should do to help children learn? What do you teach him at home? There must be a thousand things to know. Report card number one should in reality be interview number two. Since children spend every day of their lives learning, it appears impossible to anticipate the answer to the query, "What did you learn in school today?"

Disorganization

Just as we assume children will fall down and get up innumerable times when learning to walk, we can assume children will fall down many times while learning to think. The eruption of boasting or lying, stealing or cheating, and crying or fighting is considered "the falling down" process of trying to make order out of the expanded world. Children will take school home and bring home to school. It would naturally follow that their significant adults should be working together. The parents, teachers, and nurses may shift roles in a primary or supportive situation. Discovery of a problem carries a different connotation than "catching" a child at stealing. Since the focus is on the child, the discoverer calls the task force into action. Parent-teacher-nurse workshops may demand at times the restoration of a sense of humor, and all adults may need to cultivate the wonderful "art of overlooking" some problems. Children can and do work out some of their problems together. Adults can provide the freedom to do so.

Disposition

Cues that the child's world is now spinning on the appropriate axis may be first observed in the school setting. The opportunity exists for nurses to not only share these observations but also to anticipate the utilization of this newfound pride in achievement within the home setting. Many parents would rather do it themselves than to permit children to experience pride in achievement of home and family responsibilities. Knowledge of the child's abilities is no secret to the child. The sweet smell of success comes when everyone knows of it.

The ability of nurses to break through the confining barriers of mandated school health programs will depend in a large measure on the ability to acquire a strong knowledge base about middle childhood. School children do not belong to schools. The wonderful world of children can only be a reality if adults permit it to happen.

BIBLIOGRAPHY

Baldwin, A. L.: *Theories of Child Development,* New York: John Wiley & Sons, Inc., 1967.

CRM Books: *Developmental Psychology Today,* Del Mar, Calif.: Communications Research Machines, Inc., 1971.

Morris, K. S.: *Study of the Effect of Three School Environments on the Self Concept of Lower Class Negro Grade School Children,* master's thesis, New Brunswick, N.J.: Graduate School of Rutgers-The State University, 1968.

Segal, J. (ed.): *The Mental Health of the Child,* Rockville, Md.: Program Analysis and Evaluation Branch Office of Program Planning and Evaluation, National Institute of Mental Health, 1971.

Shoemaker, L. P. (ed.): *Parents and Family Life Education: For Low-income Families,* U.S. Department of Health, Education, and Welfare, no. 434, 1965.

Stamler, C., and J. O. Palmer: *Dependency and Repetitive Visits to the Nurse's Office in Elementary School Children,* master's thesis, Los Angeles: University of California at Los Angeles, 1970.

Torg, J.: Interview for *Temple Times,* 2(3):2, Oct. 14, 1971, Philadelphia: Temple University School of Medicine.

Chapter 19

The Adolescent and His Family

Rene Clark Davis

The basic requirement for nurses who plan to work with adolescents is to sincerely like and enjoy them. As cited in most theories of adolescence, this is a period of searching for self-identity, vacillating attitudes and emotions, and tremendous body development. Consequently, teen-agers are frequently unpredictable in their behavior, and nurses who care for them must be able to accept this. This is not always easy, and the nurse must be sure of his feelings before he becomes deeply involved with work that includes adolescents. As well as being likable and interesting, adolescents can also be difficult to get along with. They are not usually seeking popularity among adults. The adolescent will know if you are not sincere in your efforts. He can easily detect a "phony." The adolescent is often treated as a misfit in our society, neither adult nor child; and he must be shown that you accept him for exactly what he is at that moment, and that you want to be involved in his care.

CONSIDERATIONS IN WORKING WITH ADOLESCENTS

There are several things to be taken into consideration when working with the adolescent. Because of his labile position in most situations, the adolescent needs people and places he can go to that can be counted on for consistency. The nurse who has identified himself and his role is an excellent resource for the adolescent. He can offer him a stable relationship that can help in his search for self. If the nurse has control of the environment in which he sees the adolescent, he can also make it a stable and secure place. For instance, the adolescent in the hospital who is forced to wear a shapeless hospital gown without good reason is being forced to relinquish some of his partially acquired identity. He is therefore threatened, frightened, and shoved into feeling like a child. However, the adolescent who is allowed to wear his own clothes and pajamas has the opportunity to protect his self-esteem and remain much like the person he was when he entered the hospital. Certainly the nature of his illness would also affect his movement toward growth or regression, but anything the nurse could do to provide stability would be helpful.

In being helpful, the nurse must have a friendly, warm attitude toward the adolescent. People who seem aloof, domineering, or unreasonable to the adolescent will not be accepted. Friendliness which does not imply intimacy may be difficult for the young nurse who is close to the age of the patient. A certain amount of emotional distance is necessary for maintaining a professional relationship. This does not mean the relationship must be sterile, but only controlled enough to render it useful.

There are times when it can be of therapeutic value to sit and relax with the adolescent, talking about whatever comes to mind and is of interest to both. But the nurse must plan wisely and not allow a "buddy" relationship to develop in which the patient fails to see the nurse as a helping person with authority.

For the nurse who has difficulty establishing trust and rapport with the adolescent, topics of interest to him such as sports, music, and friends can be used as icebreakers. The nurse who has a natural interest in the adolescent world has an excellent chance of establishing a sound relationship that can be helpful to the patient.

The adolescent should be allowed as much independence and individual expression as the nurse can safely allow within the context of his work. The adolescent's parents have a great deal of influence over the amount of independence he is allowed, and the nurse should try to work within the framework set by them. If the nurse should allow more freedom than he is accustomed to, the adolescent will be confused about his role. The nurse must be careful not to create differences between the adolescent and his family, for this has the potential of damaging their relationship or abruptly ending the nurse's contact with them. Independence can comfortably be allowed in such ways as expressing himself while in conference with the nurse, setting his own schedule for the day while in the hospital when possible, and making some decisions about his plan of care.

Another important means of allowing independence is to give the adolescent the opportunity and dignity of choosing the person whom he feels could be the most helpful. If he does not seem to relate well to the nurse, he should be allowed freedom in refusing to have conferences with him and in finding someone with whom he feels more comfortable. The nurse should be prepared to accept the fact that he may not be able to establish satisfactory relationships with all adolescent patients.

Certainly, the nurse's primary responsibility to the adolescent is to meet his needs which arise from his search for identity. The basis for this can be accomplished by establishing a stable and workable relationship, providing a safe environment that allows individual expression, and allowing independence that will build self-esteem. By striving toward these goals, the nurse will have the opportunity to assist the adolescent in his problems of adjustment, whether they be problems of adjustment to the hospital, to a family situation, to a chronic illness, or to himself as an emerging adult.

THE FAMILY OF THE ADOLESCENT

Some special considerations must be given to the family of the adolescent. The two cannot be separated, although there may be times when the nurse is either forced or chooses to work only with the adolescent. Most families are genuinely concerned and interested in their teen-ager and his growth. They want him to achieve his goal of satisfactorily reaching adulthood. However, it would not be unusual for a family to be totally confused about the adolescent's behavior. They may see no reasons for his moodiness. They may feel that his rebellion against their authority and opinions is a deliberate act of malice. They may also feel that his inability to think and act with certainty is a sign of childishness, and therefore be afraid to allow independent privileges. The parents may specifically seek out the nurse for help with these problems, or they may mention these problems when the nurse is working with the family because the adolescent is ill.

Their lack of understanding may be cleared up with a factual explanation of normal adolescent growth and development as it applies to their situation, or it may become the focal point of the entire nurse-adolescent-family relationship. Severe breaks in family cohesiveness can occur as long as there are misconstrued perceptions of each other among the family members. The nurse must be able to identify the problems within the family and then decide if he is capable of handling them. He must know which ones to seek help with and what sources of additional help are available.

A case in point is one of a sixteen-year-old boy who was hospitalized with his first attack of acute lymphocytic leukemia. He and his parents both knew of the diagnosis, but they were unable to talk about it among themselves. The patient thought his parents did not care about him because they always seemed happy and jovial when they visited. Nursing intervention was planned to alleviate this lack of communication. Individual conferences were held with the patient and with his parents, allowing and encouraging them to express their feelings about the situation.

Finally, an incident occurred while the family was together that triggered the sharing of love and care for each other. The mother brought a box of candy to her son, but he said he did not care for any. Then she opened the box and asked if she could have a piece, and he replied, "Sure, go ahead, you bought it for yourself anyway, you didn't buy it for me." Immediately, the mother began to "pour out" to her son how she felt about his illness, and how concerned she was, and how much she cared. Subsequently, the family was able to talk among themselves about leukemia and what they would do when they went home. Nursing intervention guided this family toward meaningful communication that was a relief to all.

Brothers and sisters of the adolescent may or may not be brought into the nurse's plan depending on the relevancy of their involvement. In many cases, the siblings would have no effect, but consider the fifteen-year-old girl who is a heavy drug user and wants to stop, but her older sister has a free source of supply and constantly encourages the girl to use drugs. No intervention will be successful unless the older sister can be involved. This can be extremely difficult for the nurse to handle, and resources in the community may need to be tapped. However, it is clear that the nurse must decide which family members need to be involved, how to involve them, and if he is capable of helping them in order for the intervention to be successful.

ESTABLISHING THE RELATIONSHIP

Establishing a working relationship with the adolescent and his family should begin with a systematic appraisal of each of them. Through data derived from the initial interviews, the nurse can plan appropriate intervention. Some standard method of gathering information is necessary for objectivity and comprehensiveness. If the institution in which one works has a nursing history or interview outline, it should be used. If such methods are not established, the nurse should choose one which follows sound practices and is comfortable to use.

In order to let the adolescent know that he is the patient, not his parents, and that you rely and act on his word, the nurse should have a separate interview with the teen-ager and then plan a subsequent interview with the parents or other family members. This practice should build self-esteem in the adolescent, let him know that you trust him from the beginning, and give the nurse insight into the viewpoints of all family members. The adolescent may not reveal some pertinent information if his parents are present. For instance, if the adolescent smokes cigarettes without his parents' knowledge, he will try to conceal this information although he knows it may have a bearing on his health. If, however, he sees the nurse alone, he may be willing to talk with complete honesty if he knows he can trust the nurse not to reveal his confidences to his parents.

This type of interviewing helps to get a more complete family and health history. The adolescent may not be able to remember important facts about his previous illnesses or medical care. His parents can give further information and also validate what the adolescent reports if there is a question.

There are many inherent problems in the practice of separate interviewing, but the competent nurse can work to avoid some of them. First of all, it is imperative to explain the interviewing technique to the adolescent and his family together to make sure they understand. Basically, they need to know that the nurse will not violate the privacy rights of either party by divulging confidential information. However, it should be made clear that the information will become part of the patient's record and will be available to other members of the professional staff. They should also be told to expect additional separate conferences during the course of contact with the nurse. It is highly important for the family to agree to this practice or it will fail. The nurse must be willing to accept their refusal and proceed with a family interview.

A warm, friendly chat with the adolescent and his family in order to explain the hospital, clinic, or whatever institution is involved; its policies; and what to expect while there is a good way to begin the relationship. The nurse should find out what their expectations are and what previous experiences they have had with similar institutions. Misconceptions and fears can then be alleviated through nursing action. The family should be made to feel comfortable and free to ask questions. While explaining his role, the nurse can give details about the separate interviews and their purposes. By establishing some rapport first, the nurse has a better chance of gaining the family's acceptance of the interview method. If they are merely told what to do, they may feel hostile toward the nurse and put up impassable barriers to communication. Allowing the family the chance to understand the procedures first is the best means of gaining their acceptance.

The parents, particularly, may see separate interviews as a threat to their position in the family. This may occur especially in cases where the parents are overprotective of their child. They may feel their child is either too young to answer for himself or too sick to be bothered. The nurse must evaluate their feelings and decide whether it is best to continue as planned or to interview as a group.

Although separate interviews seem desirable, they may not be possible for many reasons. Whatever the method, the primary goal is to obtain adequate and reliable information in a systematic way in order to plan, institute, and evaluate sound nursing care.

THE ADOLESCENT IN THE HOSPITAL

There are some differences in the type of contact the nurse has with the adolescent depending on whether he sees him in the hospital or somewhere in the community, such as at school or in youth centers. The adolescent's behavior will be controlled to some extent by the setting in which he is seen. For instance, being a patient in the hospital may make the adolescent feel that he must behave in a certain way. He may feel compelled to assume the role of the patient as he perceives it. Therefore, some of his true identity will not be apparent to the nurse. He may act in ways he believes are expected of him, and not as he truly feels. The nurse who helps the hospitalized adolescent to feel safe and accepted will offer him the best chance for individual expression. This can be important in helping the adolescent maintain his dignity while in an unfamiliar environment.

The environment of the hospital can be modified to aid in the adolescent's adjustment. A separate adolescent unit with comfortable furniture, stereo and television, an activities room, and possibly a snack bar is the ultimate in creating a familiar environment for teen-agers. If this is not feasible, the adolescent should at least be placed with other patients his age. The adolescent without a peer group to relate to will feel out of place on either the adult or the pediatric unit.

It is almost certain that the nurse will have contact with the adolescent's family while he is in the hospital. The nursing intervention planned will usually relate to the patient's and family's adjustment to illness and the hospital. The adolescent's major need may be to learn to accept the dependency role his illness has created, and the family may need assistance in helping the adolescent maintain his independence. The adolescent may merely resign himself to the staff and the treatments and not actively participate in his care. The adolescent and his family may be too scared of the hospital and its meaning for them to be effective in helping each other. The parents may try to protect the adolescent unnecessarily while he is ill. The adolescent may be painfully self-conscious about exposing his body to nurses and doctors. All these situations can be improved if the nurse is alert to them and able to plan appropriate intervention.

There are certain rights and privileges that can be given to the adolescent in the hospital, if his condition permits, which will help him maintain his stage of development and sense of identity. These privileges could be established as standards of care for the adolescent so that they would be provided as part of the hospital routine and without extra effort for the nursing staff. The first of these is to grant a separate interview to the adolescent so that he knows he is the patient. This has already been discussed as a means of establishing a good relationship, but it truly should be used for all adolescents and their families if they agree.

Second, the adolescent should be allowed to participate in planning his daily menu, including snacks, with the assistance of the dietitian. Even if he is on a restricted diet, there are usually choices that can be offered. This would give the patient an opportunity to make some decisions about his care, to feel important about being consulted, and to gain some information about proper nutrition.

Third, it is imperative that the adolescent be allowed contact with others his age. This may mean introducing him to other teen-agers in the hospital or permitting his friends to visit frequently. The peer group is important to the adolescent for it is primarily through them that he establishes who he is in relation to others. Severe restrictions on contact with others his age may limit his abilities in adjusting to the hospital and his illness.

Fourth, it would be of benefit to the adolescent if he were allowed some special privileges, especially if he is placed on the pediatric unit. These might include wearing his own clothes or pajamas; being allowed to leave the unit with his parents, adult visitors, or staff members as long as he signed in and out in a designated place; and setting his own time for going to sleep and getting up. Each of these privileges would have to be allowed within reasonable limits and would always be dependent on the patient's condition.

These four standards of care can be used for all adolescents, with the understanding that alternate means of allowing independent thought and action can be devised to meet individual needs. When there is an exception to the standard, it should be written into the specific plan of care for that patient, so that his hospitalization can meet his needs and hopefully become a promoter of individual growth.

THE ADOLESCENT IN THE COMMUNITY

Frequently, when the nurse sees the adolescent in the community, at school, or at youth centers, it is because the teen-ager has sought him out for help or guidance. There seems to be one group of adolescents who can identify why they came to the nurse and another group who seem to have a vague sense of having some unfulfilled needs but lack the ability to identify them. Certainly there is a third group who have problems that are apparent to the nurse of which they themselves are unaware. This group is the most difficult to reach because they do not seek help. Because of the broad scope of this situation, it cannot be covered adequately in this short chapter.

However, ideas for working with the first two groups can be presented here. Adolescents seek the nurse's help either with questions about their health or with needs relating to adjustment to a particular situation. Often the two become concurrent in the contact with the nurse. An example is the fourteen-year-old diabetic girl who frequently came to school after taking her insulin but without eating breakfast. She would experience symptoms of beginning insulin shock, be sent to the clinic by her teachers, and subsequently be sent home. One such episode resulted in her hospitalization for a week. Because the mother knew of these incidents, it was natural for the school nurse to confer with her. During the course of many separate conferences with the mother and her daughter, it was discovered that refusal to eat was this teen-ager's way of rebelling against her mother's authority. Nursing intervention in this situation had to be aimed at improving their relationship in order to safeguard the girl's health. Adjustment to health and one's relations to others seem to have great bearing on one another.

The adolescent who has identified his problems and seeks help with their solutions is really looking for a sounding board. He does not truly want to be given the answers; he wants someone on whom he can test his ideas. Therefore, the wise nurse will listen more than he talks. Explanations of why things occur as they do is often his major contribution. For instance, adolescents often ask why people act as they do, and some facts about human behavior can be offered to give him guidelines for looking at himself and others. The nurse should be careful not to offer opinions, especially about the adolescent's family or friends. The adolescent just wants to know how to judge them himself, and would eventually lose faith in the nurse who offered his own values as solutions for him. Feedback to the adolescent should help him carefully examine his own ideas and decide things for himself.

A seventeen-year-old girl reported to the school nurse that her parents were "crazy." Clearly, the nurse needed to question the girl about what led her to this conclusion. As the story unfolded, it was learned that the family had been in a serious car accident and both parents had been injured. The father was in his eighth month of unemployment with little chance of returning to work in the near future. For the first time, this family was being supported by welfare. Consciously relating these facts to the nurse gave this teen-ager many plausible reasons for her parents' behavior, and she then saw a need to support them more as real people with problems. For example, she began to help more with the housework and care of her younger brother. This girl knew there was a problem, but she had not adequately identified it.

Through her own resources, brought to recognition by the nurse, the girl was able to find a solution.

Of course, it is not always this easy for the nurse to help an adolescent identify his needs and problems. Some teen-agers' abilities are limited by their own intellectual faculties or outside influences, such as drug abuse. In these instances the nurse may need to seek additional help from expert counselors. At this point, the parents might be consulted if it would not break the confidence established with the adolescent.

The nurse who sees the adolescent in the community often has no contact with the parents. Meeting with the parents is often part of the planned intervention designed to help the teen-ager. There are certain instances when the parents cannot be involved because it would harm the relationship with the adolescent. The nurse must be prepared to take the adolescent's side at times in a family situation if he wishes to be of help. This is often difficult and seems to defy the concept of nursing the family. However, priorities must be set that will be of greatest value to the patient, and not contacting the family may be a priority. The adolescent who is taking drugs and asks the nurse to help in his attempt to stop will probably request that his family not be informed. The nurse must decide whether it would be of greater benefit to the adolescent to work with him alone or with the entire family. It is possible that through continued discussion the nurse can convince the adolescent that his family is his best source of help. In every case in which the adolescent seeks help alone, the decision of whether or not to contact the family is the primary one to be made by the nurse.

Indirect means of involving the adolescent's family can be accomplished through the nurse's attendance at and participation in parents' groups, school projects, and any activities that involve parents and their children. This can provide an excellent opportunity for meeting families and beginning relationships with them.

CONCLUSION

It can be concluded that working with adolescents usually means helping them adjust to a particular situation. They, unlike children, have the energy, talents, and resources to attack their problems, but are just learning what their abilities are, and therefore need assistance. Adults do not always give adolescents credit for being able to handle most of their adjustments, and interpreting this to the family is often necessary. Each adolescent is striving to become a unique individual in his family, among his friends, and in society; and the nurse's primary responsibility to him is to aid in his search for identity.

BIBLIOGRAPHY

Erikson, E. H.: *Identity: Youth and Crisis,* New York: W. W. Norton and Co., Inc., 1968.

————: "Establishing Standards for Nursing Practice," *American Journal of Nursing,* **69**:1458–1463, 1969.

Gordon, I. J.: *Human Development,* New York: Harper & Brothers, 1962.

Greenough, K.: "Determining Standards for Nursing Care," *American Journal of Nursing,* **68**:2153–2157, 1968.

Hammar, S. L., and J. A. Eddy: *Nursing Care of the Adolescent,* New York: Springer Publishing Co., 1966.

Lamers, W. M.: "Understanding the Teenager," *Obstetrics and Gynecology,* **33**:131–137, 1969.

Lewin, K.: "The Field Theory Approach to Adolescence," in J. M. Seidman (ed.), *The Adolescent: A Book of Readings,* rev. ed., New York: Holt, Rinehart and Winston, Inc., 1953.

Wells, K. A.: "The Adolescent's Dilemma," *Texas Medicine,* **65**:60–65, 1969.

Chapter 20

The Family with an Elderly Member

Lucille Gress

While professional nursing has long been concerned with the expanding nuclear family, there has been little attention focused upon the contracting nuclear family and the problems that arise as the remaining aged family members approach the end of the life cycle. Undoubtedly, the disruption that occurs when the aged individual must change to a new environment has as much potential for becoming a crisis episode as that occurring with the birth of a child. In either case, there is a psychological reaction that creates a state of disequilibrium until the family learns ways of coping with the change and adapts to such change. Usually assistance is sought from extrafamilial health professionals during these periods of disequilibrium. When the professional nurse becomes involved, nursing intervention must be predicated upon those principles related to psychosocial needs as well as those related to physical needs if the intervention is to be appropriate and effective.

In order to provide some basis for appreciation of the role of the nurse, a general definition of nursing and a definition of gerontological nursing will be given. In a basic definition of nursing, Henderson (1966, p. 15) states:

The unique function of the nurse is to assist the individual, sick or well, in the performance of those activities contributing to health or its recovery (or to a peaceful death) that he would perform unaided if he had the necessary strength, will or knowledge. And to do this in such a way as to help him gain independence as rapidly as possible.

Referring more specifically to care of the elderly, Stone (1971, p. 1a) writes:

Gerontological nursing is the nursing care of the elderly based on scientific knowledge from the fields of gerontology and nursing. It encompasses preventive care, maintenance and rehabilitative aspects of health care. It requires an understanding of the process of aging and its relationship to nursing intervention.

These definitions give direction to the nurse practitioner and describe the locus of practice.

In addition to direction from the definitions of nursing, the professional nurse may benefit from developing and using a conceptual framework appropriate to the chosen field of practice. Such a framework may be eclectic in nature, leaving some freedom for creativity in the development of a plan for nursing intervention.

Using a developmental conceptual framework, the family may be viewed as a social system experiencing developmental stages just as individual family members do. The family may be defined as a nuclear unit including husband, wife, and children. The nuclear family ends with the death of the last spouse. This family unit functions as a dynamic social system in an interdependent relationship with extrafamilial social systems. These social systems engage in a reciprocal give and take relationship with certain shared expectations that often are not formally stated.

An example of the interdependent relationship of the social systems may occur as the aged family member approaches the end of his life cycle. Because of the increasing dependency needs of the aged family member, assistance may be sought from an extrafamilial system. The nurse often becomes involved at this point. The family expects help with one of its traditional functions, i.e., care of its aged family member. The nurse, in turn, as he interacts with the family and assumes some responsibility for care of the aged individual, expects certain behaviors of the other family members. For example, if the aged individual is being institutionalized, provision of clothing, cosmetics, and visits from the family are expected. If the nurse chooses to conceptualize the family seeking assistance as a "patient" with certain needs, rather than to limit concern to the aged family member, he may function in a role that can be supportive of the continuing developmental process of the entire family and of individual family members.

The following case study of Mrs. Rowe (fictitious name) will provide the basis for consideration of the ways in which the professional nurse might function with the aged individual and his family. The fact that a professional nurse was not formally involved with the Rowe family does not necessarily negate the need for, or possibility of, a nursing role at that point in time. Part of the problem in terms of the nursing role, is related, no doubt, to the nurse's perception of his role in continuity of care. The nurse in the emergency room functioning within the framework of family nursing might have interpreted continuity of care and needs of the family as being part of his responsibility. His role might have become increasingly visible by means of a referral made to a community nurse who could, in turn, have worked with the family. The community nurse could have perhaps been effective in listening to the expression of feelings about the change in Mrs. Rowe's condition and the need for other arrangements for her care. Pointing out available community resources and being supportive during the institutionalization process might have enabled him to alleviate some of the feelings of anxiety of the Rowe family. Not only would this kind of nursing intervention make visible the role of the nurse in a family-centered nursing approach, it would also give visibility to the nursing role of meeting needs of the aged individual and his family, as the older person experienced the last stage of his life cycle.

CASE STUDY

Mrs. Rowe, a 67-year-old widow of Catholic faith, continued to live in her own home following the death of her husband 10 years ago. There were 13 children, the youngest died at the age of one month. The ages of the living children ranged from 28 years to 49 years. These children, 4 daughters and 8 sons, lived nearby. Of these children, one son, 28 years old, was single; two sons, aged 35 and 37 years, also single were mentally retarded and institutionalized; the rest have children of their own and were living with spouses except for the 44-year-old son who was recently widowed. He and his sons continued to maintain their own home.

Busy with her family during the years, Mrs. Rowe had not developed hobbies. She had a sixth grade education and regretted not having more. She tended to be moody and to cry frequently with little provocation. Although finances were limited, especially following the death of her husband, Mrs. Rowe managed to meet her own needs and, on occasion, extended financial help to some of her married children. The children visited at intervals as circumstances permitted, but did not assume responsibility for their mother's care, or for making decisions regarding her care, with the exception of Mrs. Green [fictitious name], the oldest daughter. Mrs. Green had been the mainstay of the entire family.

In recent months, Mrs. Rowe had been hospitalized several times because of illness related to arteriosclerotic heart disease. Mrs. Green, in seeing her mother's changing health status and recognizing her mother's increasing need for supportive care, invited her to live in her home. Other family members accepted this arrangement and continued to visit their mother as usual.

Soon after going to live in her daughter's home, Mrs. Rowe began making numerous telephone calls to various family members, often calling the same individual at frequent intervals during the day. The family attempted to set limits by asking Mrs. Rowe to make only one call to each family member daily. One son obtained an unlisted number as a means of controlling the incoming calls because his wife, under treatment for emotional problems, was disturbed by the calls.

Mrs. Rowe's sleep pattern began to change. She was up frequently at night and usually went to the refrigerator to get something to eat. One night Mrs. Green, awakened by her mother's "prowling," found Mrs. Rowe sitting on the edge of her bed eating chocolates. Melting chocolate was running down her face and dripping on her gown. Mrs. Green commented that her mother looked like a child sitting there. She did not scold her mother "because there was no use." Instead, she cleaned her up and helped her back to bed.

Mrs. Green, relating her feelings about her mother's condition, said her mother looked to her more than to the others because she was more sensitive and responsive to her mother's feelings and needs. If the rest of the family were unable to help Mrs. Rowe, she always tried to help. Mrs. Green said she loved her mother and wanted to do whatever she could to make her happy. Sometimes she was concerned with the seeming lack of attention given her mother by her brothers and sisters. She acknowledged the fact, however, that they had other family responsibilities and were concerned with financial problems.

Another change in Mrs. Rowe's behavior became obvious. Several times in the absence of Mrs. Green (beautician), Mrs. Rowe called the police and an ambulance to take her to the nearby medical center. In spite of the fact that these trips were unnecessary for medical reasons, the cost was the same as for a true emergency (four times in one week totalled $120 that was paid by Mr. and Mrs. Green). At this time, Mrs. Green began to realize that her mother could no longer be left alone.

Mr. and Mrs. Green, both nearing retirement, needed to keep on working to prepare for their own future, as well as to contribute toward the support of Mrs. Green's mentally retarded brothers and their own children. It was decided, therefore, to hire Mrs. Rowe's sister to stay with her during the day. However, this arrangement soon proved unsatisfactory. Mrs. Rowe continued to insist on making frequent telephone calls and became very agitated when attempts were made to dissuade her. On one occasion, she managed to cross the street to a neighbor's home and reported that her daughter was withholding her medication and poisoning her.

In the meantime, Mrs. Green acknowledging the fact that she could no longer cope with her mother's unpredictable behavior, began looking for a suitable nursing home. She reported feelings of ambivalence as she made the search. Taking her mother outside the family for care was in opposition to the family value system and to her mother's expressed aversion to going into a nursing home. Some of the family members expressed rejection to the idea of institutionalization for their mother, but offered no alternatives. Mr. Green, anxious about his wife's mental well-being, was supportive of the plan.

Mrs. Rowe quietly accepted going to the nursing home the day of admission. Mrs. Green, on the other hand, felt more uncomfortable than ever. Lack of the "common courtesy of a greeting" from the staff necessitated inquiry as to where to leave her mother and added to the feeling of "coldness" she experienced. Overhearing an aide "threatening an elderly man with a cold shower if he became incontinent," did little to relieve her anxiety and concern for her mother's welfare. "I almost gathered my Mom up and brought her back with me," she said in recounting the experience.

Since the staff, composed of a registered nurse, licensed practical nurses and nurse aides, did not ask for any information, Mrs. Green was uncertain if they had a telephone number in case of emergency. She decided to visit her mother after work to see how things were going. In the meantime, because of her anxiety and concern, she called the social worker on the case to determine whether or not the admission procedure in this situation was the usual approach.

During the early postadmission period, Mrs. Rowe began to have crying spells. The staff was puzzled about the reason for the episodes but assured Mrs. Green that her mother was receiving good care.

Mrs. Green said that although she felt the right decision was made regarding institutionalizing her mother, she was saddened by the thought that she could not take care of her mother during her time of dependency as her mother did for her when she was a baby.

Although the role of the professional nurse is hardly visible in the case of Mrs. Rowe, functions of a nurse in the role will be explored in the analysis of the case.

THE ROLE OF THE NURSE

Perhaps a look at the role of the nurse as it developed historically is a useful way to point out why the role of the nurse is being considered. According to Virginia Stone (1970, p. 106):

> In the past nursing care of older people was delegated to the good natured, kind, ill prepared people with kind feelings toward old people.

However, because more people are living longer and are being cared for in institutional settings and because consideration is beginning to be given to a quality of life that is more satisfying, the need for nurses prepared to function in a different way is essential. Having lived longer, with the likelihood of becoming more differentiated, aged individuals have some needs that are unique in addition to those needs held in common with their fellow human beings. Rights of the aged are being recognized with societal expectation tending toward respect of those rights in terms of health care. Equal status recently given by organized nursing to geriatric nursing with other specialities, such as medical-surgical nursing, has been cited by Stone (1970, p. 108) as reflecting this trend and is indicative of the need for reexamining the role of the professional nurse.

No longer is it acceptable for nursing practice to be based upon intuition or to have those nurses who think of care of the aged as being out of the "mainstream" of nursing responsibilities, be responsible for care of the elderly. Rather, the professional nurse should be prepared to work with the elderly and their families wherever they are developmentally, or on the wellness-illness continuum. In this role, the nurse is changing from functioning as a custodian of aged individuals to functioning as a "counselor, teacher, researcher, consultant, and patient-side practitioner" (Davis, 1968b, p. 1106).

An analogue of the development of the role of the nurse might be made to the development of the aged individual. The nursing role, developing over a long period of time, is also becoming more differentiated. While there are areas contributing toward the development of specialities in nursing practice, i.e., pediatric nursing, coronary care nursing, geriatric or gerontological nursing, there are components of nursing shared with practitioners in any locus of practice. The differential in gerontological nursing arises out of the physical and psychosocial needs of the aged individual and his family, according to their individual and collective developmental levels and where they are on the wellness-illness continuum. Just as the aged individual should be viewed as a member of his family rather than a separate entity, the role of the gerontological nurse should be viewed within the context of the "whole" of nursing. In order for the nurse to function effectively with the aged individual and his family, knowledge of the developmental levels of the individual and his family and the aging process is essential.

ASSESSMENT

Regardless of whether the nurse's initial contact with the family occurs during a relatively quiescent period of development, or during a time of disruption and crisis as in the case of Mrs. Rowe, an assessment of the family and its needs should be started.

Assessment, in this case, may be defined as the process of collecting data as a means of learning about the family and acquiring information that will provide the basis for nursing intervention. Setting of priorities should be determined by the present needs of the family. Since the family is assumed to be in a continuing state of development, the need for a continuing process of assessment is implied.

Assessment in the case of Mrs. Rowe will be made within a modified developmental conceptual framework of the family. Concepts from the crisis theory will be incorporated into the framework to allow for a more comprehensive assessment. While the modified developmental conceptual framework of the family will be used here, it is well to acknowledge that other conceptual frameworks might be equally useful. The crucial factor hinges upon use of a more formalized, systematic, and deliberative approach to nursing intervention. Assessment can be an important part of formalizing the nursing process.

The focus of the assessment in this situation will be upon the psychosocial parameters. This is not to deny the need for assessment of physical parameters, but is in cognizance of the impact of institutionalization and the importance of preventing depersonalization. Usually, attention is given to the more obvious physical needs almost to the exclusion of attention to the psychosocial needs. In an institution providing long-term care for the aged, it is important to help the aged individual to retain his personal identity and his identity within the family group. This task is facilitated by assessment of the family dynamics.

In beginning assessment of the family, the nurse should observe the interaction of family members as a means of learning about the dynamics of their relationship. The level of anxiety of family members should be assessed during the process of institutionalization. Although Mrs. Rowe and her daughter were the only family members present initially, the composition of the family as a whole and where they lived could have been a part of the data obtained. Additional information about the strengths and weaknesses of the family might also have been elicited. During such an assessment process, the nurse would have an opportunity to convey understanding and empathy to the family. This interchange should be helpful in decreasing the level of anxiety and in building a trusting relationship that would enable the family to feel more comfortable in expressing their concerns verbally.

The impact of institutionalization should have been explored with Mrs. Rowe and her daughter. Institutionalization constitutes a crisis episode for many aged individuals and their families. According to crisis theory, the family should be more open to therapeutic intervention during periods of disequilibrium, therefore, the nurse-family interaction at this point may markedly influence the outcome of the crisis episode. Providing opportunity for these family members to express their feelings and offering support while they do so, should be helpful in relieving some of their anxiety and contributing toward initiation of the coping process.

It is important for the nurse to have an understanding of some of the factors contributing to the impact of institutionalization. The Rowe family, after exhausting its own resources, sought help from an extrafamilial institution. Separation anxiety occurring in the anticipated loss of privacy for family intimacy and realization of the ultimate separation by death, probably influenced the reaction of the family. Families often experience guilt feelings about institutionalizing their aged family member while the aged individual often experiences feelings of rejection and abandonment. This reaction is not unusual in spite of the fact that institutionalization seems to be the only viable alternative to care of the older person. Taking these factors into account and having knowledge of the increased mortality rate that occurs in the immediate postadmission period, the nurse should carefully examine ways in which he can interact responsibly with the aged individual and his family.

A more detailed assessment of the aged individual than of the family as a whole is necessary. Although the primary emphasis in this situation is on the psychosocial parameters, the physical parameters cannot be completely ignored. These parameters are so closely related that it is difficult to separate them for the purpose of analysis. Focus on the psychosocial dimension, in this case, is to point out the tendency to overlook psychosocial factors that also influence the well-being of aged individuals. The impact of institutionalization and the potential for depersonalization are documented in research findings. Since reaction to institutionalization occurs over time, there is need for a continuing assessment of the aged individual, including his way of coping with the major change in environment.

In most cases, a physical examination is a part of the admission requirement and provides some useful information. However, the nurse should also make some physical assessment of the older person. For example, Mrs. Rowe was quiet at the time of admission to the nursing home. Did she give any indication of hearing impairment, i.e., lip reading, inappropriate responses to questions? Sensory loss may be the result of impacted cerumen and temporary or permanent pathological change in the eighth crainial nerve. On the other hand, was Mrs. Rowe's quiet manner a reflection of feelings about institutionalization and the marked change in environment? The nurse should make an assessment with interpretation of the data and exercise judgment in determining the appropriate nursing intervention.

Physical assessment should be useful in determining capacity to perform activities of daily living such as ambulation, dressing, eating, toileting, and bathing. Such assessment of functional ability should also include attention to any help that might be necessary, or to aids needed to support ability for self-care, such as a hearing aid, a walker, or special eating utensils. Eliciting this kind of information conveys interest in the individual and is useful in helping the person make an easier transition into the nursing home setting. Observation of the individual's normal pacing of activities should be made to facilitate planning that would avoid rushing the person beyond his capacity.

Hurrying the individual sometimes leads to confusion and does not give the individual time to do what he could do for himself.

Mental status should be assessed in an effort to learn the person's ability to initiate and carry on usual activities. Orientation to time, person, and place is a part of this assessment. The amount of freedom allowed, or supervision required, is partially determined by this assessment.

Since Mrs. Rowe was a new admission, she and her daughter had a right to be oriented to the nursing home environment. During the orientation further assessment of Mrs. Rowe's mental status could have been made. Learning how she interacted with other residents would have given some idea of her ability to socialize. Simple testing of her ability to recall the location of her assigned room, and certain other areas, might have been helpful in evaluating mental ability. Additional observation of the interaction between Mrs. Rowe and her daughter could have been made during the tour of the nursing home. Other information about Mrs. Rowe's care and previous life style might have been elicited at this time.

Assessment of emotional status may be a means of picking up information regarding behavior patterns and predictability of behavior. Mrs. Rowe's history of frequent crying episodes shows a tendency toward a labile emotional status. Given this information, the nurse should explore further to try to determine what triggers this behavior and how to effectively support Mrs. Rowe. If change occurs in emotional status that may be the result of pathological processes, the family may need help in learning how to cope with the change. Effort should be made to prevent the family from becoming unduly emotional, thus diminishing its coping ability. In any case, an attempt should be made to identify any correctable problems that might be disturbing to the emotionally labile aged individual and to learn ways of dealing appropriately with the disturbed individual and his family.

Additional information about other family members to determine their reactions to the institutionalization of Mrs. Rowe might be helpful in assessing their possible need for counseling. Some family members find it hard to visit the individual in the nursing home. In some situations this may be because of problems with transportation. In others, it may be that the psychological reaction to the institutionalization is an inhibiting factor. Working within the conceptual developmental framework of the family makes it imperative to identify the problems if the nurse is to discharge responsibility for preventive care, maintenance, and rehabilitative aspects of health care of the aged individual and his family. The nurse must seek to determine ways of helping the family to learn how to use its capacities to continue development of potential for meaningful family relationships.

To assess the role of the nurse in the Rowe case necessitates calling attention to the basic developmental task of the nurse/family in the nursing home situation. This task is that of developing a trusting relationship. The fact that the role of the nurse is unclear in this case does not rule out the need for a nurse who will define and clarify the role in the interaction with the aged person and his family. If the nurse is unable to meet with the family, he should have a staff that is prepared and expected to extend a warm greeting to the family experiencing the crisis of institutionalization. This is important in establishing a trusting relationship.

One of the major nursing goals in the Rowe case, and other similar situations, should be to prevent depersonalization. This goal should pervade the total of the nurse/family interaction. Health for the older person and his family in the nursing home experience depends, to a great extent, on the continuing interaction of individual family members in a supportive and affectional relationship. The knowledgeable nurse functioning in an effective role will be sensitive to the human needs of these people. He will be seeking to promote continuing growth and development of potential for a more satisfying experience for all concerned.

The professional nurse role can be further developed in the nurse/family interchange during the crisis episode related to institutionalization of the aged family member by use of available knowledge and skills in a responsible way. To formalize and systematize a deliberative nursing approach is to take nursing out of the realm of intuition through application of principles of the behavioral, social, and physical sciences. Assessment is an important part of the deliberative nursing process. The outcome of the nursing intervention under such conditions should be the enrichment of the living experience of the aged individual and his family wherever they are in the life cycle. This process should also bring fulfillment to the nurse experiencing the nursing role in dynamic interchange with the family.

To paraphrase Schwartz (1969, p. 79), the unique function of nursing centers upon care of families seeking health care in situations in which they lack the ability or knowledge to care for themselves. If the professional nurse is to accept the challenge and act responsibly, he will need to use his knowledge and apply skills important to the humaness of the aged person and his family as well as skills important to physical well-being.

BIBLIOGRAPHY

Ackerman, W.: *The Psychodynamics of Family Life,* New York: Basic Books, Inc., Publishers, 1958.

Benjamin, F.: "The Role of the Geriatric Nurse in Health Maintenance," *Geriatrics,* **22**:58–64, 1967.

Brody, E. M., and G. M. Spark: "Institutionalization of the Aged: A Family Crisis," *Family Process,* **5**:76–90, 1966.

Brown, M. M.: "Personalization of the Institutionalized Older Patient," *ANA Clinical Sessions*, American Nurses' Association, 1969, New York: Appleton-Century-Crofts, Inc., 1969, pp. 118-124.

Davis, B. A.: "ANA and the Geriatric Nurse," *Nursing Clinics of North America*, 3:741-748, 1968*a*.

————: "Coming of Age: A Challenge for Geriatric Nursing," *Journal of the American Geriatrics Society*, 16:1100-1106, 1968*b*.

Deutsch, S., and B. Krasner: "Meeting the Needs of the Patient through Comprehensive Planning," *Journal of Geriatric Psychiatry*, 3:107-120, 1969.

Henderson, V.: *The Nature of Nursing*, New York: The Macmillan Company, 1966.

Kalis, B. L.: "Crisis Theory: Its Relevance for Community Psychology and Directions for Development," in D. Adelson and B. L. Kalis (eds.), *Community Psychology and Mental Health*, Pennsylvania: Chandler Publishing Company, 1970, pp. 69-88.

Kent, E. A.: "Role of Admission Stress in Adaptation of Older Persons in Institutions," *Geriatrics*, 18:133-138, 1963.

Knoll Pharmaceutical Company: "Psychodynamics in Extended Care of the Aged: Illness, Loss of Function: A Special Kind of Stress," *Geriatric Focus*, 6:1, 56, 1967.

Knowles, L. N.: "Nursing Care to Increase Older Patient's Potential in Potentialities for Later Living: A Report on the 17th Annual Southern Conference on Gerontology, University of Florida, February 4-6, 1968," Gainesville, Fla.: University of Florida Press, 1968, pp. 53-62.

Lawton, M. P.: "The Functional Assessment of Elderly People," *Journal of the American Geriatrics Society*, 19:465-481, 1971.

Leiberman, A.: "Institutionalization of the Aged: Effects on Behavior," *Journal of Gerontology*, 24:330-340, 1969.

Parad, H. J. (ed.): *Crisis Intervention: Selected Readings*, New York: Family Service Association of America, 1965.

Robischon, P.: "The Challenge of Crisis Theory for Nursing," *Nursing Outlook*, 15:28-32, 1967.

Schwartz, E.: "Aging and the Field of Nursing," in M. W. Riley (ed.), *Aging and Society: Aging and the Professions*, New York: The Russell Sage Foundation, 1969, p. 79.

Shaughnessy, E.: "Emotional Problems of Patients in Nursing Homes," *Journal of Geriatric Psychiatry*, 1:159-166, 1968.

Spark, M., and E. M. Brody: "The Aged Are Family Members," *Family Process*, 9:195-210, 1970.

Stone, V.: *Gerontological Nursing*, Student Syllabus, Evanston, Ill.: Video Nursing, Inc., 1971, p. 1*a*.

————: "Nursing Services to Meet the Needs of the Aged," in M. Field (ed.), *Depth and Extent of the Geriatric Problem*, Springfield, Ill.: Charles C Thomas, Publisher, 1970, pp. 106-116.

Part Three

The Family in Crisis

The chapters in Part Three illustrate a variety of crisis events that families may encounter during their life-spans. This is not to say that these are the only critical situations families experience; rather they represent a variety of critical events from which commonalities can be identified and applied to other family crisis situations.

Crisis theory as it relates to families is presented, followed by examples of its application when working with families facing stresses such as physical, mental, emotional, and behavioral handicaps.

Chapter 21

Theories of Family Crisis

Carolyn Brose

Increased interest has been focused in the last few years on crisis and crisis intervention. Much attention has been given to psychological and mental health crisis since the consequences of crisis management often have significant and long-lasting effects on the level of a person's mental functioning (Bloom, 1963, p. 498). Crisis theorists have shown that crisis situations have predictable outcomes and that timely intervention will greatly influence the predicted result. Not only can intervention affect the outcome of the actual crisis, but also it can influence the adaptation or maladaptation that the person will continue to make to the situation. For some people, the changes wrought by crisis may mean increased health and maturity; while for others the changes may be the beginning of incapacity to deal effectively with life's problems.

From the physiological point of view, crisis intervention may entail life and death situations. Death from trauma, especially in our age of increasing power and speed potential, added to acute, life-threatening medical emergencies such as myocardial infarctions, accentuates the need for crisis intervention. Despite the movement of the medical health systems in the direction of preventive medicine versus acute, episodic care, one cannot negate the need for a functional crisis-oriented system to provide life support for the physiological crisis. Immediate action must be taken in the true physiological crisis if the organism is to survive. The biggest problem seems to be one of a gap between knowledge and its application.

CRISIS DEFINITIONS

Today, *crisis* is almost a household word. We hear of the political crisis, the international crisis, the economic crisis, and the drug crisis, to mention only a few. Often we hear *crisis* used interchangeably with *stress* (Selye, 1956) because both terms imply actual or potential disruption of the stable state of those involved.

A leading crisis theorist, Gerald Caplan, and his colleagues have described crisis as an "upset in the steady state" (Caplan, 1964, p. 40; Parad, 1965). They believe a crisis is produced when a person finds his usual methods of problem solving ineffective when coping with an obstacle to important life goals. Fink defines crisis as "an event in which the individual's normal coping abilities are inadequate to meet the demands of the situation" (1967, p. 592). Miller and Iscoe present crisis as "the experiencing of an acute situation where one's repertoire of coping responses is inadequate in effecting a resolution of the stress" (1963, p. 196). Bloom states that crisis will vary in severity as determined by the degree of reorganization required to cope with the situation and that a crisis represents a turning point in one's life. The crisis, therefore, necessitates a reorganization of some of the important aspects of the individual's structure (Bloom, 1963, p. 498).

McHugh (1960, p. 227) describes a crisis as an event which disturbs the equilibrium of social relationships in a situation. Erikson (1965) expands the definition by classifying crises as *developmental* (maturational) or *situational* (accidental). A situational crisis is an external event or stress, such as illness or death of a loved one. Developmental, or maturational, crisis is a normal and expected occurrence in the process of one's psychosocial development. Puberty, courtship, marriage, pregnancy, and menopause are examples of developmental times of increased susceptibility to crisis. Developmental and situational crises may occur simultaneously, as in the case of the adolescent facing hospitalization. It appears evident that crisis may assume different forms to different persons or even to the same person at different times. Although these definitions vary, we might generalize to say that crisis involves a threat, either real or implied, to the person or persons involved, even though the threat may take different forms.

RESPONSE TO A CRISIS SITUATION: THE BYSTANDER

It is important that the nurse have an understanding of the actions and reactions that may occur in a crisis. If the nurse understands possible response mechanisms, their causes and meanings, he is better equipped to cope with his own responses as well as those of the victim, family, and bystanders. He may also better understand the effect of crisis on the victim and his ability or inability to make decisions for himself, and perhaps use other resources available to him.

To fully appreciate crisis responses, we should look at both the bystander's and the victim's points of view. A great deal of the bystander's behavior can be explained by listing the characteristics of an emergency situation (Latanè and Darley, 1969). Threat is inherent in an emergency, perhaps to one's well-being, life, or property. Rewards for successful intervention in an emergency, such as self-satisfaction, public recognition, or even financial reward, are possible but may be difficult to assess in value. On the other hand, one must consider that the rescuer often must put his own life in danger, if he is to aid the victim. A man standing at the water's edge, hearing the call for help from a drowning man, must decide within himself the potential cost. Will he take the risk of losing his own life in an attempt to save another's? Does he consider the possibility of endangering his own family's support if he is drowned in the attempt? At the scene of an auto accident, will he attempt to give care to the injured, even though he may be sued for his well-intentioned actions? Witnessing a mugging, will he go to the aid of the victim and perhaps be required to appear in court as a witness against the assailant? How much time, effort, and funds will such follow-up activities take? Would it be easier to not get involved? Is he prepared in the first place to intervene?

An emergency is a rare event. Statisticians have presented evidence that truly critical medical emergencies may occur only once or twice to a person during his lifetime. Other statistics indicate that, on the average, a person may encounter fewer than six serious emergencies of all types in his lifetime. It becomes obvious that the individual is poorly prepared to meet these emergencies. Man, who is used to adapting to new situations by recalling previous situations, will find he has limited reference experience to guide him in a new crisis. He is much like the actor who is thrust onto the stage to perform a new role without the benefit of rehearsal.

Another basic characteristic of emergencies is that they differ in type and character. Problems presented to the rescuer of the drowning man and those presented to the rescuer of a potential suicide victim are vastly different. The nurse faced with a patient on a bad LSD trip finds different problems than the nurse caring for a patient who has been severely burned. Just as the situations are different, so are the actions to be taken.

Emergencies are unforeseen events which arrive suddenly, with little or no warning. Time to think through feasible courses of actions and alternatives is denied. Immediate action is a necessity. Time to consult with others of greater knowledge and experience cannot usually be taken. The individual *must* act if the condition is to be rectified. Stress will begin to influence him. How then will he perform? Will the effect of the stress spur him to greater action, or will the stress level be of such a degree that he will become immobile under its influence? This depends a great deal on the individual and his previous exposure and manner (coping mechanisms) with which he has been able to function under other stresses.

Another important element in the understanding of reactions to crisis is the decision-making processes that are inherent in each situation. Before a person can intervene in a crisis situation, he must in fact recognize that a crisis exists. That is, he must be aware that an event is taking place and must also decide if something is awry.

As you hurry down a busy street crowded with shoppers, do you notice the young man leaning in the doorway of a building, clutching his abdomen and moaning? Or, is your mind crowded with the pressures of the day, and the young man goes unnoticed in the crowd? Let us assume that you have seen him. You must now decide if there is something wrong. In our culture, we are hesitant to be too observing of others, especially strangers. For example, have you ever felt the flush of unexplained embarrassment when you realize that you are unwittingly caught staring at another, or vice versa? It is not polite to stare or gape at another person. It is not proper to examine another, especially a stranger. Another factor that may influence your decision is the young man's mode of dress. Is he clean-shaven and neatly dressed in a suit; or is he a hippie with beard, beads, and long hair? Maybe he is on dope or on a "bad trip." Maybe he is pretending to be ill to lure a victim to him, whom he will then assault. Even if you have decided that something is wrong, will you next make the decision to take on the responsibility of action? If you do, you must next decide what form of aid is needed and how its implementation will be carried out. Finally, you must decide where your responsibility for the young man ends.

As has just been demonstrated, a series of decisions must be made if one is to intervene in a crisis. A logical sequence of decisions is rarely made. The bystander may overlook some decisions, or he may simultaneously make several decisions and vacillate between possible actions and outcomes before he actually initiates intervention. The bystander, therefore, is not an objective observer. He is caught up in the crisis. His emotional level is probably high.

Social determinants also will strongly affect the decision-making process and, therefore, the intervention or lack of intervention that occurs. An individual will be strongly influenced by the decisions he perceives others to be making. Let us return to the young man in the street. If, while he leans against the building and moans, people hurry by him with only side glances and indicate by their behavior that nothing is out of the ordinary, you are apt to follow suit. This behavior is demonstrated by one who goes to a very formal dinner with copious quantities of silverware on the table. He will watch the behavior of others—what spoon or fork is picked up first and used in what manner. In strange situations, we check others for cues of how we are expected to perform. As a result, in our case of the young man, the inaction of other passersby may present the situation as less serious than perhaps you would determine if you were alone.

Not only will the perceived decisions that others are making influence your actions, but also the knowledge that others are watching your behavior will affect your decision. To be a "good nurse" you must remain calm and poised in the face of crisis. To show emotion or undue concern would possibly open the door to ridicule and weaken your professional image. In the hospital setting, emotion or undue concern may be equated with inexperience or lack of knowledge. Therefore, it is very possible, even in the hospital, to misjudge the seriousness of a crisis when behavioral cues alone are taken. One needs to remain calm and collected to function effectively, but too much calm can be calamitous for the patient.

There is safety in numbers, or is there? Research has shown that when faced with a stressful situation, most people do seem less afraid when they are in the presence of others than if they are alone. (Latanè and Darley, 1969, p. 266; Latanè, 1969, pp. 61-69; Latanè, 1968, pp. 142-146). Who does not find comfort in the fact that there are many others moving about the street on a dark, misty night? What nurse has not found comfort in the knowledge that his supervisor and peers from other units can come to his aid if he calls? We may feel our chances for assistance are greater with a greater number of people around us. Research has disproven this (Latanè and Darley, 1969, p. 249; Darley and Latanè, 1968; Latanè and Darley, 1968).

Take, for example, the reports in the newspapers in 1963 of a young woman in New York City coming home from work in the early hours of the morning and being attacked by a maniac. Her cries for help attracted a total of thirty-eight neighbors and witnesses, surely enough people to overpower her attacker and rescue the victim. These people watched for over half an hour while the maniac slowly killed his victim. Such incidents have spurred research into bystander apathy. These studies have shown that the greater the number of people who witness a crisis situation, the less likely the victim is to receive aid. This information has also filtered into the lay literature (Blank, 1970, p. 73).

We have already presented some of the possible causes of the reluctance to offer aid in the presence of others. Real or potential threat to his own life, fear of litigation against him for his efforts, unwillingness to "appear against" the wrongdoer, and the inaction of others can encourage a person not to become involved. However, other factors should also be considered. In a large crowd of onlookers, who has the responsibility of stepping forward and taking charge? Should the bystander in a crowd rush to a phone to summon an ambulance or the police, or has someone already called for help? Are his efforts necessary or will they be wasted? While responsibility can be delegated to an individual, for example, to the surgical resident in the emergency room who is responsible for the management of all cases of serious trauma, who is responsible when the designated person is absent? No one, everyone, or someone else?

The sins of omission and commission are equally important in the action that a person takes in face of an emergency. This is still a persistent concern to physicians and nurses despite the Good Samaritan Laws which have been passed in many states (Chayet, 1969, pp. 275-294). If a person witnesses an emergency situation alone, he then bears the total responsibility for his action or inaction. But, if there are others who also witness the emergency, the blame is diffused and not focused on any one person. Courts may decide such cases on the basis of what was "wise and prudent" for a person of his training and experience to have done. A nurse, who has been trained to give care, is held more responsible for providing such care than a person without such training. He may have been off duty at the time of the emergency, but he is, nevertheless, a nurse, on duty or off.

Research has shown that people are more willing to take the chance of exposure and action when in the presence of friends than when in the presence of strangers (Latane and Darley, 1969, p. 263). If the emergency is witnessed by a group of friends rather than by a group of total strangers, the victim will be somewhat more apt to receive aid. In view of the decisions that one must make and the forces that impinge upon the decision-making process in the face of a crisis situation, it becomes almost a miracle that intervention ever occurs.

RESPONSE TO CRISIS FROM THE VICTIM'S POINT OF VIEW

Fink (1967, p. 592) has presented a theoretical model of changes which he feels occur in the person who is experiencing a crisis situation. This model is a useful one, for it provides the professional with a systematic organization of events that otherwise appear chaotic and incomprehensible. As such, this model offers information on what behavior the rescuer might expect from the victim, as well as the type of aid that would best be given and its timing.

The model consists of four sequential phases: (1) shock, (2) defensive retreat, (3) acknowledgment, (4) adaptation. Each of these phases is described in terms of self-experience, reality perception, emotional experience, and cognitive structure (see Table 21-1).

Table 21-1 Psychologic Phases of Crisis

Phase	Self-Experience	Reality Perception	Emotional experience	Cognitive structure	Physical parallels	Social parallels
Shock (impact)	Depersonalization	Sharp, clear; "objective"	None; possible euphoria; indifference	Organized; automatic functioning	Shock; emergency reactions	Individual centering; associality; docility
Realization	Collapse of existing structure	Reality seems overwhelming	Panic; high anxiety; helplessness	Inability to plan, reason, or understand situation	Objective somatic damage requiring immediate care	Breakdown of ordinary social controls; chaos
Defensive retreat	Attempt to reestablish previous identity	Avoidance of reality; wishful thinking; denial	Indifference or euphoria except when challenged, in which case, anger	Progressive rigidity; situation-bound thinking; resistance to change	Recovery from acute phase; rapid improvement. Treatment plans solidify	Authoritarian control; tightening of structure; use or organized force
Acknowledgment	Disintegration; self-depreciation	Reality "imposes itself"	Depression; apathy, or agitation, or bitterness. If overwhelming, suicide	Disorganization; reorganization in accord with altered reality perceptions	Physical plateau. Rate of improvement slows	Recognition of inadequacies in old system; re-evaluation of structure; plan for change
Adaptation; change	New identity appears; new sense of personal worth	Reality testing; mastery efforts	Anxiety decreases; satisfaction increases	Stabilization of reorganization; integration with earlier structure	"Functional improvement" with no change in actual disability status	Repatterning of behavior and environment to cope with or avoid future similar crises

The shock phase represents the individual's first moments of encounter with the crisis situation. This phase may last only a few minutes or may extend over a period of hours.

Shontz (1964) has divided the shock phase into two periods. The first period is the *impact phase,* in which the person understands that "something is wrong." For example, the mill worker reaches full realization that his hand has just been severed by his machine, yet he may not panic or express overwhelming anguish at what has just happened. Rather, he appears to become emotionally numb. He clearly understands that he has just lost his hand, but he is unable to formulate a plan of action to cope with the situation. He is at a prime stage for help and will be submissive to the will of others. Depersonalization will begin, and he will not see himself as the one who has just lost the hand. It is obvious that the victim should not be required nor expected to make decisions regarding his care or well-being. Someone else must formulate a plan of action and communicate this plan to the victim, if the situation is to be managed efficiently.

The second period of the shock phase, as reported by Shontz, is *realization,* when panic begins to set in. At this point, the victim may be overwhelmed by what has happened to him because the situation may appear totally hopeless. His anxieties may soar. Although he may begin to feel the need to plan a course of action, he is unable to do so because of his clouded perceptions and high level of anxiety. At this stage, he will usually be very open to suggestions. Help might need to be presented to him in a very firm and decisive manner in order for him to control his own behavior and cooperate with the rescuer's efforts. During this stage, attention is focused upon the damage and its repair. It is during this stage that the victim is usually first seen by the nurse or physician. The total phase of realization may last for weeks or be reasonably brief.

The next stage into which the individual will move is that of *defensive retreat.* This stage can be compared with the "fight or flight" behavior exhibited by an organism under attack. The victim will seek ways in which to lower the stress he feels at the moment. Reality will become an element which he will attempt to avoid. He may express anger, and denial may begin.

Denial should be considered in the victim's response to a crisis as it is very much a part of one's reaction to the stressful event. Denial becomes a useful tool, which the victim uses in attempting to maintain some degree of equilibrium during a period of disorganization. As such, denial becomes a normal and inevitable response to a crisis. Just as a crisis event will vary in severity, so will the degree of denial that may be exhibited.

With a serious crisis, however, denial cannot be maintained. According to Shontz, a person has three alternatives: (1) withdraw entirely from the situation, (2) express anger or despair, or (3) yield, or succumb, to the disorganization and disruption imposed by the situation. If the victim withdraws, he then must find gratifications and his being in a fantasy world. If he expresses anger or despair, he will have resorted to destructive emotions; and a constructive solution to the situation will not be forthcoming. If the victim yields, he has at least broached upon the vital element of realism.

It is during the response of yielding that many medically trained persons lose grasp of what is happening to the victim. If the victim "yields" by hysterical outbursts of crying, the physician or nurse may see this as unacceptable and annoying behavior. This behavior is, in fact, acceptable for the victim at that particular time. The victim, by yielding, has let reality overwhelm him. The passive, very quiet, stoic patient might be completely denying and avoiding all contact with reality. This reaction is obviously not healthful and should not be allowed to continue. The nurse and/or physician must try to see the crisis from the patient's point of view, rather than viewing it in coldly objective reality.

Take, for example, a young woman who is brought into the emergency room after sustaining facial lacerations in an auto accident. Despite reassurances that her injuries are not serious, she continues to cry hysterically. The emergency room staff becomes increasingly annoyed with the patient because she is not responding correctly as gauged by the reality of the situation. Unknown to the staff, however, this young woman is a model, and she equates the facial lacerations with scarring and potential loss of her livelihood. She is overwhelmed and cannot think in rational terms, such as plastic revision of any scarring.

Unless the victim totally maladapts, he will not be able to forever suppress reality. Finally, he will move into the stage of *acknowledgment*. This becomes a period of increased stress for the victim, as he not only *recognizes* reality but also is forced to *accept* reality. This phase is a gradual one which may last a period of years, and perhaps the rest of the victim's life.

The final phase is that of *adaptation*. Shontz emphasizes that adaptation necessitates a change, not a resumption of preexisting structure. A reorganization, a restructuring, and a new approach to management of life's demands constitute adaptation to a crisis situation.

GENERALIZATIONS

If one were to combine the previously mentioned observations of crisis theory and intervention with other related studies, four major generalizations might be made. The first is that whether a person emerges stronger or weaker as a result of crisis experience is not based so much on his previous character makeup as on the kind of help he receives during the actual crisis (Caplan, 1964, p. 53). This fact places great responsibility upon the nurse who is faced with the patient and/or family who is in a crisis situation. He must recognize that a crisis exists and attempt to understand the impact on the family. He must render "crisis care" or call upon others to assist him with the patient and/or family. It is important to realize that there may be others, for example, a social worker, physician, or minister, who may be more effective as the "crisis manager." This utilization of others should not be a mode of escape, however, for the nurse who would rather evade responsibility for crisis management.

The second generalization is that people become more amenable to suggestions and open to help during the actual crisis (Brandon, 1970, p. 631; Robischon, 1967, p. 29; Caplan, 1964, p. 53). In the hospital setting, this fact means that the responsibility for dealing with the crisis is assumed by the emergency room nurse, by the intensive care nurse, and by the floor nurse. As time passes, even the community health nurse should assume some of the intervention role. The ideal opportunity and time to render aid is now.

Family support is also very important. The person who is in crisis needs the support and encouragement of those closest to him. The family can help the person by acknowledging that he is in trouble and that they are concerned (Caplan, 1964, pp. 44-47). It must be emphasized that the family may need support from the nurse or others in order to recognize this need and to cope with it effectively. The basic strength of the family must also be considered. If the family is crisis prone, consistently passing from one crisis to another, resolution and opportunity for growth and maturation may never be realized. Maladaptive behavior may be encouraged by this type of family because they have not yet learned effective ways of coping with the stress of life. Cultural factors are also relevant. The person's cultural heritage may have prepared him to be able to deal with the more complex problems (Brandon, 1970, p. 628).

The need for the nurse to be keenly aware of the family and to assess the family as well as individual patient should be self-evident if optimum crisis care is to be realized. Take, for example, the family of a sixteen-year-old boy who was brought to the emergency room by the police after he was apprehended during an armed robbery attempt on a bank. The staff's primary concern was quickly directed to physical care, since the youth had sustained a gunshot wound resulting in a sucking chest wound. After the physical crisis was stabilized, attention could then be diverted to the psychosocial crisis, considered from both developmental and situational crisis standpoints. Here was an adolescent (developmental crisis-prone time) facing a life-threatening physical crisis as well as a situational crisis, a felony charge. The family situation was assessed as malignant. The mother came into the emergency room where she was first detained and questioned by FBI agents. When she was allowed to see her son, she stood at a distance from the cart for several minutes in stony silence. Her only comment was, "Who was in on this with you?" The boy stared at the ceiling and yelled, "No one!" At this point, the mother left the room and refused to accompany her son to the hospital unit. Brief assessment of the family from an interview with the mother yielded the following information. This was a crisis-prone family. Their life was a long series of one crisis followed by another, none of which appeared to result in maturation or growth for the family. The family was of a lower-socioeconomic level and daily faced crucial financial problems of providing the essentials of living. There had been no stable father figure in the home. All the children over fourteen years of age had dropped out of school. One older son was in prison, convicted of assault with a deadly weapon. It is obvious that this family will most likely be unable to cope with the new crisis in an acceptable manner. The addition of the act of crime, subsequently resulting in the injury, further isolated the victim from some type of family support. The identical injury, if it had been sustained accidentally, might have mobilized greater support.

The nurse in the emergency room will not be able to deal with all the problems involved; however, he should be aware of their presence and base his involvement upon assessment of the patient and family. He should then convey his information, along with the need for additional information, to the floor nurse and others needed to cope with the crisis resolution. The crisis for this family will not be resolved in a short period of time. It may take many weeks, months, or years, and many people assisting the family and boy to adjust. Hopefully, the emergency room nurse will start the intervention to help this family learn to better cope with the crisis and emerge as a more healthy entity.

A third generalization is that with the onset of a crisis situation, old memories of past crises may be evoked. If maladaptive behavior was used to deal with previous situations, the same type of behavior may be repeated in the face of the new crisis. Another example of this behavior was reported by Hiatt and Spurlock (1970, p. 53) as what they term *geographical flight*. This behavior is a "pattern of travel wherein motionless and geographical fleeing has become a chronically episodic way of coping—characteristic of a way of life or life style." The onset of the flight coping mechanism appears to begin in childhood, for example, in the runaway child.

A fourth generalization is that the only way to survive a crisis is to be aware of its existence. This generalization is reinforced by the work done by Lindemann on the Coconut Grove fire and the process of grieving (1965, pp. 7–21). He concluded that people who adjusted stoically to their loss (denied the loss to a degree) were, in the long run, the ones who suffered the most, as evidenced by the decline in their mental health in the following years. Lindemann pointed out the need to face the fact of death and to go through a grieving process.

Related to the preceding generalizations, Cadden (1964, pp. 288-296) has listed seven ways which she feels a person can help another who is in crisis:

1 Help the victim to confront reality. Help him to speak of his unspoken fears. Help him to cry.

2 Help the victim to confront reality in manageable doses. Rest is important, but do not misgive drugs to induce excessive sleep when the person needs assistance to look at reality.

3 Help the victim to find the facts. Fantasy is always much worse than fact. The nurse can assist greatly in this area by being truthful with the patient and his family as well as promoting communications between doctor and family.

4 Do not give false reassurances.

5 Do not encourage the victim or family to blame others.

6 Help the victim to accept help.

7 Help the victim and family with the everyday tasks of living until resolution or stabilization is attained.

CONCLUSION

The intricate blend of the psychological and physiological factors make it impractical, if not impossible, to consider the patient on only a physiological basis. The psychological crisis involving the realization of an injury and the impending medical care, its costs, and the potential loss of income and rearrangement of family structure, even on a temporary basis, may well overwhelm the patient with even a minor illness or injury. The professional nurse, therefore, needs to consider the patient as a whole being rather than "the fracture in room nine" or "the stroke in the medical room." Perhaps the nurses who should be most aware of these problems, by nature of their work in acute episodic care areas, are the least sensitive to the more subtle crisis which a patient and his family may feel. With an understanding of the many factors that may influence the patient's response and reactions to crisis, the professional nurse will, it is hoped, take the additional step in providing more comprehensive crisis care.

BIBLIOGRAPHY

Augilera, D. C., J. M. Messick, and M. S. Farrell: *Crisis Intervention: Theory and Methodology,* St. Louis: C. V. Mosby Company, 1970.

Blank, J. P.: "Rescue on the Freeway," *Reader's Digest,* **97**:73-80, 1970.

Bloom, B. L.: "Definitional Aspects of the Crisis Concept," *Journal of Consulting Psychology,* **27**:498-502, 1963.

Brandon, S.: "Crisis Theory and Possibilities of Therapeutic Intervention," *British Journal of Psychiatry,* **117**:627-633, 1970.

Cadden, V.: "Crisis in the Family," in G. Caplan (ed.), *Principles of Preventive Psychiatry,* New York: Basic Books, Inc., Publishers, 1964.

Caplan, G.: *Principles of Preventive Psychiatry,* New York: Basic Books, Inc., Publishers, 1964.

Chayet, N. L.: *Legal Implications of Emergency Care,* New York: Appleton-Century-Crofts, Inc., 1969.

Darley, J., and B. Latanè: "Bystander Intervention in Emergencies: Diffusion of Responsibility," *Journal of Personality and Social Psychology,* **8**:377-383, 1968.

Eastham, K., D. Coates, and F. Allodi: "The Concept of Crisis," *Canadian Psychiatric Association Journal,* **15**:463-472, 1970.

Erikson, E. H.: *Childhood and Society,* New York: Penguin Books, Ltd., 1965.

Fink, S. L.: "Crisis and Motivation: A Theoretical Model," *Archives of Physical Medicine and Rehabilitation,* **48**:592-597, 1967.

Hiatt, C. C., and R. E. Spurlock: "Geographical Flight and Its Relation to Crisis Theory," *American Journal of Orthopsychiatry,* **40**:53-57, 1970.

Latanè, B.: "Gregariousness and Fear in Laboratory Rats," *Journal of Experimental Social Psychology,* **5**:61-69, 1969.

────── and J. Darley: "Bystander Apathy," *American Scientist,* **57**:244-268, 1969.

────── and ──────: "Group Inhibition by Bystander Intervention in Emergencies," *Journal of Personality and Social Psychology,* **10**:215-221, 1968.

────── and D. C. Glass: "Social and Non-social Attraction in Rats," *Journal of Personality and Social Psychology,* **9**:142-146, 1968.

Lindemann, E.: "Symptomatology and Management of Acute Grief," in H. J. Parad (ed.), *Crisis Intervention: Selected Readings,* New York: Family Service Association of America, 1965.

McHugh, M.: "The Management of Crisis in Human Situations," *The Canadian Nurse,* **56**:227-229, 1960.

Miller, K.: "The Concept of Crisis: Current Status and Mental Health Implications," *Human Organizations,* **22**:195-201, 1963.

Parad, H. J. (ed.): *Crisis Intervention: Selected Readings,* New York: Family Service Association of America, 1965.

Robischon, P.: "The Challenge of Crisis Theory for Nursing," *Nursing Outlook,* **15**:28-32, 1967.

Selye, H.: *The Stress of Life,* New York: McGraw-Hill Book Company, 1956.

Shontz, F. C.: "Reactions to Crisis," paper presented at Speech and Hearing Workshop, Kansas City: University of Kansas Medical Center, May 14, 1964.

Chapter 22

Family Habilitation: A Child with a Birth Defect

Mary J. Tudor

During the lifetime of any family unit, several crisis situations will arise. Although many may actually be stress situations, a state of crisis can also possess "growth-promoting potential" (Rappaport, 1965, p. 24). The birth of a child is seen as a crisis having growth-promoting potential. The birth of a defective child is seen as a stress-producing crisis situation.

A birth defect, as defined by the National Foundation–March of Dimes, is a "structural or metabolic disorder present at birth, whether genetically determined or as a result of environmental influence during embryonic or fetal life" (Lipton, 1969b, p. 40). It is said that birth defects account for the greatest wastage of human life, including perinatal and prenatal deaths. Nearly 500,000 deaths occur before birth each year. Over 250,000 babies are born with birth defects each year, 700 per day, or one every 2 minutes. More children are hospitalized from birth defects than from infectious disease. Three out of five children with birth defects who live past two years of age will require special medical, rehabilitative, educational, or custodial care (Lipton, 1969a).

The presentation of these figures is not an attempt at sensationalism but is made in order to stress the magnitude of needs that are presented by defective children by mere number alone.

BIRTH DEFECT: A CRISIS EVENT

Many families each year experience in the birth of a defective child, a crisis situation quite unique and yet quite similar to those covered more extensively in the literature. One element of uniqueness is the long-term effects that this event precipitates. The similarity lies in the approximation of stages seen in reaction to and coping with the crisis situation.

Caplan (1965, p. 24) has defined crisis in its simplest terms as "an upset of a steady state"—a state of crisis is a state of disequilibrium. As the human body during illness strives to regain homeostasis, so a family in a crisis situation strives to reinstate equilibrium by utilizing formerly successful coping mechanisms. The manner in which a family deals with the stress of disequilibrium of the crisis which a defective child represents, and their success in coping, is unique to each family.

Hill (1958) identifies three variables affecting the dynamics of a crisis situation: the event itself, the family's resources in dealing with a crisis situation, and the meaning given to the event by the family.

The birth of a defective child is viewed as catastrophic by our culture. As health, beauty, intelligence, and physical prowess are primary goals for oneself and one's children, a child who is unlikely to reach or who is handicapped in reaching these goals is a source of despair. A variable of the event is the degree of disfigurement and/or handicap caused by the particular type of defect. However, the amount of stress of the family cannot always be measured by the severity of the defect of the child. Other variables, such as values of the parents, goals they have conceived prenatally for the child, and their perceptions of requirements for a successful life, will influence their perception of the event.

Some of the resources available to the family are coping mechanisms utilized and proved successful in previous crisis situations. The previous crisis need not have been a totally disruptive or negative experience in order to provide resource potential. Other resources are seen as a stable marriage, economic stability, support from the extended family and the community, and the ability of the family to adapt.

In only a few cases do families experience having a defective child for the second time. Thus, specific means of coping with such an event are not readily available. Crisis events such as marriage, death, loss of employment, and others are perceived as more likely or expected to occur. In most instances, a family never truly foresees the possibility of having a defective child. Prenatally, the parents begin to idealize their child and all the perfection of this new life. The values they hold determine their perception of the child before he is born. None value imperfection and thus do not perceive their child as defective.

Children are believed to be seen by their parents as extensions of themselves; they idealize the child not only as they perceive themselves but also as they would like to be perceived. An unstable self-concept on the part of one or both parents can be further threatened by a child who is imperfect.

The definition the family gives the event is also critical. Again, values play a vital role in placing meaning to their child's defect. An intellectually oriented family might experience a greater degree of stress if their child were mentally retarded than if he were orthopedically defective. Parents putting high priorities on beauty would find hardship in accepting a child who to them is aesthetically unpleasant to look at or to touch. Studies have shown that fathers have greater difficulty in working through their negative feelings when the child is male. Assets of virility, strength, and leadership often are not possessed by their defective sons.

It can be seen that each family is unique, and their defective child is unique. When the two meet and begin to learn about and interact with one another, a unique situation occurs. No one can generalize the specific dynamics of all crisis situations, the stress factors, the course of events, or the outcome. One must look upon each situation as unprecedented, observe the dynamics of the situation, and then draw upon what is known about the crisis event to begin to evaluate what intervention must be taken. Then consistent reevaluation of the situation and the intervention must be made.

PARENTAL REACTIONS TO THEIR DEFECTIVE CHILD

Much has been written on the initial reactions of parents to the birth of a defective child. The bulk of this literature deals with mental retardation but is applicable to all other types of birth defects.

Gonzalez (1971) lists the stages of adjustment said to be experienced by parents of a defective child which are representative of most theories found in the recent literature. She includes the stages of shock, disbelief, anger, guilt, despair, and grief leading to a stage of acceptance.

Love (1970, p. 27) stresses the individuality of parental responses by noting that their personality makeup and patterns of reacting to "critical life events" (crisis situations) will greatly influence their responses to the stress situation. Love lists six stages that all parents are said to experience whether or not it is realized by them. These he describes as:

1 *Shock* "The initial emotional reaction of the parents to the handicapped child is a brief period of pure emotion" (1970, p. 28).

This reaction is said to occur because of the sudden end to the parents' plans or goals for their idealized child.

2 *Refusal*   "Refusal. . .acts as a defense mechanism for the stress situation" (1970, p. 28).

Included in this stage is the "shopping around" behavior occasionally seen as parents go from one physician to another. They are said to be refusing the diagnosis of a defect and searching for either a diagnosis of normality or perhaps a cure. Some feel that such behavior is neurotic and others that such responses are needed in order to proceed through the adjustment phases.

3 *Guilt*   "Guilt and shame have their roots in basic human nature" (1970, p. 29).

The parents need to find a cause or rational reason why their child is defective. Many times this guilt will be placed on oneself for imaginary reasons or fallacious correlations between a personal weakness and the defect of the child. Occasionally it is seen that an older mother attributes her age to the child's defect when, scientifically, there is no basis for this assumption. The father too can feel guilty for actions he did or did not take that he feels led to the child's defect. Further guilt feelings develop when the parents find themselves reacting with ambivalence toward the child.

4 *Bitterness*   "The reaction of bitterness springs up in the family when the parents see the child as an obstacle interfering with personal, family and social desires" (1970, p. 30).

Bitterness, or anger, often remains covert as such feelings are not acceptable to the parents. Anger may result from feeling as though a stigma is forced upon them. Continually needing to readjust their perceptions and goals for their child, as it becomes more and more evident through his on-going development what capabilities the child possesses, may result in feelings of anger.

5 *Envy*   "The parents become envious and jealous of those who do not have an exceptional child" (1970, p. 31).

This reaction is closely correlated to and may result in further anger or bitterness. Extreme envy may also alienate those who could lend support to the family.

6 *Rejection*   "Rejection finds its origin in the personalities of the parents, reasons for having the child and preconceived ideas concerning the youngster before he is born" (1970, p. 31).

Again, the parents have formed perceptions of their child prenatally; the defective child does not fit these perceptions and thus is rejected. Rejection, if not worked through, may lead to different degrees of either neglect or overprotection. Guilt, again, can result from wanting to reject the child which, in turn, intensifies anger as a response to being made to feel guilty.

Feelings of ambivalence are often described as parents feel resentful or rejecting while at the same time feeling love and the need to protect their child.

Those more psychoanalytically oriented have a slightly different approach to viewing parental responses to a defective child. Solnit and Stark (1961) describe initial stages of numbness and disbelief correlating with states described by Love. They recognize depression, guilt, and anxiety as possibly leading to one of two extremes, complete attachment to or complete rejection of the child through the employment of defense mechanisms. The cause of such reactions is designated as *object loss,* loss of the idealized child. After these initial reactions, the parents are said to go through a mourning process when awareness of the reality situation along with the acute feelings of disappointment and loss are experienced. This mourning state is said to be accompanied by observable physical and behavioral symptoms. In the last phase of grief reaction, an intensified experiencing of the crisis situation "gradually reduces the hypercathexis of the wish for the idealized child" (Solnit and Stark, 1961, p. 535). The last phase of acceptance, they believe, must be reached to achieve a state of mental health.

Miller (1968) describes three stages of parental adjustment. The first is *disintegration,* when dealing with their emotional reactions demands the parents' strength and leaves little time for realistically dealing with the environment or situation. *Adjustment,* the second stage, is when the parents are said to suffer "chronic sorrow" (Olshansky, 1966) and have achieved only partial acceptance. At this point they are looking for a cause for their circumstances and try to restore an equilibrium. Finally, it is hoped they reach the final stage of *reintegration,* where they begin to function more effectively and realistically. The child and his defect are seen in the proper perspective and appropriate reactions occur. Miller states that this more often remains a goal rather than becoming a reality.

Much emphasis has been placed on the grief process, as grieving behavior may be seen initially, through the first few weeks of adjustment and continuing as the child matures. Lindemann (1944, p. 141) describes acute grief as "a definite syndrome with psychological and social symptomology.... This syndrome may appear immediately after a crisis; it may be delayed; it may be exaggerated or apparently absent."

Olshansky (1966) describes chronic sorrow as an unending extension of an acute grief reaction. He believes that initial reactions are understandable in view of a tragic fact. He disagrees with Solnit and Stark in that their descriptions of parental reactions tend to imply that a neurosis is present if guilt or grief is not overcome and a state of acceptance is not reached. Olshansky states that a more appropriate goal is "increased comfortableness in living with and in managing a mentally defective child day by day" (Olshansky, 1966, p. 22). Such increased comfortableness is said to be reached by the provision of concrete services to the family. He stated that chronic sorrow on the part of parents is a justifiable reaction to having a defective child and that professionals should neither make parents appear neurotic for experiencing such sorrow nor try to eradicate this sorrow.

Parents will be more or less acutely in grief initially and grieve overtly for greater or lesser lengths of time. Again, each family is unique in their emotional makeup and their readiness to express their emotions. The topography and length of the grieving process is less important than other factors in dealing with these families. It is vital that any grief or sorrow should not be scoffed at or labeled as unnatural. It must be dealt with, however, if it interferes with the family's ability to begin intervening in behalf of their child's welfare.

As some theorists focus on grief as the pervasive emotional reaction, other authors have placed it as one among the many reactions. It is doubtful that responses seen can be so neatly categorized or weighed as to importance. Such mental computations are not as meaningful unless the main concern is then establishing modes of treatment and formulation of goals.

Menolascino (1968) provides a very vital and long-needed operational approach to dealing with parents of mentally retarded children. It is mentioned because of its applicability to children with all types of defects, its usefulness in dealing with large ranges of parental reactions, and its implications for nursing intervention. Through description of these stages, direct relationships are made among family responses, needs of the family, and intervention taken with the family.

It is evident that a great deal of literature had been compiled concerning parents' initial reactions to a defective child. Less information is available concerning long-term comprehensive support of the family and intervention to meet their needs, especially as related to the nursing profession. This chapter deals mainly with the needs of the parents initially and as the child matures in relation to professional nursing intervention.

IMPLICATIONS FOR NURSING

Initial Intervention

Education Initial intervention starts before a defective child is conceived. There is a great need for education of the general public on the incidence, probability, types, and prevention of birth defects. More information is currently appearing in the popular literature concerning genetic counseling, amniocentesis, and viral and pharmacological agents known to cause teratogenesis. This is a start, but more instruction and counseling must be made available.

The professional nurse should be oriented to case-finding in being able to ascertain whether there is cause for investigation concerning potentially defective offspring. A working knowledge of genetics, the causes and patterns of defects, and diagnostic tests available are necessary for the professional nurse in any position of employment. A history of any defect in the immediate or extended family, repeated miscarriages, or stillbirths should immediately alert the nurse to the possibility of the birth of a potentially defective infant.

Neonatal Period   Any nurse functioning in a delivery room, on a postpartum floor, or in the newborn or intensive care nursery will undoubtedly observe the very initial reactions of parents to a defective child. Such observations are not pleasant as the reactions are quite the opposite of those seen most frequently following the birth of a normal infant. No one can comfortably witness acute shock and sorrow.

Needs of both the mother and the father are great at this time. They are attempting to assimilate a fact that is completely foreign and devastating to them. They will need to speak about it, to test reality by asking questions, and to know that someone is aware of their tragedy. When they are silent, there is a need for silent support.

It has been advised by some that both the mother and the father be allowed to see the baby as soon after delivery as possible. As Rubin (1967) identifies the "taking-in" phase of acquiring the role of a mother, emphasis was placed on the necessity of first identifying the object of her taking in. Kapke (1970, p. 313) suggests, in view of Rubin's article, that "normalizing" or "overnormalizing" may occur unless the parents remain in touch with the reality of their child's defect. This realization should begin at the time of birth.

It is suggested that normal postpartum procedures be followed as closely as possible without danger to the child. If the mother is awake, the physician will, hopefully, briefly and simply explain the child's defect; and the mother will be allowed, if customary, to see and hold her child, unless it is seen that this is not desired by her. The mother's concept of her idealized child will remain intact unless a conflicting concept arises. A normal labor and delivery will begin to confirm a normal product, the child. At the time of delivery, many have heard a mother ask if the child is normal. At this time she is more open to the possibility that the child is not normal. If told that the child is "fine," the mother incorporates this into her perceptions and begins to experience having given birth to her idealized, normal infant. More devastating is the loss of trust in the professionals in charge of her care when she later discovers that her child is indeed not "fine."

The nurse caring for the child will witness the parents', especially the mother's, reactions to touching and looking at the child. As many of these infants require special care from the time of birth, it is difficult to keep the mother and child "in touch" with one another physically as well as emotionally. All efforts should be made to allow the mother to assist in some care of the child. She should never be prevented from viewing her child and asking questions.

Honesty must be employed with these parents. If the child is hydrocephalic and the father asks the nurse if the child's head appears large to her, she must respond in the affirmative. He realizes the child is not normal in appearance but is attempting to find a concrete basis for denial.

It is quite difficult to respond to such questions as, "Will she live?" or "Do you think he will be mentally retarded?" or specific questions about cause, medical treatment, and the like. Usually, the parents at this stage are not yet able to ask these questions. If such circumstances arise, however, the nurse cannot respond directly to all questions. She can, however, respond to the anxiety and doubts evidenced by them and lend herself to allowing further emotional expression. She should be able to offer sympathy but not in a maudlin or pitying manner. She should refer the parents to the physician and then follow-up to make certain the parents did in fact discuss their questions with the doctor.

The parents will assimilate all the information given them by the nurses and physicians slowly and only as they are able. Repetition may be necessary in explaining the child's defect. Many weeks or months will pass before the parents actually realize what has occurred and the meaning of this crisis situation to them. One should not attempt at this time to educate them completely. Support and understanding are greater needs initially.

The nurse should ask the parents if they have questions or concerns if they have not expressed any. Many times they may feel hesitant to "interfere" or do not know where to begin.

Whenever possible, the nurse should point out the abilities of the child such as, "He is sucking well," or "She has a nice, strong cry." Such comments should be truthful and not spoken to avoid discussing the defect or inabilities of the infant. Later, as the child grows, the parents will be learning to work with and capitalize on the child's abilities.

At the time of discharge, it should be the responsibility of the nursing staff, in consultation with the physician, to instruct the mother as to special, as well as routine, infant care and to arrange for comprehensive follow-up through referral.

Long-term Intervention

Clinic or Agency   The President's Panel on Mental Retardation in 1963 set up guidelines to ensure continuum of care for mentally retarded children and their families. It is stated that "There should be available in every community a 'fixed point of referral and information' which provides a life consultation service for the retarded child. The 'point' should be 'fixed' in relation to the retardate and his ongoing needs."

The large university settings offer the most comprehensive and ongoing services. These facilities however are too few and are, as a result, over-crowded. Here too much needs to be done to provide the type of continuum of care described.

The nurse's role in affiliation with any agency serving these families will vary according to the location, size, services offered, and the population of the children seen.

Initially, the parents will need to learn and relearn the facts about their child's defect. The causitive factor, if known, the treatments he will be receiving, the child's eventual prognosis, and more are all concerns at this time. Thus, education remains a very major part of the nursing role. The families are beginning to ask and be concerned about day-to-day care of their child and perhaps may doubt their capabilities in meeting his special needs.

At this time an assessment should be made of the parent's present emotional status, the reality of their perceptions of the situation, and their strengths or weaknesses in coping. As no reactions occur uniformly or in the order they were presented above, one may see denial occurring after feelings of rejection were evident. Unless the assessment of the parents' emotional and coping status is done with treatment or intervention methods in mind to deal with them, it is meaningless to assess.

Much of the parents' anxiety can be alleviated by helping them to realize that reactions such as confusion, disappointment, embarrassment, guilt, and others are natural for parents in their circumstances. In an atmosphere of acceptance, the family is more likely to work with the professional team in a therapeutic and goal-directed manner.

The family must be considered and worked with as a unit. Often, one parent or, more often, the child becomes the focal point of intervention. Parents must work together and they must be able to resolve their conflicting views. Mandlebaum and Wheeler (1961) describe the situation in which the mother takes upon herself full responsibility for the child. She begins to resent this difficult task and becomes angry with her husband. The father, in turn, withdraws and leaves the mother feeling as though she has been deserted.

Hill (1958) describes the family in crisis as seeking a "source of the trouble." One parent may designate himself or his mate as being the source of the child's defect, especially in genetically based birth defects. This place-ment of blame can result in lessening the strength of the family unit and demoralizing the parents. Thus, communication between family members must remain open and each parent be included equally in consultation ses-sions and treatment to help prevent a breakdown of their best resource for coping, a strong family unit.

The nurse in a clinic setting has many responsibilities in working with parents of defective children. He can no longer consider weighing, measuring, and seating the families his main duties. A nurse in the congenital defects clinic must have a contemporary, comprehensive, and sound knowledge of the defects and their ramifications presented by the children in his population. With this background, he can anticipate what difficulties the parents may have in day-to-day care of their child. He must be treatment-oriented as well as informative and supportive. It is important for the nurse to have a time set aside to discuss with the parents such routine but vital questions as eating and sleeping habits, interaction with siblings, play patterns, and motor and verbal behaviors. The discussion should be free and relatively unstructured by allow-ing the parents to verbalize questions or concerns they have. No question can be considered trivial or irrelevant if it exists.

Assessment of development is a vital part of the information-gathering process. Both observation of the child and discussion with the parents should give the nurse the opportunity to spot developmental lags. By using the Denver Developmental Screening Test, a more concrete rating of develop-ment can be made. Assessment alone is not enough. Means of providing stimulation to encourage behavior in the deficit areas should be developed and discussed with the parents.

The nurse will be called on to reinforce and instruct the parents in carrying out prescribed treatments such as brace care, special diets, medica-tion, and the like. He must educate parents as to symptoms that would call for immediate medical attention, such as vomiting, increased head size, and seizures in a child with hydrocephalus.

The nurse has a preventive, supportive, and educative role in discussing with the parents what they are likely to observe in their child in appearance, behavior, development, and disabilities in the future. While keeping them oriented to reality, the nurse should encourage discussion and observation of the child's abilities and potentials.

Should the child need follow-up care in the home setting, it is the respon-sibility of the nurse in the clinic or agency to see that such follow-up is done. Problems in mobility, feeding, stimulation, and discipline often become more obvious and readily dealt with in the natural environment.

If the child is hospitalized for elective surgery, diagnostic tests, an emer-gency or any other reason, the clinic or agency nurse should be aware of such hospitalization. This nurse can then be of great value to the staff nurses by discussing with them the child's defect; special needs; the care he is receiving in the clinic; and facts that make caring for the child, working with the parents, and continuum of care more successful.

Very soon, the question of education must be considered. If the child has not had formal psychological testing and is a potential candidate for regular or special education, this should be done. Many defective children are not mentally retarded. Some will be able to attend a regular school while others cannot because of physical limitations. The educational setting that will be most advantageous for the child should be sought. The nurse should be aware of whether such action is being taken.

The nurse, when necessary for comprehensive treatment and continuum of care, should set in motion referrals to such professionals as speech, physical, and occupational therapists; public health nurses; medical social workers; psychologists; nutritionists; and the like. In the ideal situation, the clinic or agency employs a team of professionals who work together for long-term, comprehensive treatment. The nurse may find himself in the situation in which he must rely upon his own knowledge and skills to try to compensate for a profession that is not available for consultation.

Hospital Most children with congenital defects will be hospitalized at least once, and often repeatedly. In the pediatric ward, these children will have special needs. A mentally retarded child will not always be able to seek his own amusement or make his needs known. He may need stimulation and toys brought to him that are appropriate for his mental age. Orthopedically, visually, or auditorally handicapped children may require more care in self-help skills than other children. While the nurse must realize when he needs assistance, he should also encourage independent behaviors that the child is capable of performing.

As with any hospitalized child, the nurse should discuss with the parents the routine of the ward, ascertain their knowledge of the reason for hospitalization, and be available for any questions they may have. The nurse may find that the parents' actual knowledge of their child's defect or normal child development is lacking. He should provide such information.

Any special methods utilized by the nurses in taking care of these children and means of providing stimulation and encouraging desired behavior should be discussed with the parents, especially if they have expressed frustrations or difficulties with such activities in the home.

The nurse has an excellent opportunity to observe the motor, verbal, and social skills of these children; their ability to carry out self-help skills; and their interaction with their parents. Developmental lags, abnormal behaviors, and abilities should be recorded. If follow-up is seen as needed, an investigation of those presently involved with the family should be made and action taken to fill gaps discovered in the continuum of care.

Community As the natural environment for the family is the home situation, this area of public health is of great concern. It is in the home setting that parents meet with day-to-day problems in managing a defective child. Childrearing is an involved and demanding occupation. Parents of normal children experience frequent problems and anxieties. These experiences are magnified when the child is defective. Children who cannot walk; who cannot see, speak, or hear; who cannot be reasoned with; who have difficulty learning and obeying are constant challenges in daily living. If they have siblings, the parents have added responsibilities.

The first concern is meeting the child's needs to sustain health and life. The second is to promote development to the child's optimal potential.

The public health nurse's role in promoting health is defined by the type of defect of each child. Depending upon the specific defect, they may be susceptible to infection, decubiti, fractures, seizures, or other threats to health.

In promoting development, the nurse must work with the parents in building up their child's behavior in areas of motor, verbal, social, and self-help skills. One concern is that the child is not totally dependent upon the parents. Blodgett (1968) has described the situation of "circular dependency" in which an older, handicapped child remains completely dependent upon the parents. The parents, to avoid the frustrations of attempting, at this later date, to initiate independent behaviors, give total care and thus become dependent on meeting the infant-level needs of their child.

The parents must be cognizant of their child's behavior in relation to those of normal children of the same chronological age. Utilizing this knowledge, the parents can nurture the child's developmental potential and avoid becoming accepting of unnecessarily retarded development. The nurse must intervene, however, should he recognize that the parents are expecting behavior that the child is unable to perform.

Of extreme importance is that the family realize their child, although exceptional, has the same basic needs as all children, with or without a defect. Love, a sense of autonomy, freedom to explore his world, and freedom to experiment with himself in relation to that world are some of the needs that every child possesses. An exceptional child may have additional special needs; however, these do not negate those inherent in childhood.

By identifying the strengths of both child and family, the nurse can act as a catalyst in joining the two for optimum development.

As well as a comprehensive knowledge of normal development, the parents must be aware of the developmental patterns of defective children. Waechter (1970) gives an excellent description of the difference in development between normal and physically disabled children. She designates two problems encountered in physical deviancy. First, limitations are posed by the defect itself; and, secondly, obstacles are imposed by society.

> Children with either physical or sensory deficits are often retarded in intellectual development, are more emotionally liable, are retarded in the development of autonomy and independence, are often less sensitive in perceiving human relationships and in social interaction have difficulties in structuring their world, are more continuously absorbed in bodily interests, are retarded in the development of body image, are more dependent on people in their environment than objects, and have greater difficulty in defining their sex roles (Waechter, 1970, pp. 91-92).

Waechter continues by describing difficulties encountered at the various developmental levels through the school years. A clear picture of the impact of a defect at each level of development is given.

Increasingly, children who are mentally retarded are being kept at home with the family rather than being institutionalized. One reason for this is the overcrowding and thus the decreased assets offered by the institutions. Concurrent with this has been the development and proved success of operant conditioning theory as a means of teaching a child behaviors acceptable to society and desirable for the child's welfare. For a child with behavioral deficits, whether mentally or physically retarded or both, no other therapy has proved as effective in building those behaviors which allow the child to become a more integrated member of the family and society in general. Through operant conditioning, unacceptable behaviors can be eliminated and desirable behaviors brought into the child's repertoire.

The greatest contributions in bringing the operant learning theory into nursing practice have been made by Linda W. Peterson (Whitney, 1966; Peterson, 1967; Whitney and Barnard, 1966) and Kathryn Barnard (Whitney and Barnard, 1966; Barnard, 1968). This theory is truly "a framework deserving nursing investigation" (Whitney, 1966, p. 229). If attainment of the highest potential for health and development is the concern and purpose of nursing intervention with defective children, then the combination of traditional knowledge and care in health promotion, the knowledge of normal child development, and the tools of operant conditioning make a very potent weapon against wastage of human life.

General Considerations

It must be reemphasized that the needs of these exceptional children and their families exist for a lifetime. Major concerns spring anew as the child matures. Parents have expressed grave concerns about their children when they begin attending school and meeting their peer groups, whether defective or normal. At each point in the child's life when he meets a new task, is expected to perform new and more complicated behavior, discovers an inability or exclusion from normal activities, the family and the child undergo a new stress situation. The situations possible are numerous, and thus the nursing intervention will change with the changes in the family and child. The basic tools described thus far will be applicable throughout the initial nursing intervention and for the extended intervention throughout the child's life.

Parents will verbalize concerns about their children as adolescents. The child is likely to be cognizant of his uniqueness and stigmas that may become evident as he ventures into the social world. Sexual maturation, the possibilities for employment, marriage, and general achievement not only concern the parents but also concern the adolescent himself. Another very important consideration for many of the parents, especially those of more severely defective children, is who will care for their children when they are no longer living.

Siblings of defective children have concerns about their own chances for having children affected as their brothers or sisters. They also must deal with their peer groups in explaining and protecting their defective siblings. Siblings should be included in discussions, care, and goals for the defective child but not beyond their capabilities or to the exclusion of their own desires and activities.

Institutionalization remains a consideration for any family of a mentally retarded child. The ultimate decision should definitely rest with the parents. It should be clear to them what potential the child has for development, the advantages and disadvantages of both the home and institutional settings in meeting the child's particular needs, and the ability of the family to cope and work with their child. Financial considerations must also be taken into account. If the parents have researched and are aware of these facts, they are capable of making and carrying out the decision.

Patterson and Rowland (1970) offer an educational model in nursing care of institutionalized children. Nursing intervention, utilizing this model, is built around teaching or guiding purposes and aims toward human development and habilitation goals. They contend that "The medical model appears to reinforce and augment the dehumanization of retardates" (Patterson and Rowland, 1970, p. 534). The nurse's medical function is not excluded, but his role is broadened by utilizing the educational model as well.

The nurse in the public school system also is in contact with children that have defects other than mental retardation. He has a great responsibility to be alert for difficulties the child may have in adjustment, learning, peer relations, and self-help skills.

CONCLUSION

Perhaps the needs of families of defective children can best be expressed by the parents themselves. Dorothy Murray (1969, p. 6) has given professionals great insight into the feelings, needs, and goals of these families. She delineates six problems: acceptance of their child's defect; financial concerns; increasing emotional tension; theological conflicts; planning for lifetime care; and "inept, inaccurate and ill-timed professional advice."

> The greatest single need of parents of mentally retarded children is constructive professional counseling at various stages of the child's life which will enable the parents to find the answers to their own individual problems to a reasonably satisfactory degree.
>
> In the early stages of our initial adjustment to life with a retarded child we need someone who can and will explain to us in lay language some of the numerous factors relating to mental retardation; we need someone to help us understand our own attitudes and feelings in relation to our handicapped child. We need someone to give us guidance in the simple, basic processes of home training. We need someone who can put us in touch with the various community and state agencies that can help with constructive management of the child. We need guidance from someone who can help us see that this thing which has happened to us, even though it may be a "life-shaking" experience does not of necessity have to be a "life-breaking" one.
>
> Several years later we need guidance from those who can help us decide upon and provide a training program for the child. In later years we need guidance and help in making plans which will provide permanent care for our child when we are gone.

In considering the ever-expanding roles of nursing, each of the needs stated above must and can be met or lessened by professional nursing interventions described in this chapter. Too long these needs have gone unrecognized and even longer the potentials for nursing action in meeting them have not been perceived.

SUMMARY

The birth of a defective child is seen as a crisis situation. The meaning and outcome of this crisis are dependent on factors unique to the family and the intervention taken with the child and his family. Utilizing both theory of crisis intervention and knowledge of initial parental reactions to this specific crisis, the role of the professional nurse is delineated.

Nursing intervention in the initial stages of the crisis, in the clinic, agency, hospital, community, institutional, and school settings, and in long-term care is generally described.

The tools of technical nursing care, knowledge of normal growth and development, specific knowledge of birth defects, their implications and ramifications, the ability to give support and understanding as well as to educate, and techniques in behavior analysis and modification are seen as necessary for comprehensive and effective nursing intervention with families of defective children.

An attempt has been made to correlate the needs of families of defective children to potential nursing intervention. More specific guidelines could and must be laid out for each type of defect and each area of nursing. No longer can we in the nursing profession be indifferent to the 750,000 families yearly that experience the all-encompassing and potentially devastating crises of miscarriage, stillbirths, and births of defective children. In no other area is the privation for nursing intervention, both in intensity and duration, quite so evident.

BIBLIOGRAPHY

Barnard, K.: "Teaching the Retarded Child Is a Family Affair," *American Journal of Nursing,* **68**:309–311, 1968.
Blodgett, H. E.: "Helping Parents in the Community Setting," in W. Wolfensberger and R. Kurtz (eds.), *Management of the Family of the Mentally Retarded,* Follett Educational Corporation, 1969, pp. 197–203. (Reprinted from *Counseling Parents of Children with Mental Retardation,* Langhern, Pa.: The Woods Schools, 1968, pp. 74–85.)
Caplan, G.: Formulated by Caplan in seminars at the Harvard School of Public Health. Reported by Rappoport, 1965, p. 24.
Gonzalez, M. T.: "Nursing Support of the Family with an Abnormal Infant," *Hospital Topics,* **15**:68–69, 1971.
Hill, R.: "Generic Features of Families under Stress," *Social Casework,* **39**:139–150, 1958.
Kapke, K. A.: "Spina Bifida: Mother-child Relationship," *Nursing Forum,* **9**:310–319, 1970.
Lindemann, E.: "Symptomatology and Management of Acute Grief," *American Journal of Psychiatry,* **10**:141–148, 1944.
Lipton, M.: "Birth Defects Today: Their Impact upon the Family, the Patient and Society," *Journal of School Health,* **39**:642–645, 1969*a*.
———:"The Problem of Birth Defects Today," *Journal of School Health,* **39**:40–42, 1969*b*.
Love, H. D.: *Parental Attitudes toward Exceptional Children,* Springfield, Ill.: Charles C Thomas, 1970.
Mandelbaum, A., and M. E. Wheeler: "The Meaning of a Defective Child to Parents," *Social Casework,* **42**:78–83, 1961.

Menolascino, F. J.: "Parents of the Mentally Retarded: An Operational Approach to Diagnosis and Management," *Journal of the American Academy of Child Psychiatry,* 7:589-602, 1968.

Miller, L. G.: "Toward a Greater Understanding of the Parents of the Mentally Retarded Child," *Journal of Pediatrics,* 73:699-705, 1968.

Murray, D.: "Needs of Parents of Mentally Retarded Children," in W. Wolfensberger and R. Kurtz (eds.), *Management of the Family of the Mentally Retarded,* Follett Educational Corporation, 1969, pp. 68-70. (Reprinted from *American Journal of Mental Deficiency,* 63:1078-1088, 1959.)

Olshansky, S.: "Parent Responses to a Mentally Defective Child," *Mental Retardation,* 4:20-25, 1966.

Patterson, E. G., and G. T. Rowland: "Toward a Theory of Mental Retardation Nursing: An Educational Model," *American Journal of Nursing,* 70:531-535, 1970.

Peterson, L. W.: "Operant Approach to Observation and Recording," *Nursing Outlook,* 15:28-32, 1967.

President's Panel on Mental Retardation: "A Proposed Program for National Action to Combat Mental Retardation," Washington, D.C.: U.S. Government Printing Office, 1963.

Rappaport, L.: "The State of Crisis: Some Theoretical Considerations," in H. J. Parad (ed.), *Crisis Intervention: Selected Readings,* New York: Family Service Association of America, 1965, pp. 23-31. (Reprinted from *The Social Service Review,* 36:211-217, 1962.)

Rubin, R.: "Attainment of the Maternal Role: Part I, Processes," *Nursing Research,* 16:237-245, 1967.

Solnit, A. J., and M. H. Stark: "Mourning and the Birth of a Defective Child," *Psychoanalytical Studies of Children,* 16:523-537, 1961.

Waechter, E. H.: "Developmental Correlates of Physical Disability," *Nursing Forum,* 9:90-107, 1970.

Whitney, L.: "Operant Learning Theory: A Framework Deserving Nursing Investigation," *Nursing Research,* 15:229-235, 1966.

——— and K. E. Barnard: "Implications of Operant Learning Theory for Nursing Care of the Retarded Child," *Mental Retardation,* 4:26-29, 1966.

Chapter 23

The Nurse's Role in Genetic Counseling

Lorraine Wolf

Genetic counseling is a relatively new aspect of clinical medicine and nursing. Until the 1940s, the field of genetics was concerned primarily with basic scientific research. Subsequently, the science of genetics has expanded to the area of clinical practice. This development is related to two influences: (1) the accumulation of scientific information and (2) governmental concerns. First, the accumulated knowledge regarding the universal biochemical structure of living organisms, the establishment of cytogenetics, and the reduction and control of pathogenic organisms as causes of disease have focused attention on the role of genetics in human growth and development. Second, impetus for clinical application comes from the health promotion and disease prevention priority set by the Department of Health, Education, and Welfare and the current concern about the potential for genetic abberations and birth defects resulting from drugs, pesticides, fertilizers, and other teratogenic agents.

The scientific aspects of genetics deal with differential diagnosis, estimation of the probability that a defect will occur, and legal and ethical implications. The practice of genetic counseling in early detection concerns interpretation of the findings, recommendations, and alternatives; and guidance and support of the family in reaching an acceptable solution to the problem. Although the medical and legal aspects of counseling remain with the geneticist or family physician, this does not preclude the nurse from contributing to early detection, counseling with patients, and follow-up care. In fact, if the health care needs of the consumer are to be met, the nurse needs to go beyond the traditional function of assessment of current health status involved in observation and limited predetermined checklists. In support of the expanded role of the nurse, Mereness (1970, p. 33) stated, "The traditional use that has been made of the abilities of the professionally prepared nurse has been short sighted and wasteful of talent and manpower."

As nurses expand their roles in health promotion and health maintenance, the *patient health history* becomes a critical tool in genetic assessment. (The term *patient health history* is preferable to the term *nursing history* which appears in the literature. The latter is a misnomer since it is neither a history of nursing nor a history of the nurse's recording.) Presently, the patient health history does not typically contain questions relevant to genetic factors in the patient's background. The inclusion of a section on genetics is mandatory if a complete health evaluation is to be done. This will necessitate, however, that nurses be well informed in the areas of genetic principles; genetic diagnostic methods; probability of occurrence of the most common genetic defects; and ways in which they can contribute to intervention, information provision, and counseling. This chapter is not designed to prepare the nurse practitioner as a genetic counselor, but rather to present basic information that can be incorporated into a family practice in any setting.

PRINCIPLES OF HUMAN GENETICS

The genetic or hereditary substance, desoxyribonucleic acid (DNA), is carried by the chromosomes. Each human cell has forty-six chromosomes arranged in twenty-three pairs. One chromosome of each pair is received from the male, the other from the female. Twenty-two pairs are the same for male and female and are called autosomes. The remaining pair is the sex chromosome and is identified as XX for the female and XY for the male (see Figure 23-1). The female contributes only XX chromosomes, whereas the male may contribute an XY (produces a male child) or an XX (produces a female child). Within the DNA of each chromosome are segments identified as genes. These are the units of heredity, with each human cell containing some 100,000 genes. As the chromosomes are paired, so are the genes; and the pairs, or alleles, determine specific hereditary traits.

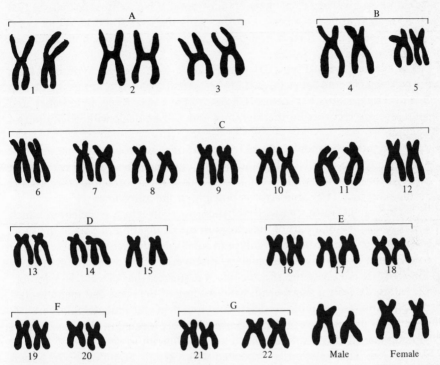

Figure 23-1 Karyotype of a chromosome set.

Cytogenetics

Knowledge about the number of chromosomes and their behavior during cell division (mitosis and meiosis) was greatly enhanced by the discoveries of Barr in 1949 and Lejeune in 1959. Barr identified the staining properties of the chromatin body in one of the two chromosomes of the female. The normal female has one Barr body, while the normal male has no sex chromatin body since he has only one X chromosome. Schimke (1968, p. 3) further elaborated, "In other words, the number of Barr bodies equals the number of X chromosomes minus one." The patient with Klinefelter's syndrome (XXY) has a single Barr body, although presenting a male phenotype (outward appearance); and the "super female" XXX would have two Barr bodies, but would be prone to menstrual irregularity, amenorrhea, and early menopause. Diagnosis of intersex states and fertility problems are now possible by studying buccal smears for the presence or absence of Barr bodies. There currently is interest in the relationship between young males presenting an XYY pattern (forty-seven chromosomes) and delinquent behavior. These males usually are tall and aggressive. They may or may not be mentally retarded. Sexual development appears normal, and they are able to reproduce. While still a controversial issue, further research may identify genetic implications for human behavior.

Lejeune (1959) discovered that children with Down's syndrome have forty-seven chromosomes instead of the normal forty-six and this opened up a new era in human genetics. Chromosomal abberations in number and structure are recorded in the literature and will be dealt with briefly in this chapter.

The most commonly referred to variations in chromosome number are those related to anaphase lag and nondisjunction. These errors occur after segregation and the daughter cell lags or fails to incorporate the chromosome in the new cell. The same error is possible in the autosomes.

One of the most common abberations in structure is deletion, which refers to the loss of a part of the chromosome. A deletion of part of the short arm of a 5 chromosome will result in the abnormality identified as *cri du chat* (see Figure 23-1). This syndrome was discovered by Lejeune and named by him because the cry of the affected infant resembles that of a cat. In addition, the infant exhibits a small head, wide spacing of the eyes, and mental retardation. Another example of deletion is found in the Philadelphia chromosome. This is a deletion of the long arm probably located in chromosome 31; although, as in Down's syndrome, it may be difficult to determine if 21 or 22 is involved. This deletion is associated with chronic granulocytic (myeloid) leukemia. Both of the above conditions are examples of autosomal abberations. Other abberations in structure are duplications indicating a transfer of material from one chromosome to another as seen in the condition of partial trisomy. Translocations indicate interchanges between two chromosomes where part or all of the chromosome is displaced to another. Some forms of Down's syndrome are now identified as 21/22 translocations and also may be noted as 15/21. Other chromosomal variations are described in the literature for the reader who wishes to explore this area in more depth.

Mendelian Inheritance

The discoveries of Mendel in 1865 regarding the principles of heredity went unrecognized until the beginning of the twentieth century. The significance of his contribution to the clinical practice of genetics was not recognized until the early 1940s. In explicating the principle of simple inheritance, Schimke (1968, p. 4) stated:

> A point mutation in a single gene occurring in a germ cell may be inherited, depending on whether or not that particular germ cell is involved in fertilization. If it is, the genotype of the resultant individual will carry the abnormality and

all subsequent generations therefore having a finite risk of being similarly affected. With this simple, single factor, or Mendelian inheritance, the proportion of offspring affected with a given trait is predictable and follows the law of probability.

The four types of simple inheritance are autosomal dominant, autosomal recessive, (sex) X-linked dominant, and X-linked recessive. Table 23-1 lists some of the genetic diseases under the two types of inheritance (i.e., autosomal or sex-linked) and the association mode of inheritance (i.e., dominant or recessive).

Autosomal Dominant   The location of the defective gene is on one of the autosomes, and as pointed out by Schimke (1968), "a single dose in a defective dominant gene is sufficient to cause the disorder." Criteria for determining this type of inheritance are listed in Thompson and Thompson (1966) as follows:

1   Trait appears in every generation.
2   Trait is transmitted by affected parent to half of his children (on the average).

Table 23-1   Examples of Genetic Disorders and Their Mode of Inheritance

Autosomal dominant	Autosomal recessive	X-linked disorders
Arachnodactyly	Adrenogenital	Agammaglobulinemia
Achondroplasia	syndrome	Aldrich syndrome
Brachydactyly	Albinism	Color vision anarubin
Congenital cataract	Alkaptonuria	Diffuse
Ehlers–Danlos syndrome	Cretinism (familial)	angiokeratoma
Gaucher's disease (adult)	Cystic fibrosis	Hemophilia A
Holt–Oram syndrome	Diabetes mellitus	Hemophilia B
Huntington's chorea	Ellis–van Creveld	Hurler's disease
Multiple polyposis	syndrome	Hypoparathyroidism
Myotonic dystrophy	Fanconi syndrome	Ichthyosis vulgaris
Neurofibromatosis	Friedreich's ataxia	Microphthalmia
(von Recklinghausen's)	Galactosemia	Muscular dystrophy
Osteogenesis imperfecta	Gaucher's disease	(Becker)
Retinoblastoma	(infantile)	Muscular dystrophy
Sickle-cell trait	Homocystinuria	(Duchenne's)
Tuberous sclerosis	Limb-girdle muscular	Nephrogenic diabetes
	dystrophy	insipidus
	Maple syrup disease	Ocular albinism
	Sickle-cell disease	
	Tay–Sachs disease	

3 Unaffected persons do not transmit the trait to their children.

4 The occurrence and transmission of the trait are not affected by sex; males and females are equally likely to have and transmit the trait.

Autosomal Recessive   Both alleles must be abnormal for the individual to be affected. Thompson and Thompson (1966) list the criteria for this type of inheritance as follows:

1 Trait characteristically appears only in sibs, not their parents, offspring, or other relatives.

2 On the average, one-fourth of the sibs of the propositus (affected person) are affected.

3 Parents of affected child may be consanguineous (blood relatives).

4 Males and females are equally likely to be affected.

X-linked Dominant   This pattern resembles the autosomal type of inheritance; however, the male-to-male transmission is absent. Females are affected when the male parent has the disorder, and both male and female children may have a 50-50 chance of being affected when the female parent has the disorder. According to Thompson and Thompson (1966), the criteria are:

1 Affected males transmit the trait to all of their daughters.

2 Affected females who are heterozygous transmit the condition to half of their children of either sex. Homozygous females transmit the trait to all of their children.

3 Transmission by females follows the same pattern as shown in autosomal dominance, and cannot be differentiated from autosomal dominance. This can be done when the male is affected.

X-linked Recessive   The female parent carrying the trait on one X chromosome will not express the disease. Depending on which chromosome is transmitted, the males may be affected, the females may be carriers, or children of both sexes may be normal. If the male parent is affected, his daughters will be carriers and the sons will be normal. Criteria for assessing this type of inheritance are listed by Thompson and Thompson (1966) as follows:

1 Incidence of the trait is much higher in males than females.

2 Trait is passed on from affected male through all his daughters to half of their sons.

3 Trait never is transmitted from father to son.

4 Trait may be transmitted through a series of female carriers, and if so, the affected males in a kindred are related to one another through females.

This author has found the criteria listed by Thompson and Thompson (1966) very useful in understanding not only the various genetic diseases, but also the risk factor for a family as well.

Multifactorial Inheritance

Some genetic conditions do not relate to a single gene, rather they are related to an interaction between both the genetic material and the environment. These genetic abnormalities do not follow strict Mendelian inheritance. The risk factor is less than with single-factor inheritance; and statistics are available regarding the chance of recurrence of congenital deformities such as congenital dysplasia of the hip, clubfoot, or cleft lip or palate. Schimke (1968, p. 6) stated, for example,

> The chance of recurrence of cleft lip with or without cleft palate if no one in the family is affected has been calculated to be less than 5 percent, or one chance in twenty. If previous child or parent had the affliction, then the recurrence risk is in the neighborhood of 10 percent.

Pedigrees

In taking a genetic history it is important that the recording of the data yields information that will assist in the determination of the type of genetic disorder presented, the number involved, and a base for prediction. These are usually done by developing a pedigree chart using standard symbols to indicate generation, relationship, sex, number, and status of each member regarding the disorder(s) (see Figure 23-2). The information obtained from the history is then translated into symbols relevant to the family involved and provides quickly retrievable information useful to all family and health care members. The following case history (the case history presented in this chapter is a composite) and the accompanying pedigree chart illustrate the effectiveness of this method (see Figure 23-3).

CASE HISTORY

This 7-year-old white male was brought to clinic for evaluation. The mother reports he is having increasing difficulty walking.

History: Child passed milestones of growth and development until he was 3 years old. Since that time he has had difficulty getting up and down, and in the past year has exhibited difficulty in walking and speaking clearly.

Family History: Maternal brother diagnosed as having Duchenne's muscular dystrophy at age 9 years. Died at age 17 years. One maternal sister living and well. One nephew, age 6, has a "muscular" problem. One niece, age 8, living and well. Present family includes mother, father, one daughter, age 9, and two sons, age 7 and 6 months. Only the 7-year-old son manifests any physical problems at this time.

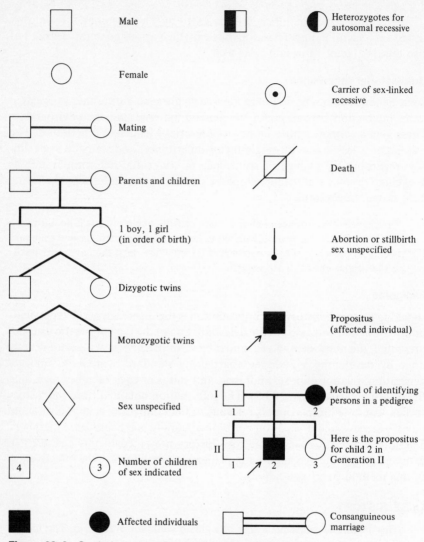

Figure 23-2 Symbols commonly used in pedigree charts.

Diagnosis: Following a multidisciplinary examination, the diagnosis of Duchenne's muscular dystrophy was made, and the family referred for genetic work-up and counseling.

NURSING INTERVENTION

By making use of the above basic knowledge, the nurse can involve himself in clinical genetics in the areas of prevention, early detection, and treatment

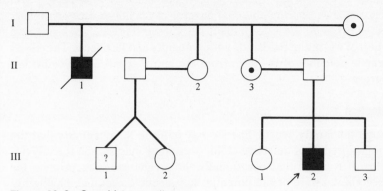

Figure 23-3 Case history pedigree.

referral. Thus, his role is extended beyond that associated only with the more common medical defects and diseases now occupying his attention. The role of the nurse in each of these areas will now be elaborated, and there will be comments about the nurse's participation in the medical management of those individuals who manifest genetic disorders that lend themselves to medical intervention.

Prevention

The collection of data through a family genetic history may indicate to potential parents the risks involved in having children with a genetic defect, the future problems associated with a genetically defective child, and the value of counseling concerning alternatives to childbearing. Concerning the previously mentioned case study (see Figure 23-3), if the health care team had focused on the risk for the patient's mother to produce a child with muscular dystrophy, following the diagnosis of her own brother, perhaps the alternatives to childbearing could have been more clearly defined in keeping with the family's wishes. In this context, opportunity should be provided for open and honest discussion regarding the risk of having children similarly affected. The nurse should then have provided comprehensive information on family planning and the use of contraceptives in keeping with the individual's values. Possibilities of adoption, resistance to adoption, and the value for further counseling regarding alternatives to childbearing may have been explored. At this point in the family development, the focus for the nurse will be on the present generation, with the realization that two more children will not survive to adulthood.

Any discussion of prevention would be incomplete without pointing out that prenatal counseling by the nurse should be focused on helping the woman become aware of the potential hazards of infections such as rubella, the impact of drugs on the fetus in the first trimester (especially aspirin), and the pollution of water and foodstuffs with pesticides and fertilizers. The effects on the genetic potential of the fetus from the above agents are documented in literature.

Early Detection

Even though the family genetic history may indicate the possibility that the parents might produce a defective child, pregnancy may still be the individual's choice. It is noted that occasionally the pregnancy exists prior to the parents becoming aware of the potential for genetic defect, i.e., having another defective child.

Prenatal detection of several defects is now possible through transabdominal amniocentesis and should be discussed with the couple. In order to minimize complications for both mother and fetus, i.e., homorrhage, amnionitis, abortion, and fetal puncture, the most advantageous period to perform the procedure is 12 to 14 weeks after conception. Sex chromatin identification, biochemical studies demonstrating mucopolysaccharidosis, Marfan's syndrome, Pompe's disease, galactosemia, and alysosomal acid phsophatasia are among the identified problems which can be determined by amniocentesis. If, subsequent to the amniocentesis, it is determined that the woman is carrying a defective child, the parents have the option, in many states, to seek a therapeutic abortion or to have the child. Utilizing the data from the family genetic history for problem identification, the nurse now can make the parents aware of the alternatives available, possible hazards, and probable outcomes of both abortion and continuation of the pregnancy, and then support the decision they make. It is also at this point that the nurse reinforces the information given by the physician and answers questions that arise from the doctor-patient interaction. Should the parents need to decide whether or not to complete this pregnancy, the nurse in family practice is in a position to offer counseling and support as the parents work through feelings of guilt, anxiety, or grief. When a decision has been made, the nurse supports the parents' rights to these alternatives.

Referral for Treatment

The need for a thorough assessment of the newborn, including a screening examination, is evident in view of our increased knowledge relevant to health promotion through disease prevention. The physician has the responsibility, therefore, of examining the newborn and determining the state of his health. The nurse must also do a detailed assessment, including a physical screening, in order to provide baseline data for identifying needs and predicting potential deviations from normal growth and development. Detection of abnormalities such as a single umbilical artery, low-set ears, or defects of the genitalia will alert the nurse to possible genetic defects. Length, weight, and head and chest circumferences plotted on a growth and development grid may provide data indicating that the infant is a risk, thus leading to further assessment of genetic implications for the problems presented, i.e., inborn error of metabolism. The nurse in family practice, therefore, is in a unique position to identify early genetic problems because of his focus on states of wellness and illness and his commitment to continuity of care.

Nursing assessment, problem identification, and nursing intervention in relation to birth defects and genetic disorders do not stop when the child passes infancy. Some disorders such as Duchenne's muscular dystrophy, diabetes, or Huntington's chorea do not show up until later in childhood, in early adulthood, or in the middle years of life. Early detection and referral are imperative to prevent the disabling consequences of these disorders. Where intervention is not effective, as in Huntington's chorea, the family will require a great deal of support in making the necessary adjustments to the fact that the father and wage earner will become permanently disabled. Similar problems may confront the family when the diabetic father develops secondary complications of visual and renal deficits in his forties or fifties, and is no longer able to assume responsibility for his growing family. In this instance, his adjustment as well as his family's may be facilitated by the nurse planning with this couple prior to childbearing. An assessment of the financial resources, as well as the status of the disease, would provide a basis for developing the necessary resources in the event of permanent disability of the wage earner.

Nursing Aspects of Medical Therapeutics

The last aspect of nursing intervention to be discussed is the remediation process. Most of the recommendations for treatment will be made by the physician. In the nurse's expanded role, however, he will be expected to participate more actively in remediation of genetic disorders. Remoin (1970) listed the following therapeutic methods now available or soon to be available for the treatment of genetic disorders or their complications:

1 Elimination diets
2 Supplementation of the missing end product
3 Replacement of the missing gene product
4 Enzyme induction
5 Coenzyme supplementation
6 Metabolic suppression
7 Elimination of body toxin

8 Avoidance of drugs
9 Organ replacement
10 Surgical removal of tissue
11 Reconstructive surgery and physical medicine
12 Genetic engineering

The first eight items listed by Remoin have both physiological and psychological components. The need to follow the prescribed regimes may be well understood by the physician and the nurse, but, unless the patient and his family also understand and concur, the disease may progress untreated with profound results. It would seem, then that the parents, family, and individual himself (if capable) must become very knowledgeable about the genetic disorder, the interventions possible to correct the defect or minimize the disability, self-care goals, and limitations requiring adaptation.

The nurse, in sharing his knowledge with the family, encourages them to continue seeking information that will aid in determining the care they will need. Continuous assessment of the psychosocial state of the parents and/or the affected individual is essential to determine the adaptation process in the life style of the family. The adolescent with diabetes may be on a suicide trail with cokes, candy, and desserts as a result of denial of his disease process, or in response to the family's overt or covert suggestions that special diet and daily medication are a burden.

The next three items (9 through 11) listed by Remoin may involve relatively minor procedures such as removing extra digits or the more complex procedures of multiple-stage plastic surgery for cleft lips and cleft palates, surgery for cardiac defects, and sex determination. The family nurse practitioner provides continuity of care through preparing the family for the hospital experience, providing relevant information about the patient and family to the health care team in the hospital, being available and supportive to the family during the hospitalization, and planning with the health care team and family for the return home. Additionally, he may coordinate needed services or refer the family to such agencies as social welfare, Crippled Children's Bureau, or parent resource organizations. When home care is required, he may refer the family to other health care members or agencies within the community, or provide the care himself. While the author recognizes that the nursing functions listed above are currently carried out by a variety of nurses, this care is viewed as fragmented and lacking the coordination, continuity, and family focus provided by the family nurse practitioner in meeting the health needs of the family.

The last point listed by Remoin, genetic engineering, is not yet available. There are many moral and ethical questions surrounding this issue. Regarding the resolution of these questions, Joshua Lederberg, Nobel Prize-winning geneticist, talking before the House Appropriations Subcommittee in June 1970, stated:

> Geneticists are not a group of power-mad lunatics just waiting for an opportunity to control the world. It's sick to think so. They are a group of scientists who through laboratory experiments have learned how to change genetically the direction of simple living forms. The ability to change man's genetic make-up, even subtly, is not just around the corner.

The implications for the practice of nursing are not clear at this point. However, this is an issue that nursing will have to address itself to in the near future.

SUMMARY

As the role of nursing expands, the inclusion of all aspects of clinical genetics will be mandatory to meet the needs of the consumer in health promotion and health maintenance as well as required intervention and rehabilitation. The family nurse practitioner may indeed become the genetic counselor of the future by working with families across all life cycles and in all states of health. Whether this is realistic or not will be determined by the practitioner himself; but the utilization of the basic knowledge presented in this chapter should enhance nursing assessment, problem identification, and nursing intervention in current practice.

BIBLIOGRAPHY

Bergsma, D. (ed.): *Birth Defects: Original Articles Series,* vol. VI, no. 1, *Genetic Counseling,* Baltimore: Williams & Wilkins Company, 1970.

Eggen, R. R.: "Chromosome Studies: Who Needs Them?" *Post Graduate Medicine,* **50**(5):283–287, 1971.

Gerbie, A. B., H. L. Nadler, and M. V. Gerbie: "Amniocentesis in Genetic Counseling," *American Journal of Obstetrics-Gynecology,* **109**(5):765–770, 1971.

Gluck, L., M. V. Kulovich, R. C. Borer, P. A. Brenner, G. G. Anderson, and W. N. Spellacy: "Diagnosis of Respiratory Distress Syndrome by Amniocentesis," *American Journal of Obstetrics-Gynecology,* **109**(3):440–445, 1971.

Hsia, D. Y-Y.: *Human Developmental Genetics,* Chicago: Year Book Medical Publishers, 1968.

Lejeune, J., M. Gautier, and R. Turpin: "Étude des chromosomes somatique de neuf enfants mongoleins," *Comptes Rendus Hebdomadaires des Seances de l'Academie des Sciences* (Paris), **248**:1721–1722, 1959.

McKusick, V. A.: *Human Genetics,* Englewood Cliffs, N.J.: Prentice-Hall, 1969.

Mereness, D: "Recent Trends in the Expanding Roles of the Nurse," *Nursing Outlook,* **18**(5):30–33, 1970.

Nadler, H. L., and A. B. Gerbie: "Role of Amniocentesis in the Intrauterine Detection of Genetic Disorder," *New England Journal of Medicine,* **282**(11):596–599, 1970.

Nitowsky, H. M.: "Prenatal Diagnosis of Genetic Abnormality," *American Journal of Nursing,* **71**(8):1551-1557, 1971.

Remoin, D. L.: "The Medical Genetics Clinic and Community Health," *Birth Defects: Original Articles Series,* vol. VI, no. 1, *Genetic Counseling,* Baltimore: Williams & Wilkins Company, 1970.

Schimke, R. N.: "Heredity for Clinicians: Genetics and the Practicing Physician," *Journal of the Kansas Medical Society,* **69**(1):1-9, 1968.

Stanburg, J. B.: *The Metabolic Basis of Inherited Disease,* New York: McGraw-Hill Book Company, 1966.

Thompson, J. S., and M. W. Thompson: *Genetics in Medicine,* Philadelphia: W. B. Saunders Company, 1966.

Whipple, D. V.: *Dynamic Development: Euthenic Pediatrics,* New York: McGraw-Hill Book Company, 1966.

Chapter 24

Behavior Modification
in the Family

Edward R. Christophersen*

Robins (1966), in a longitudinal analysis of children referred to a child guidance clinic, emphasized that there is an apparent relationship between early-
appearing antisocial behavior and later patterns of deviant behavior. Moreover, she emphasized the importance of developing intervention techniques to
deal with these childhood behavior problems. Traditionally, child guidance
clinics have utilized a variety of psychotherapeutic techniques, ranging from
psychoanalytic to nondirective to eclectic, both in individual and group treatment programs. However, as Eysenck (1960) and Levitt (1957, 1963) have
indicated in their extensive reviews of most of the published reports which
have attempted to evaluate the effectiveness of psychotherapy, these traditional child guidance procedures have not been demonstrated to be effective
in ameliorating child behavior problems. In fact, both Eysenck and Levitt

* The author was supported during the preparation of this manuscript by a grant from the National
Institute for Child Health and Human Development (HD 03144–03) to the Bureau of Child Research,
University of Kansas, and a grant from the National Coordinating Center, National Program on Early
Childhood Education (OEC-3-7-070706-3118) to the Kansas Center for Research in Early Childhood Edu-
cation.

315

report, in the studies reviewed, that on the average, approximately 65 percent of the patients undergoing psychotherapy showed at least partial improvement, whereas in the control populations (no-treatment groups), approximately 70 to 75 percent of the patients showed at least partial improvement. [It should be noted that Strupp (1963) and others have criticized Eysenck's report on the basis of (1) his comparing patients who underwent psychotherapy with patients who either received no treatment at all or were treated by general practioners; (2) his discussion of criteria for discharge and spontaneous recovery; and (3) his suggestion that patients in psychotherapy should, if psychotherapy is effective, show greater improvement than patients that have never been in psychotherapy. Eysenck counters these arguments by stating that if psychotherapy were an effective intervention technique surely a favorable comparison would have been made by now.]

Recently, evidence has increasingly shown that a behavioral approach can be effective in dealing with child behavior problems. A number of interesting case studies have been published which deal with child behavior problems. Several of these will be briefly reviewed prior to a discussion of more comprehensive approaches to management of child behavior problems. Williams (1959) reported a decrease in a child's crying at bedtime from instructing the parents to ignore all crying once the child had been put to bed and his door closed. Within 2 days the child's crying had decreased from almost 45 minutes at bedtime to less than 10 minutes, and at the end of a week the crying no longer occurred at bedtime. Russo (1964) reported a similar procedure in which the mothers of two children were encouraged to ignore inappropriate behavior such as violent outbursts and rudeness. In addition, however, the mothers were encouraged to pay particular attention to their children when they were engaging in appropriate behavior like sociability and friendly conduct. Although Russo does not report any data from these two families, he does indicate that the parents were satisfied with the gains shown by the children.

Hawkins, Peterson, Schweid, and Bijou (1966) reported a study where the parents were instructed to alter their attention toward their child. However, in this case the therapists were actually present in the home and instructed the parents, using three prearranged hand signals to indicate that the mother should (1) tell Peter to stop whatever objectionable behavior he was engaging in; (2) immediately place Peter in his room and lock the door; or (3) give Peter attention, praise, and affectionate physical contact. The data in this study indicated that the program was effective with Peter. His objectionable behavior decreased from about sixty times in a therapy hour to less than ten times in only 2 days. This study represents a real contribution in the sense that it is one of the earliest behavioral studies to report a scientific analysis of the child's behavior. After Peter's objectionable behaviors had decreased, the therapist stopped signaling the mother and instructed her to respond to Peter the way that she had been responding prior to any interaction with the therapist. When the mother did this, Peter's objectionable behavior increased. Then the therapist started signaling the mother again, and the objectionable behavior decreased again. The authors also discussed the inherent weakness of relying on observers' reports of a child's behavior. They pointed out that such reports would be much more believable if two observers were to independently record what a child does. The two reports could then be compared to arrive at the interobserver reliability. Any time that human observations are included in a report (e.g., interviews, diagnostic work-ups, nurse's notes), an occasional interobserver reliability check lends credulity to the observation. [For further discussion of the importance of interobserver reliability checks, see Baer, Wolf, and Risley (1968) and Bijou, Peterson, and Ault (1968).]

O'Leary, O'Leary, and Becker (1967), in a study similar to Hawkins et al. (1966), showed parents how to alter three general classes of behavior: deviant, cooperative, and isolate. The therapist instituted a procedure whereby the children received candy and praise for being cooperative; and the parents were instructed to ignore crying, screaming, and temper tantrums. Later on, the parents began isolating the children in the bathroom for 5 minutes for each time that they engaged in any deviant behavior. The data presented showed that these procedures were effective in that the children's cooperative play was increased from approximately 40 to 90 percent. As in the Hawkins et al. (1966) study, the procedures were temporarily removed and then reinstituted, and the authors reported on their interobserver reliability. The Zeilberger, Sampen, and Sloane (1968) study is essentially a replication of Hawkins et al. (1966). When a 4½-year-old boy, Rorey, acted aggressively or was disobedient, the parents were instructed to take him to a designated bedroom and leave him there until he had been quiet for a minimum of 2 minutes. They were also instructed to pay attention to Rorey and to praise him each time that he engaged in cooperative play. Implementing this program resulted in Rorey's (1) following instructions much more readily, (2) engaging in much less aggressive behavior, and (3) engaging in much less yelling and bossing. All the observations were done in the home by professional observers. Frequent checks were made of interobserver reliability.

Wahler, Winkel, Peterson, and Morrison (1965) described a set of procedures whereby the therapist went into the home on several occasions prior to any intervention in order to obtain an accurate picture of the current parent-child interaction. Also, this period prior to any intervention was used as an opportunity to revise the observation techniques until they were reliable. That is, until the two observers recorded *exactly* the same behavior at least 90 percent of the time. During the initial intervention sessions, the therapist gave verbal instructions to the mother before and after the playroom sessions, plus signal light communications to her during the sessions. Initially, the signal light was used to tell the mother when to respond in a certain way. Later it was used to tell the mother that she had behaved appropriately. Thus, in this study, behavior modification procedures were used to teach the mother how to modify her child's behavior. The mother was instructed to ignore her child's deviant behavior and to respond to her child in a socially approving manner when he was not engaging in any deviant behavior.

Using these procedures with Danny, a six-year-old boy who frequently issued verbal commands to his mother and who seldom cooperated with his mother's instructions, resulted in a considerable drop in Danny's commanding behavior and a sharp increase in his cooperative behavior.

Similar data were reported for another child, Johnny, age four. However, for a third child, Eddie, age four, these procedures were not very effective until the mother was also instructed to isolate Eddie immediately following any oppositional behavior. The data from these three families indicate that it is possible to analyze a particular parent-child interaction and to develop a set of instructions for the parent in order to teach the parent how to modify the child's deviant behavior.

Wahler (1969), using a set of procedures somewhat similar to those applied in Eddie's case, demonstrated substantial decreases in the oppositional behaviors of a six-year-old boy and a five-year-old boy. These data indicated that, as the parents became more skillful in their ability to isolate the child for oppositional behavior, the child spent progressively less time in isolation.

BEHAVIOR FEEDBACK

Bernal (1970) and Bernal, Duryee, Pruett, and Burns (1968) have developed a unique program utilizing behavioral feedback and parent education for training parents in child management. Initially, home observations and video tapes of parent-child interactions were used to analyze how the parents were reacting to the child and to look for ways that the parents might have been inadvertently encouraging the child to misbehave. This analysis then served as a basis for designing clear and simple step-by-step instructions for the parent to respond socially to the child at the time he behaved in specified ways. For example, the therapist might have set out to teach the parents to reduce or eliminate what they said to their child when he misbehaved. The instructions were given in very brief form, out of concern that too much instruction at one time might have been confusing to the parent. The exact nature of the instructions was tailored to the unique features of the particular relationship. During the first session, a video tape was made of the parent interacting with the child at the clinic. Each session thereafter consisted of the clinician playing excerpts from the previous week's video tape and discussing with the parent the ways the parent might alter her behavior in order to modify the child's behavior. For example, if the parent had been ignoring the child when the child was engaging in appropriate social behavior, the clinician might suggest that when the child is behaving appropriately the parent should attend to the child and praise him. Following the discussion between the clinician and the parent, another video tape was made of the parent interacting with the child. Before the next meeting, the week's tape can be viewed as often as necessary by the clinician; such immediate replay facilitates evaluation both of the parent's performace and of the effects of the instructed parental behavior upon the child. Replay also permits the clinician the freedom to revise his treatment plans as he sees new parent-child behaviors emerge. Immediate feedback to the parent can be provided following each instructed interaction session. During the actual taping of the parent-child interaction, varying signals such as a buzzer and lights, as well as a walkie-talkie, can be used to help the parents follow the instructions. The use of videotaping permits the clinician to give the parents extensive feedback on whole patterns of parent-child interactions.

An example of these procedures is described by Bernal (1969). Jeff, an 8½-year-old boy, was referred because he had frequent temper tantrums and physically attacked his mother, his teachers, and his peers. Observations were initially made in both the home and the clinic to provide data for the behavioral analysis. Jeff appeared to be controlling his mother's behavior with threats of hitting, screaming, smashing his glasses, etc. His mother confessed that she did not like Jeff and was terrified of him.

A program was designed to teach the mother (1) how to reduce her verbal output and to selectively ignore Jeff's abusive behaviors, (2) how to punish Jeff when the need arose (e.g., "Tell him you're angry with him and why; if he continues, look angry and give him one hard spank"), and (3) how to respond warmly to Jeff and to praise him when he behaves properly.

The program was carried out in seven intervention sessions. During these sessions, the mother and the clinician met without Jeff for about 30 minutes to view the video tapes and to discuss what the mother should do. Then Jeff and his mother interacted for approximately 15 minutes. A brief tone was played over the intercom to cue the mother when she was to stop talking and turn away from Jeff.

The following is an excerpt from the fifth intervention session:

> To exert control over (Jeff), you can intervene as follows: Tell him what you want him to do or stop doing. Then give him time to shape up. If he doesn't shape up, tell him again what you want him to do or stop doing. Tell him clearly what

it is you wish or you disapprove of and be angry about it. Give him time to shape up. If he doesn't, repeat your angry statement, and smack him hard on the rear end. Keep it up until you get results, again pairing the spanking with an angry explanation. Don't be nice to him again until he deserves it (Bernal, 1969, p. 378).

As Figure 24-1 shows, using procedures similar to that just outlined resulted in Jeff's general abusiveness decreasing from approximately twice a day prior to any intervention to about once every other day after approximately 6 weeks. Jeff's physical abusiveness decreased from about once every other day to about once every 2 weeks.

Bernal, Williams, Miller, and Reagor (1971), using procedures like those described above, reported that it had been possible to produce considerable reduction in deviant child behaviors in five different children using from five to eight intervention sessions.

Generally, Bernal reports the most success has come when (1) both parents participate, (2) the parents are cooperative, and (3) the parents have

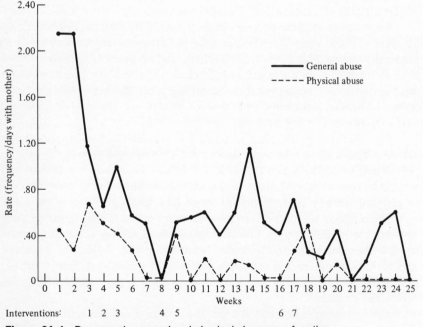

Figure 24-1   Decrease in general and physical abuse as a function of clinical intervention using video-taped feedback to train the parent. *(Source: M. E. Bernal, "Behavioral Feedback in the Modification of Brat Behaviors," Journal of Nervous and Mental Disease, **148:** 375–385, 1969.)*

an essentially stable and satisfying marriage. For the five children reported, their ages ranged from 2½ to 8½ years, and all the children behaved in the clinic much as they did at home which allowed ample opportunity for the clinician to train the mother.

REPROGRAMMING THE SOCIAL ENVIRONMENT

Patterson, McNeal, Hawkins, and Phelps (1967) have suggested that, for some deviant children, their environment is such that on those occasions when the child displays a socially adaptive or appropriate behavior, the parent or the peer tends to ignore the adaptive behavior. In these cases, they suggest that the environment should be reprogrammed in an attempt to teach the parent to attend to the occurrence of socially adaptive behaviors and to provide praise and attention when these behaviors occur. Further, they make the point that the only suitable place for such reprogramming is not the clinic or the hospital, but the home, and perhaps the school.

Patterson, Cobb, and Ray (1972) describe their procedures for intervention in the homes of families with very aggressive boys between the ages of six and thirteen. During the intake interview, the program is described to the parents, and, after some discussion, the parents are asked to sign release forms allowing the investigators to obtain information from other community agencies. Prior to any intervention, the families are observed for approximately 10 hours in the home with all the family members present (usually 1 hour each evening, five evenings per week). The observers record such behaviors as crying, laughing, playing, ignoring, and attention.

Patterson, Cobb, and Ray (1972) describe the observation technique they have used to obtain data on parent-child interactions. Observations were taken in the home 1 hour a day, generally between 4 P.M. and 7 P.M., when the entire family was present. Each observer was provided with the names of family members listed in random order. The observation hour was divided into 5-minute periods, and each family member was sampled as a subject for a 5-minute interval. When data had been taken on each member, the whole series was replicated until the observation hour had ended. Each observer was equipped with a clipboard containing a timing device that set off a light and a tone through earphones every 30 seconds. The observer was provided with a list of twenty-nine categories which described behavioral events. The events were catagorized as responses (such as command, cry, whine, yell, touch, etc.) and consequences (such as ignore, approve, disapprove, etc.). The observer took data on the subject's behavior and how the other family members reacted to it for the 5-minute period by writing down each behavioral event(s) that occurred in the 30-second interval. The data from observers were compared event by event for agreement during each 30-second interval. The agreement on events should be 80 percent or better before the data can be considered reliable. By taking this kind of intricate data, the clinician can observe, among other things, the sequence of behaviors and infer which behaviors seem to be maintaining other behaviors.

During the first 10 to 12 weeks of intervention, all families participate in a similar program. The parents must start out by learning the basic social learning framework upon which the intervention procedures are based. They do this by successfully completing a programmed textbook on child management (Patterson and Gullion, 1968). Then the parents are taught how to select and record their children's behavior. After they demonstrate that they can keep accurate records on their children's behavior, they are invited to join a parents' group. They are usually in the parents' group for about 10 weeks. If a family has particular problems not covered in the group, arrangements are made to work individually with the parents. [The actual intervention procedures are clearly and comprehensively described in Patterson, Cobb, and Ray (1972), so no attempt will be made here to incorporate the detailed procedures.]

Patterson, Cobb, and Ray (1972, pp. 79-80) reported that these intervention procedures "seem to be effective for between half and two-thirds of the families at a cost of roughly 32 hours of professional time. While as yet incomplete, the findings do underline the feasibility of training persons who live in the client's world to accept the major responsibility for changing deviant behaviors. Rather than send the child or the spouse, to 'some other place,' such as a hospital or clinic, family members can be trained to accept responsibility for each other's behavior."

BEHAVIORAL CONTRACTING

Stuart (1971) has proposed the use of behavioral contracts to change parent-child interaction. The behavioral contract he has described is composed of five major elements: a statement of privileges, a statement of responsibilities, a system of sanctions, a provision for bonuses, and a monitoring system. First, the statement of privileges must be described in specific behavioral terms (that can be easily observed), and each privilege must be the kind of positive activity which can be granted by another family member. Stuart gives an example of this kind of privilege as that of an adolescent wanting to be with his friends during certain hours of the evening or that of a parent wanting to know when his child will return home.

A statement of responsibilities which must be met in order to earn each privilege should be included in every contract. Each responsibility is to be paired with a privilege and must not exceed the scope of that privilege. (If the responsibility is too great, it may not be worth it to the child to work for the corresponding privilege.) Another element to consider in choosing responsibilities is that each responsibility must be one which can be checked on by the parent. An example of a responsibility which fits the above criteria is that a parent may permit his daughter to go out in the evening if she arrived home on time the prior evening. In this case, the responsibility is her returning home on time the prior evening, and the privilege paired with it is that she could go out the following evening; her return home was specific and observable enough that the parent could check it himself.

The third element of the behavioral contract is a system of sanctions (penalties) for failure to meet responsibilities. Building sanctions into the contract adds incentive for compliance with the terms of the contract and provides a stable means of responding to violations of the contract. One example of such a sanction would be that when a child arrives home late, his parents could set an earlier curfew for the following evening.

The fourth element of the contract is the provision for bonuses. Bonuses are in the form of extra privileges (such as an hour or two of extra late-night free time, or permission to go on a trip, etc.) and are to be given to the adolescent when he has followed the terms of the contract for a long period of time. (A sample of a behavioral contract is included in Figure 24-2.)

The final component of the contract is a monitoring system: a written record of privileges, responsibilities, sanctions, and bonuses. By writing down every responsibility fulfilled and every privilege granted, each child knows exactly where he stands relative to the agreement; thus the contract can proceed as smoothly as possible.

The procedure for developing such a contract can be deduced from Stuart's work (1971). In an initial interview with the parents, they should be asked to list specific behaviors which they want their child to maintain and certain behaviors which they wish to eliminate in their child. The list of behaviors, which must be observable and monitorable, constitutes the statement of responsibilities. Next, Stuart apparently asks the child to write a list of privileges, each privilege corresponding to a particular responsibility. Together the parents, child, and therapist work out a final list of responsibilities, privileges, sanctions, and bonuses that is acceptable to both the parents and the child. The last step of the procedure is to work out written monitoring sheets as needed. For example, a monitoring sheet might list all the days of the week and a space to fill in which behaviors (responsibilities) were performed each day in a column on the left-hand side of the page, and on the right-hand side, a column for the privilege (if any) that was used after the completion of the corresponding responsibility. The monitoring sheets should be written up with the help of the parents and child, so that it will be in the most readable form for them. (A sample of a monitoring form is included in Figure 24-3.)

Figure 24-2   A Sample of a Behavioral Contract Which Includes a List of Privileges with Their Accompanying Responsibilities, a List of Bonuses and Sanctions, and a Provision for Monitoring

Privileges	Responsibilities
General	
In exchange for the privilege of remaining together and preserving some semblance of family integrity, Mr. and Mrs. Bremer and Candy all agree to	concentrate on positively reinforcing each other's behavior while diminishing the present overemphasis upon the faults of the others.
Specific	
In exchange for the privilege of riding the bus directly from school into town after school on school days	Candy agrees to phone her father by 4:00 P.M. to tell him that she is all right and to return home by 5:15 P.M.
In exchange for the privilege of going out at 7:00 P.M. on one weekend evening without having to account for her whereabouts	Candy must maintain a weekly average of "B" in the academic ratings of all of her classes and must return home by 11:30 P.M.
In exchange for the privilege of going out a second weekend night	Candy must tell her parents *by* 6:00 P.M. of her destination and her companion, and must return home by 11:30 P.M.
In exchange for the privilege of going out between 11:00 A.M. and 5:15 P.M. Saturdays, Sundays, and holidays	Candy agrees to have completed all household chores *before* leaving and to telephone her parents once during the time she is out to tell them that she is all right.
In exchange for the privilege of having Candy complete household chores and maintain her curfew	Mr. and Mrs. Bremer agree to pay Candy $1.50 on the morning following days on which the money is earned.
Bonuses and Sanctions	
If Candy is 1–10 minutes late	she must come in the same amount of time earlier the following day, but she does not forfeit her money for the day.

Privileges	Responsibilities
If Candy is 11–30 minutes late	she must come in 22–60 minutes earlier the following day and does forfeit her money for the day.
If Candy is 31–60 minutes late	she loses the privilege of going out the following day and does forfeit her money for the day.
For each half hour of tardiness over one hour, Candy	loses her privilege of going out and her money for one additional day.
Candy may go out on Sunday evenings from 7:00 to 9:30 P.M. and either Monday or Thursday evening	if she abides by all the terms of this contract from Sunday through Saturday with a total tardiness not exceeding 30 minutes which must have been made up as above.
Candy may add a total of 2 hours divided among one to three curfews	if she abides by all the terms of this contract for two weeks with a total tardiness not exceeding 30 minutes which must have been made up as above and if she requests permission to use this additional time by 9 P.M.

Monitoring

Mr. and Mrs. Bremer agree to keep written records of the hours of Candy's leaving and coming home and of the completion of her chores.

Candy agrees to furnish her parents with a school monitoring card each Friday at dinner.

_____

_____

_____

Source: R. B. Stuart, "Behavioral Contracting within the Families of Delinquents," *Journal of Behavior Therapy and Experimental Psychiatry,* **2**:1–11, 1971.

Days of month

	1/17	2/18	3/19	4/20	5/21	6/22	7/23	8/24	9/25	10/26	11/27	12/28	13/29	14/30	15/31	16/--
Chores																
Set table, etc.																
Dishes, kitchen, etc.																
Bathroom																
Vacuum front room, living room, halls																
Cat boxes																
Other																
Other																
Curfew																
Time leave afternoon																
Phone after school																
Time arrive home from school in afternoon																
Time leave in evening																
Destination approved																
Time return in evening																
Time leave afternoon																
Lateness																
Lateness made up																
Bonus time																
Bonus 1 earned																
Bonus 1 spent																
Bonus 2 earned																
Bonus 2 requested																
Bonus 2 spent																

Figure 24-3 A sample of a monitoring form with provisions for indicating chores and curfews met on particular days along with a place to indicate bonus time. (Source: R. B. Stuart, "Behavioral Contracting within the Families of Delinquents," Journal of Behavior Therapy and Experimental Psychiatry, **2**:1–11, 1971.)

Stuart indicates some general rules that should be employed when utilizing the behavioral contract: (1) statements of privileges, responsibilities, sanctions, and bonuses must be described in very specific behavioral terms, and in enough detail so that each member of the family has a clear understanding of each behavioral description; (2) the four items stated above should be reasonably in balance with each other; (3) each of the items stated should be monitorable by the parents; and (4) privileges should not be abused, i.e., when a privilege is earned it must be granted by the parent. Stuart gives an example of using a behavioral contract as the primary treatment procedure for a sixteen-year-old girl who was referred by the local juvenile court. Candy had been hospitalized as an in-patient at a local psychiatric hospital following alleged promiscuity, exhibitionism, drug abuse, and home truancy. Her parents also reported that Candy engaged in "chronically antagonistic exchanges" within the family and had for a year done near-failing work in school. A behavioral contract was drawn up which stated specific privileges, responsibilities, bonuses and sanctions, and monitoring form (see Figures 24-2 and 24-3). Stuart reported that when this contract was put into effect, Candy's rate of compliance was very high, and her behavior continued to improve as time progressed. It was also stated that the behavioral contract served as a useful means of structuring a constructive interaction between Candy and her parents. When Candy and her parents did have arguments, they tended to negotiate by using the options available through the contract.

According to Stuart, the use of a behavioral contract between parents and their children is a highly effective, readily applied technique for use in efforts to promote appropriate behaviors and to eliminate inappropriate behaviors. In the case of Candy, it appears to have laid the groundwork for a more effective interaction in and of itself. In other instances, behavioral contracting might profit from interaction training for the parents, tutoring or vocational guidance for the adolescent, or financial assistance for the family. The decision about any additional techniques is optional, but Stuart suggests that behavioral contracting be made a part of every plan to improve the interaction between an adolescent and his parents.

BEHAVIOR RESEARCH PROJECT

Tharp and Wetzel (1969, p. 62) have outlined their work at the behavior research project with 147 different cases over a 2-year period. In their program, the supervising psychologists worked with "behavior analysts" (young, bright, individuals whose sole training was a 3-week seminar and on-the-job training) who, in turn were responsible for all the interaction with parents or teachers, who in turn effected the reported changes in the adolescents referred to the program.

Assessment   During the assessment phase, there are two requirements. The first is that of selecting and carefully defining the behavior that is to be changed. For example, although a child may be referred for hyperactivity, in the classroom setting this may translate to out-of-seat behaviors and talking-out behavior. Then, prior to any intervention, the behavior must be observed in the setting in which it is reported to be a problem and in which a change is indicated. This may be either at home or at school or in both places. This behavioral assessment, unlike diagnostic tests and historical assessment, actually indicates not only what the problem behaviors are, but also exactly at what frequency the behaviors are occurring. In this way it is possible to assess whether or not a given treatment technique is effective by noting whether the behavior in question improves (either increases or decreases depending on the referring complaint). In addition, observing the behavior in the natural environment allows the clinician to observe upon what occasions a child misbehaves. It is also important to note, as we have earlier in this chapter, what effect a child's behavior has on his environment. For example, some of the parents that Wahler (1969) described were actually encouraging their children to misbehave by providing attention and social interaction only when the child misbehaved.

Next, Tharp and Wetzel suggest interviewing the parent or teacher to establish what items or activities are attractive to the child. There are two ways of verifying that a child actually will work for a particular item or activity. One is to ask the child what he would like to have. Preferable to this, however, is to observe the child in his natural environment and record how often he works for each desired activity. It is also important to ascertain, as accurately as possible, not only *what* a child will work for but also for *whom* he will work best. This is usually based, in part at least, on what kind of interaction the child has with the person and also, in part, on what items and activities are mediated by the person. For example, if a child plays football as often as possible, a good mediator might be either a football coach or a recreation director.

Intervention   According to Tharp and Wetzel (1969), the basic paradigm for intervention is a simple one, and virtually invariant: rearrange the environment in such a way that desirable behavior pays off (i.e., obtains items or activities desired by the child) and undesirable behaviors have no effect or a negative effect on the environment. Tharp and Wetzel include a discussion of activities, materials, and people that can be used to increase desirable behaviors of a child, as well as a section discussing several ways of developing new behaviors in a child.

Evaluation   Tharp and Wetzel discuss several ways of evaluation in their research including: (1) change in the behavior that resulted in the court's referring complaint, (2) school achievement, (3) the parents' ratings of the changes in the child, and (4) the behavior analyst's ratings of the changes in the child. In terms of change in the referring behavior, approximately 99 percent of the referring complaints were reduced to at least half of what they were prior to any intervention, while 21 percent of the referring complaints were completely eliminated. In terms of school achievement, no significant changes in grades occurred. In terms of court contacts, "of the 77 intervened cases, 26 committed some offenses, and the vast majority were prior to termination. Five committed one or more offenses following termination, [e.g., 5 out of 77 pre-delinquents, and 3 of these 5 were subsequently committed to institutions" (p. 173)]. In terms of the parents' ratings of change in the referring complaints, approximately 82 percent of the behaviors were rated as either improved or very improved (very improved—approximately 20 percent). And finally, in terms of the behavior analyst's ratings, they indicated "that the overall effects have been to reduce the probability of the (child's) undesirable behavior" (p. 176).

HOME POINT SYSTEMS

Christophersen and Arnold (1971) and Christophersen, Arnold, Hill, and Quilitch (1972) have reported a set of procedures for training parents in the home to manage their children's behavior problems. The primary component in the procedures is a point system modeled after the work of Ayllon and Azrin (1968) and Phillips (1968). The parents are shown how to set up an economy, based on points, that is analogous to our monetary system. The children can earn points for engaging in appropriate behavior; they lose points for engaging in inappropriate behavior; and they can spend whatever points they have left at the end of a day in order to purchase privileges naturally available within the home. The point system differs from our monetary system in that there is no provision for deficit spending (i.e., no credit). There is also no provision for borrowing or lending, although the children do earn interest for saving their points, and it is practically impossible for a child to accumulate an excess of points.

During the first meeting between the therapist and the parents, the parents are questioned about the responsibilities they think each child should have and the privileges they think the child would like to have. Also, the parents are questioned about what behaviors they consider undesirable in their children. Whenever the parents suggest a responsibility or an undesirable behavior, they are encouraged to make their descriptions in terms of observable behaviors. For example, no child can ever be expected to "be good around the house"; however, he can be expected to "make his bed," "put his clothes away," and "empty the garbage." When working with older children, eleven to fourteen years, the children are asked to participate in deciding upon the appropriate responsibilities and privileges.

During the second meeting with the parents the actual point system is finalized. The list of responsibilities, privileges, and undesirable behaviors is compiled. Point values are assigned to specific behaviors, and the parents and the therapist decide on the cost of each of the privileges. Figure 24-4 shows an example of a partial list of the behaviors that earned and lost points and some of the privileges and their costs. The point values are assigned such that the child should be able to purchase most of the privileges he wants by doing most of his routine chores around the house and by losing a minimum of points for undesirable behaviors. In most of the systems that have been implemented thus far, the majority of a child's points are earned by what we call "maintenance behaviors" (e.g., household chores such as emptying the garbage, making the bed); and most of the points are lost from fines levied

Figure 24-4 A Partial List of Behaviors and the Number of Points They Gained or Lost and a Partial List of the Activities for Which Licenses Were Available and the Price in Points

Licenses available			Price in points
Basic privileges			60
Drive-in movie			200
Picnic			50

Behaviors that earned and lost points			Points earned or lost
George	1	Make beds	10
	2	Hang up clothes	10
Keith	3	Empty trash	20
	4	Make bed	20
Dollie	5	Feed cat	20
	6	Bathe	20

Behaviors that earned points		Points earned
1	Sweep rug	10
2	Clean bathroom	20
3	Answer telephone	15

Behaviors that lost points		Points lost each occurrence
1	Bickering	10
2	Teasing	10
3	Whining	10

Source: E. R. Christophersen, C. M. Arnold, D. W. Hill, and H. R. Quilitch, "The Home Point System: Token Reinforcement Procedures for Application by Parents of Children with Behavior Problems, *Journal of Applied Behavior Analysis*, 5:71–83, 1972.

against social behaviors like crying, cursing, and coming home late. The privileges are such everyday things as watching TV and riding bikes.

The parents are instructed that they should only warn a child once for each undesirable behavior—not once each time, but a total of one time. After that initial warning the child should be fined each time the undesirable behavior occurs. Also, the parents are instructed not to nag at the child. In fact, in several families the children earn points each time one of the parents nags at them.

Usually, the therapist goes out to the home several evenings during the first week that the point system is in effect. These meetings are used to discuss various aspects of the system and to give the parents feedback on their use of the system.

Christophersen, Arnold, Hill, and Quilitch (1972) described the application of the point system with three different families. One of these applications will be described here briefly, as an example of this technique.

Subjects

The three subjects in this family were all members of the same family: a nine-year-old boy (George), an eight-year-old girl (Dollie), and a five-year-old boy (Keith).

The nine-year-old boy was a good student academically but had some problem behaviors both at school and at home. He had begun skipping school, he rarely followed directions at home, and he had become particularly sassy toward his mother.

The eight-year-old girl had mild cerebral palsy and was in an educable mentally retarded class in the public school system. She had had extensive speech therapy and occupational therapy by the Doman-Delacatto method. At home, she was described as hyperactive, occasionally engaging in tantrum-like behavior.

The five-year-old boy presented a few behavior problems. The parents' major complaint was his whining.

All three children engaged in bickering on frequent occasions. Bedtime was an occasion for giggling, talking, and general horseplay by the two boys who shared a bedroom.

Target Behaviors

Target behaviors were selected in maintenance (e.g., household chores) and social areas considered to be important by the parents. The target behaviors were defined in writing and posted for each child. Figure 24-4 shows examples of behaviors which gained and/or lost points and the privileges available. Each child had a 5- × 7-inch note card on which his points were added and subtracted (see Figure 24-5). The card was divided in half, with points earned

Name.....George............. Date.....6-6-71.............

Points made	Description	Who gave points	Points lost	Description	Who made points
10	MAKE BED	DH	-10	BICKERING	DH
10	CLEAN ROOM	DH	-10	"	DH
10	HANG UP CLOTHES	WH	-10	SASSY	DH
10	SWEEPING RUG	WH			
20	CLEAN BATHROOM	WH	-30		
20	HELPING DAD	WH			
20	CHURCH	DH			
10	FIXING SANDWICHES	DH			
110					

Privileges

...... Allowances

...... Snacks

...... Stereo

...... Telephone

...... Free time

Weekend

...... Weekend bank

...... Bond bank

60 Basics

Todays Point Totals

110 Earned

-30 Lost

80 Difference

Figure 24-5 Example of a 5 x 7 card used for keeping track of George's points gained and lost. At the end of this day, George had earned 80 points and spent 60 on privileges, so 20 points were put in the bank.

on the left side along with what the points were earned for and who gave them. The right side contained similar information for points lost. At the end of the day, the points were totaled and the basic privileges were purchased before any others. This assured a daily expenditure of points. If extra points were earned, they could be spent on other activities or placed in the bank for large activities such as a movie or camping out. In an attempt to evaluate the efficacy of the point system, several of the children's behaviors were recorded for several weeks prior to the introduction of the point system. After the system was instituted, the children's point gains and losses were recorded on a "point card" similar to that shown in Figure 24-5.

Initially the point system was put in only on maintenance behaviors. That is, only maintenance behaviors could gain and lose points. Although

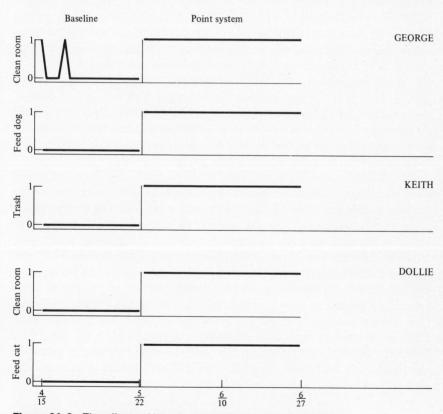

Figure 24-6 The effects of introducing a point system for maintenance behaviors of three children (five, eight, and nine years old) simultaneously. *(Source: E. R. Christophersen, C. M. Arnold, D. W. Hill, and H. R. Quilitch, "The Home Point System: Token Reinforcement Procedures for Application by Parents of Children with Behavior Problems," Journal of Applied Behavior Analysis, 5:71–83, 1972.)*

social behaviors were being recorded, only one, whining, was in the system when it was originally put into effect. Figure 24-6 shows the effects of the point system on the three children's maintenance behaviors. For each of the children, maintenance behaviors were practically nonexistent prior to introducing the point system. On May 22, when the system was introduced, all the children began doing their assigned maintenance jobs.

After the point system had been in effect on maintenance behaviors for almost 2 weeks, the point fines were introduced for one social behavior at a time, at 2-week intervals. This is a multiple-baseline or time-series analysis design (Baer, Wolf, and Risley, 1968). The parents recorded all the social behaviors between May 16 and July 22. A point fine was introduced for just bickering for George, while getting up after bedtime and teasing his younger siblings went unpunished. On June 17, George started getting fined for both bickering and getting up after bedtime. Then on July 7, George started getting fined for all three social behaviors. As Figure 24-7 indicates, each of the social behaviors remained relatively unchanged until the point fine went in for that specific behavior. Then, and only then, did the behavior change.

Christophersen, Arnold, Hill, and Quilitch (1972) reported the use of a point system as the prime intervention technique with two sets of parents, with a total of five children between the ages of five and ten. Data are reported on the measurement and modification of fifteen problem behaviors in one family, and six in the second family. All twenty-one behavior changes were rated as significant improvement by the parents.

It should be noted here that none of the parents using the point system were given any academic training. No effort was made to teach the parents any new vocabulary or any general behavioral principles. The entire training program consisted of teaching the parents how to use the point system. Also, for the most part, the point system was restricted to behaviors which were relatively easy to observe, rather than complex social interactions. This technique is used for two reasons: (1) many previous investigations have reported difficulty in reliably observing complex social interactions and (2) the point system is designed to be a training technique—a technique which demonstrates to the parents the efficacy of behavioral control in child management. Each of the parents who have employed the point system, to date, have gradually expanded the system on their own, to cover a variety of behaviors too complex to study with presently available observation techniques, e.g., logical thinking and problem solving.

HOME TOKEN SYSTEM

Alvord (1971) has described the use of a home token economy with families seen at a private psychiatric clinic. Of the twenty-eight families originally

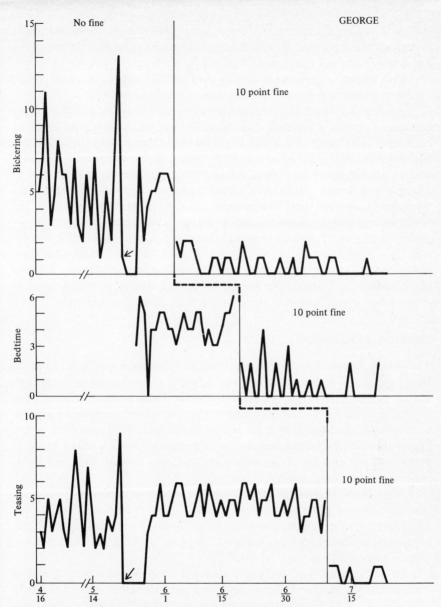

Figure 24-7 Multiple baseline analysis of the effects of introducing point fines on social behaviors of a nine-year-old boy. The arrows indicate when the point system was instituted for maintenance behavior. *(Source: E. R. Christophersen, C. M. Arnold, D. W. Hill, and H. R. Quilitch, "The Home Point System: Token Reinforcement Procedures for Application by Parents of Children with Behavior Problems," Journal of Applied Behavior Analysis, 5:71–83, 1972.)*

starting out with the system, Alvord reports that twenty-six sets of parents attempted to use the system, with four parents unable to enforce it due to the age and size of their children.

Two 1-hour sessions were usually used to teach the parents how to use the token system; the first session was spent discussing any behavior problems in the home and discussing relevant principles of behavior. Beginning with the second session, a contract sheet was filled out which listed and specified ten desirable behaviors by which the child could earn tokens (poker chips), five specific undesirable behaviors which resulted in the withdrawal of tokens, and ten ways in which tokens could be exchanged for privileges obtainable in no other way. Figure 24-8 shows a hypothetical example of a contract sheet for Suzy Q, age thirteen. The contract sheets provide (1) a place to list desirable and undesirable behaviors, privileges, and behaviors for which the parents must pay; (2) a place to record the occurrence of the listed behaviors; and (3) a convenient way to keep track of the child's daily token balance. Using one of these contract sheets enables the parents to keep track of the entire system for 2 weeks. Dr. Alvord is currently analyzing various aspects of the token system and will be reporting these data at a later time.

GENERAL DISCUSSION

The studies reviewed here have described and discussed a variety of behavioral approaches to intervention when a family is confronted with children having moderate to severe behavior problems. These procedures have been utilized with children from 2½ years of age up to the late teens and with behavior problems ranging from refusal to do household chores to severe aggressive and destructive behaviors. The intervention has taken place in both the home and the clinic, with parent training varying from cuing and instructions to formal academic training.

Most of the studies reviewed have two aspects in common. The first is that they depend upon cooperative parents. If the parents will not use the procedures, no therapeutic gains can be realized. The second aspect is that behavioral observations were made of the parent-child interaction to document whatever effects were reported.

It is often said that deliberate attempts to modify children's behavior with techniques similar to those described in this chapter constitute "bribery." Bribery is an emotionally charged term, difficult to specify, often associated with paying off those in governmental offices to perform personal favors. In relation to children's behavior, "bribery" seems to denote a relationship between parent and child in which the parent "pays off" the child for doing something that he "ought to want to do anyway," such as helping with chores around the house, doing his homework, and so on. This raises the

Home Token Economy

for **Suzy Q.**   age **13**   for weeks ending **6 - 6** & **6 - 13-71**

Desirable behavior

	Payoff	S	M	T	W	T	F	S	Events	S	M	T	W	T	F	S	Events
1 Folding & putting away clothes	2		2					2	2		4			2			3
2 Make bed	1	/	/	/	/	/	/	/	6	/	/	/	/	/	/	/	7
3 Brush teeth x 3	1	2	3	3	2	/	3	1	15	3	3	3	/	2	/	/	14
4 Room pass inspection	3	3	3	3		3	3	3	5	3		3		3		3	4
5 Breakfast cleanup	2	2	2		2	2	2		5	2	2	2	2	2	2	2	7
6 Brush hair	1	/	/		/	/	/	/	5	/	/		/	/		/	3
7 Take bath	2		2	2		2			3		2		2		2		3
8 Feed dog	1	/	/	/	/	/	/	/	6	/	/	/	/	/	/	/	7
9 School papers A=6 C=2 B=5 D=1			5		2	10			3			2					1
10 Play piano per ½ hr.	5			10	5	5			4	5			5				2
Tokens		10	19	21	14	26	11	3	54 / 104	11	18	13	7	16	8	8	57 / 81

Undesirable behavior

	Fine	S	M	T	W	T	F	S	Events	S	M	T	W	T	F	S	Events
1 Yelling	15						15		1	15							1
2 Crying	10																
3 Coming home late	20	20							1								
4 Lying	20				20				1								
5 Angry replies to requests	10																
		20		20		15			3 / 55	15							1 / 15

Privileges

	Cost	S	M	T	W	T	F	S		S	M	T	W	T	F	S	
1 Wear short skirt	2		2		2	2			3	2		2		2		2	4
2 Wear makeup	2	2		2		2			3	2	2	2	2	2	2	2	7
3 Phone rent per week	5	5							1	5							1
4 Dates - double only	5					5			1						5	5	2
5 Overnighters	2						2		1								
6 New records	10		10						1		10						1
7 T.V. per half hour	1		2		4	/	/		3		2	3					2
8 Snacks	1	/	/	/	/	/	/		4	/		/	/				2
9 Out after dinner	1		/		/	/	/	/	4	/	/		/	/		/	4
10 Special events																	
		8	0	17	2	10	9	3	21 / 49	10	3	14	5	9	7	10	25 / 58

Parents pay

		S	M	T	W	T	F	S		S	M	T	W	T	F	S	
1 failure to enforce economy	10																
2 Mother yelling	5																
3 Father cussing	5																

Token balance (bring forward)   2 / / 5 17 13 15 0   / / / 0 2 9 10 8

Note: No bankruptcy   No credit   No advances   No millonaires – Please read instruction booklet.

Figure 24-8 Example of a contract sheet for Suzy Q, age thirteen, showing her desirable and undesirable behaviors as well as her privileges and the three parental behaviors for which Suzy gained points. The Token balance at the bottom of the sheet indicates how many tokens Suzy has on any particular day. *(Source: J. R. Alvord, "The Home Token Economy," Journal of Corrective Psychiatry and Social Therapies, 17(3), 1971.)*

question of why children want to do anything. Common experience seems to indicate that children act in much the same way as their parents; i.e., they do things which are in their self-interest. Children want to go to see a movie that they think they will like; parents see a play they think they will like. Perhaps part of our job, as therapists and parents, lies in constructively arranging children's environments so that they *want* to do what society (and their parents) *demand* that they do. Children left to their own desires might as easily become child-guidance clinic clients as not. Those who would suggest that we let children develop freely do not take into account the fact that children, as their parents, are constantly subject to a variety of environmental and social controls. Perhaps it eventually becomes a question of whether we choose to deliberately raise our children to standards we think are reasonable, or whether we choose to turn these choices over to an accidental arrangement whereby, as likely as not, we teach children that noisy behavior pays off better than quiet, or hitting a kid brother gains more attention than does cooperating with one's siblings.

One further point that needs to be considered is that behavioral psychologists are not in the business of deciding what behaviors to expect from a child. Rather, we are developing procedures with which we can *assist* parents in developing behaviors in a child which the parents consider important. When parents seek professional help because they are concerned about their child, we can help them. We can train them to modify their own child's behavior, or we can modify the child's behavior and teach the parents how to maintain the behavior once it is modified. In every family mentioned in this chapter, the parents sought effective professional help in handling the problem behaviors—and they received it.

BIBLIOGRAPHY

Alvord, J. R.: "The Home Token Economy: A Motivational System for the Home," *Journal of Corrective Psychiatry and Social Therapies,* **17**(3):1–8, 1971.

Ayllon, T., and N. H. Azrin: *The Token Economy: A Motivational System for Therapy and Rehabilitation,* New York: Appleton-Century-Crofts, 1968.

Baer, D. M., M. M. Wolf, and T. R. Risley: "Some Current Dimensions of Applied Behavior Analysis," *Journal of Applied Behavior Analysis,* **1**:91–97, 1968.

Bernal, M. E.: "Behavioral Feedback in the Modification of Brat Behavior," *The Journal of Nervous and Mental Disease,* **148**:375–385, 1969.

——: "Training Parents in Child Management," in R. Bradfield (ed.), *Behavior Modification and the Learning Disorders,* San Rafael, Calif.: Academic Therapy Publications, 1970, pp. 41–67.

——, J. S. Duryee, H. L. Pruett, and B. J. Burns: "Behavior Modification and the Brat Syndrome," *Journal of Consulting and Clinical Psychology,* **32**:447–455, 1968.

————, D. E. Williams, W. H. Miller, and P. A. Reagor: "The Use of Videotape Feedback and Operant Learning Principles in Training Parents in Management of Deviant Children," in R. Rubin (ed.), *Advances in Behavior Therapy*, vol. III, New York: Academic Press, Inc., 1971, pp. 19-31.

Bijou, S. W., R. F. Peterson, and M. H. Ault: "A Method to Integrate Descriptive and Experimental Field Studies at the Level of Data and Empirical Concepts," *Journal of Applied Behavior Analysis*, 1:175-191, 1968.

————, ————, F. R. Harris, E. K. Allen, and M. S. Johnson: "Methodology for Experimental Studies of Young Children in Natural Setting," *Psychological Record*, 19:177-210, 1969.

Christophersen, E. R., and C. M. Arnold: "Behavior Modification Program for Parents of Children with Behavior Problems," American Psychological Association, in *APA Proceedings*, 1971.

————, ————, D. W. Hill, and H. R. Quilitch: "The Home Point System: Token Reinforcement Procedures for Application by Parents of Children with Behavior Problems," *Journal of Applied Behavior Analysis*, 5:71-83, 1972.

Eysenck, H. J.: "The Effects of Psychotherapy," in H. J. Esyenck (ed.), *Handbook of Abnormal Psychology*, New York: Basic Books, Inc., 1960.

Hawkins, R. P., R. F. Peterson, E. Schweid, and S. W. Bijou: "Behavior Therapy in the Home: Amelioration of Problem Parent-child Relations with the Parent in a Therapeutic Role," *Journal of Experimental Child Psychology*, 4:99-107, 1966.

Levitt, E. E.: "Psychotherapy with Children: A Further Evaluation," *Behavior Research and Therapy*, 1:45-51, 1963.

————: "The Results of Psychotherapy with Children: An Evaluation," *Journal of Consulting Psychology*, 21:189-196, 1957.

O'Leary, K. D., S. O'Leary, and W. C. Becker: "Modification of a Deviant Sibling Interaction Pattern in the Home," *Behavior Research and Therapy*, 5:113-120, 1967.

Patterson, G. R., J. A. Cobb, and R. S. Ray: "A Social Engineering Technology for Retraining Aggressive Boys," in H. Adams and L. Unikel (eds.), *Georgia Symposium in Experimental Clinical Psychology*, vol. II, Springfield, Ill.: Charles C Thomas, Publisher, 1972.

————, and M. E. Gullion: *Living with Children: New Methods for Parents and Teachers*, Champaign, Ill.: Research Press, 1968.

————, S. McNeal, N. Hawkins, and R. Phelps: "Reprogramming the Social Environment," *Journal of Child Psychology and Psychiatry*, 8:181-195, 1967.

Phillips, E. L.: "Achievement Place: Token Reinforcement Procedures in a Home-style Rehabilitation Setting for Pre-delinquent Boys," *Journal of Applied Behavior Analysis*, 1:213-223, 1968.

Robins, L. N.: *Deviant Children Grown Up*, Baltimore: The Williams & Wilkins Company, 1966.

Russo, S.: "Adaptations in Behavior Therapy with Children," *Behavior Research and Therapy*. 2:43-47, 1964.

Strupp, H. H.: "The Outcome Problem in Psychotherapy Revisited," *Psychotherapy: Theory, Research and Practice*, 1:1-13, 1963.

Stuart, R. B.: "Behavioral Contracting within the Families of Delinquents," *Journal of Behavior Therapy and Experimental Psychiatry,* **2**:1-11, 1971.

———: "Behavioral Control of Delinquency: Critique of Existing Programs and Recommendations for Innovative Programming," in L. A. Hamerlynck, F. Clark, and L. Acker (eds.), *Innovative Services to Youth,* Calgary: University of Calgary Press, in press.

Tharp, R. G., and R. J. Wetzel: *Behavior Modification in the Natural Environment,* New York: Academic Press, Inc., 1969.

Wahler, R. G.: "Oppositional Children: A Quest for Parental Reinforcement Control," *Journal of Applied Behavior Analysis,* **2**:159-170, 1969.

———, G. H. Winkel, R. F. Peterson, and D. C. Morrison: "Mothers as Behavior Therapists for Their Own Children," *Behavior Research and Therapy.* **3**:113-134, 1965.

Williams, C. D.: "The Elimination of Tantrum Behavior by Extinction Procedures," *Journal of Abnormal and Social Psychology,* **59**:269, 1959.

Zeilberger, J., S. E. Sampen, and H. N. Sloane: "Modification of a Child's Problem Behaviors in the Home with the Mother as Therapist," *Journal of Applied Behavior Analysis,* **1**:47-53, 1968.

Chapter 25

The Family That Fails to Thrive

Ruth F. Stewart

The failure to thrive of children without organic disorders is an indictment of society, and yet one that occurs frequently. The maternal deprivation associated with the syndrome is often part of a complex cycle of inadequate mothering breeding a succeeding generation of inadequate mothers. This malady will be perpetuated if professional recognition of a need for help occurs only with a major health crisis. Identification of high-risk families and early therapeutic intervention are critical aspects of health care. Nurses' involvement with the situational and interpersonal factors affecting family wellness puts them in a strategic position to help families who fail to thrive.

THE FAMILY

Reproduction and nurturance of the young are virtually universal responsibilities of the family. Other functions vary somewhat with the culture, but commonly provide economic and psychosocial support, as well as for sexual needs for adult members (Ackerman, 1958, p. 16). The dominant family pattern of Western societies assigns primary responsibility for childrearing to the biological mother. Her charge is to cultivate the societal ideal in the helpless and need-engrossed infant she has borne. It is her duty to satisfy the physical and emotional needs of her child, as well as to provide the training and discipline necessary to his adaptation to society. The mothering process, however, is not an automatic response to parturition, but depends on a variety of individual, as well as cultural, determinants.

Success and satisfaction as a woman are related to motherhood in United States culture. Because of this, there are women not maternally inclined who are nonetheless pressured into the mothering role. Others may succumb to the cultural persuasion despite their inability to meet the demands of an infant (Anthony and Benedek, 1970, p. 102). Motherhood is often embarked upon with far less rational consideration than that given to marriage, although its ramifications are far more pervasive. It results, also with no conscious decision for or commitment to it, through accidental impregnation.

Problematical, too, is that training for motherhood is inadequate in the modern, urban United States. Small families and mobility have altered the traditional pattern of learning the mothering process and practices within the family milieu. Institutional efforts to provide this are limited to high school courses in home economics and family life and to public health nurses' involvement with expectant or new families. Even these opportunities are limited, as policy or mores often restricts participation to families in low-income groups. Society, whose future is assured only through the health and well-being of its young, must give serious consideration to motherhood as a skilled and essential craft.

MATERNAL DEPRIVATION

The need of infants for a mothering relationship was demonstrated in thirteenth century Germany when Frederick II, King and Emperor of the Holy Roman Empire, decreed the separation of infants from their mothers. The infants died. Scientific awareness in the twentieth century brought about study of the relationship of developmental retardation to maternal deprivation. The earliest studies focused on children who were institutionalized, and thus physically separated from their mothers. World War II produced additional studies of children dislocated because of war-related incidents. Later studies have identified the maternal deprivation syndrome in families that are physically together but psychologically distanced. The distancing may be initiated because of the mother's insufficient or distorted relationship with her child, or by the child's inability to respond to the mothering attempts. These dimensions of maternal deprivation, i.e., discontinuity, distortion, and insufficiency, are all encompassed by Ainsworth's definition as "insufficiency of interaction between a child and a mother-figure" (1962, p. 98).

Deprivation Outcomes

The accumulated data leave little question of the adverse effect of maternal deprivation on infant development, despite inadequate understanding of the dynamics involved. The reversibility of developmental damage resulting from this deprivation can be viewed from several theoretical positions, including learning theory, psychoanalytic theory, and "critical periods." Ainsworth (1962, p. 152) believes that these can be compatible, and explains:

> Some impairment (is) . . . overcome through learning after deprivation has been relieved, while some impairment resists reversal to a greater or lesser degree . . . while still other impairment may persist because the sensitive phase has passed.

The age at which deprivation occurs and is relieved is undoubtedly a pivotal variable, though little is understood of this (Ainsworth, 1962, p. 153). Studies of children separated from their mothers have indicated that a child is most vulnerable from three months until about five years of age, with the last half of the first year a particularly critical period (Ainsworth, 1962, p. 21; Spitz, 1946, p. 338). At this time a child is normally differentiating himself from his mother, and developing a primitive body image. An impaired relationship with his mother during this period may interfere with this ego differentiation (Ainsworth, 1962, p. 21).

The extent of the deprivation is also related to the permanency of its effects. Any problems brought about by a single and short-term deprivation experience can be reversed almost completely, though a child is more susceptible thereafter to threats of separation. Longer or more severe deprivation, however, increases the possibility of continuing consequences (LaMarre, 1967, p. 584). Genetic differences are possibly a factor in the impact of deprivation on a child, though this is conjectural at present (Ainsworth, 1962, p. 23; Clarke, 1968, p. 1074; Schaffer, 1966, p. 595).

Language and abstraction are particularly vulnerable developmentally in a deprived child, with a resulting effect on intellectual maturation. Personality may be hampered by an inability to control impulses in the interest of long-term goals and from difficulty with interpersonal relationships (Ainsworth, 1962, p. 119).

FAILURE-TO-THRIVE SYNDROME

The failure-to-thrive picture is remarkably similar to the classical description of mourning and melancholia, with silent despair the overriding depression

(Spitz, 1946, p. 320). The child's expression may be soberly watchful (Leonard, 1968, p. 468), apprehensive (Spitz, 1946, p. 326), searching, or frozen. Little interest is evidenced in toys or his own body, and he may ignore activity going on around him. Warding off of stimuli occurs through averting his face (Spitz, 1946, pp. 313-314) or covering it with his hands or clothing (Leonard, 1968, p. 468; Barbero and Shaheen, 1967, p. 640). He will often remain immobile, with his body either rigid or flaccid (Barbero and Shaheen, 1967, p. 640). In contrast, though, some children cling tenaciously to any adult, and look woebegone when left behind (Spitz, 1946, p. 326). An obsessional need to stroke soft, silky materials when under stress may be manifested when the need for human warmth has been unsatisfied (Freudenberger and Overby, 1969-1970, p. 302).

Physical development is impaired, with weight more affected than height (Leonard, 1968, p. 469; Barbero and Shaheen, 1967, pp. 639-640). Gross motor development is delayed, as well (Barbero and Shaheen, 1967, p. 640; Leonard, 1968, p. 470; Spitz, 1946, p. 328). Other problems may include anorexia, vomiting, diarrhea (Barbero and Shaheen, 1967, p. 640), and insomnia (Spitz, 1946, p. 313). Deprived children are extremely susceptible to infections, and react more acutely to ordinarily minor ailments than would be expected. In Spitz's foundling home groups, thirty-four of the ninety-one children died within a 2-year period, from such illnesses as respiratory and gastrointestinal infections, measles, and otitis media (Schaffer, 1966, p. 313).

PROGENITORS TO FAILURE TO THRIVE

The ability of the family to meet its responsibilities to its members and to society is precarious at best. Comparing the family to other systems in society, Reuben Hill (1965, pp. 33-34) points out the handicaps imposed by family organization. He notes that the age composition is heavily weighted with dependents, and the weak or incompetent members cannot usually be expelled. Acceptance results from membership, with no additional requirements. It is a puny work grouping and awkward for decision making. Despite burdensome responsibilities, its structure is not organized to withstand stress. Stress, though, is a frequent occurrence in family life, deriving from situational or interactional factors. The disorganization of the family may be minor and transitory, but can quickly become a crisis. Manifestations of family disorganization, minor or major, are varied. Failure to thrive is one expression of this.

Situational Progenitors

Situational factors common to modern family life that are stressful include changes of job or residence, movement upward or downward in social status, illness, and increase of members. Additional strain is imposed by inadequate food supply, poor housing, indebtedness—constants in a life of poverty. An abundance of children multiplies the family expenses and magnifies its deficits. This often necessitates "moonlight" efforts of one or both parents in the attempt to support the family. One-parent families result in the assumption by one individual of most of or all parental functions, ideally shared. Physical or intellectual handicaps of any family member alter the usual role or task performance of all family members. Considerable pressure results when knowledge or skill is inadequate for implementing family or societal roles. Identification of any of these situations in a family suggests a high level of vulnerability to disorganization at that time.

Interactional Progenitors

The family, an "arena of interacting personalities" (Nye and Berardo, 1966, p. 100) can be viewed from an interactional frame of reference when considering its level of organization or disorganization. A child's failure to thrive, when pathology or malnutrition are ruled out, indicates interactional problems between that child and the mothering person. Basic to this, however, are interactional difficulties within the mother's family of orientation and within the current family of procreation.

The childhood relationships of the mother influence her perceptions of the roles in family life, and her ability to fulfill those roles assigned to her. Gender identity is a major facet of stable personalities and is learned from identification with the parent of the same sex. This identification may result in distorted psychosexual development if there are variances in the parents' sex roles. These may be manifested in overt role reversals, or by an incapacity to adequately fill the expected role. A cold, unyielding mother is particularly detrimental to her daughter's gender identity (Lidz, 1968, pp. 59-60), and this may foment masculinity and humiliation at being female (Anthony and Benedek, 1970, p. 398). On the other hand, a child's perception of insufficient mother-love creates the same results, even when this was not the case. This can occur when rivalry with siblings for maternal attention or love remains unresolved.

The mother-child relationship must also be viewed relative to other current family role reciprocities, such as husband-wife and father-child. The role of wife usually precedes, chronologically and affectionally, that of mother, and the achievement in the first role affects achievement in the other. Dissatisfaction with any of the processes involved in marital life, including sex, influences the mothering. Performance as a mother is related to the performance of the father in his role as well. Values held by the family regarding children, ranging from their number and timing to their sex and coloring, influences the maternal reaction to them (Ainsworth, 1962, p. 18; Rhymes, 1966, p. 1973).

A child's own behavior can be the initiating factor in his subsequent deprivation. He may be an "overactive" or "colicky" baby who creates sufficient stress that resentment and, subsequently, rejection may result. The phlegmatic infant courts deprivation because of this low-response level to maternal overtures, thus depriving his mother of positive reinforcement of her mothering role (Bullard, Glaser, Heagarty, and Pivchik, 1967, p. 688).

PREVENTING FAMILIES WHO FAIL-TO-THRIVE

"Give me good mothers and I will give you a good society," challenged Huxley. This society, as evidenced above, needs to heed the challenge and systematically promote better mothering. Nursing, whose focus is the individual, his health-related situation, and his perception of it, provides a critical mode for this within the health care system. The nurse has been traditionally accepted as a helping person, with less threat or stigma to the family than often associated with other health team members (Rhymes, 1966, p. 1975). A deliberative nursing process is an appropriate frame of reference for operationalizing the nursing intervention, with the goals falling within one of the three levels of prevention. *Tertiary prevention* (prevention of complication in an irreversible condition) will be instituted when the process begins with identification of a child with the failure-to-thrive syndrome, and where there is no apparent malnutrition or organic pathology. The child may have irreversible developmental damage, so that nursing goals will be focused on promoting sufficient family interaction and mothering that further deterioration may be averted, and infections prevented. [*Mothering* is defined for the purposes of this chapter in accordance with Freudenberger and Overby as "a process that may be performed either by men or by women. By the mothering process we mean a capacity to care for and relate to another in terms of the *other's* needs—especially as this process applies to the care of children by adults" (1969-1970, p. 299).]

Secondary prevention (early diagnosis and treatment) is involved where the inferential nursing diagnosis indicates mild to moderate family disorganization and poor mothering, but where there are no observable symptoms of failure to thrive in a child at the time. The goal in this situation is to promote family interaction and mothering conducive to the well-being of the progeny (present and potential) and to the prevention of symptoms.

Primary prevention (avoidance of the condition) is the level appropriate to families currently well-organized, with maintenance of this equilibrium and the mothering process as the goal. Child care practices aimed at primary prevention are the ultimate in family health patterns, but are only cursorily noted in this chapter. A primary aim, herein, is to suggest that problem families can be identified and assisted before the child and the family organization suffer irreparable damage.

The early identification of a family who has a potential for failing to thrive requires independent and sophisticated assessment by the nurse, as there is no observable physical pathology. It necessitates collection and analysis of data that encompass the parental attitudes and values related to family life and motherhood, as well as to each other. Collection of pertinent data can be instituted through inclusion in a guide for the nursing history or assessment. Other data may be revealed directly or indirectly through discussion between the nurse and the family members, through family interaction, and from nonverbal behavior. Limited contact with the family necessitates collecting only samplings of family interaction, such as how a woman holds and responds to her baby, how a spouse describes his marriage, or how a decision is made regarding health care. A woman's attitude toward a possible or existing pregnancy may be predictive of her interaction with her child in the future. Should these samplings suggest the need, methods should be instituted for further data collection. If the initiating nurse cannot follow this through, a referral should be made to a community-based nurse.

Nursing Process: Initiating Event

The initiating event for prevention of failure-to-thrive families is the coming together of a nurse with a family, or any of its members, in the early stages of family development. This may be at the stage of betrothal, honeymoon, prenatality, natality, or early childrearing. The predictability of problems with childrearing in this society should suggest to the nurse the data to be collected in order to assess the family for a possible need for help toward parenthood.

Nursing Process: Data Collection

The data necessary for assessment of a family's potentiality for failure to thrive are determined from the research discussed above. The data should be organized in a way that they can be easily used by all health team members, and specific history or assessment systems (i.e., family sociocultural assessment, individual client assessments) simplify the organization.

Situational variables, the tangible facts of daily life, can be gathered by routine interview. Sociocultural data that are useful include:

Household composition
  Head of household
  Relationship and ages of family members
  Nonfamily members living in household
  Family members not living in household
Educational level(s)

Ethnicity and language(s) spoken
Religion and involvement level
Employment: type(s) and duration
Financial factors
   Income and other resources
   Indebtedness
   Insurance, including health
Housing status
   Utilities available
   Soundness and size
Transportation

Health status is another fact of daily life, and the family's perception of this (realistic or not) is an important facet of the data. These data should reveal the family's view of:

Current health status of members
Past illnesses, health problems, deaths
Expectations regarding size of family
   Contraceptive practices
Health care facilities used, regularly or occasionally

Interaction of members is a crucial index of the organizational strength of the family. The interactional conceptual framework views this through the dynamic relationships relative to needs, behavior patterns, and adjustment processes. If the nurse-family relationship exists over a period of time, the processes to be studied include:

Communication patterns
   Who talks to whom
      how frequently
      conditions involved
      response to
   Who does not talk to whom
      regularly
      occasionally
   Who speaks for family to outsiders
   Nonverbal communication
      touch
      eye contact
      other
   Clarity of communication
      to nurse observer
      to family members

Handling of anger
  verbally
  nonverbally
  conditions involved
Decision-making patterns
  Egalitarian family
  Parent only
  Husband only
  Wife only
  Influence on by extended family
  Consistency of perceived to real patterns
Role relationships
  Consistency with societal expectations
  Acceptance of assigned roles
  Competency in assigned roles
  Role conflicts

Other processes of interaction that might be identified relate to family norms, recreation, and child socialization.

Nursing Process: Ordering and Selection of Data

The data need to be organized so that deficiencies or irrelevancies, as well as priorities, are revealed.

Nursing Process: Inferential Nursing Diagnosis

This step of the process involves "the active, conscious, deliberate consideration of the meaning of the data"—forming a hypothesis or hunch (Bregg, 1971, p. 6). The success of the nursing intervention hinges on the validity of the inferences. The inference necessary here concerns the adequacy of the family organization and the ability of the (current and/or potential) mothering individual to meet the nurturance needs of the (present and/or potential) children.

Nursing Process: Setting Goals

Goals established for nursing intervention necessarily rest on the previous steps of the process. To be operational, the goals cannot be an ideal, or wishful thinking, but must reflect the realities of such family and nurse resources as interest, energy levels, abilities, and time. They may require modification as the family progresses or regresses in its functional adequacy. In order to evaluate any change in the family, the goals need to be stated in behavioral and temporal terms.

Long-term (3 to 6 months) goals and short-term (each contact period, or a series of contacts) goals are necessary to provide direction for and to suggest methods of intervention.

Nursing Process: Intervention

Nurse-Family Relationships   The relationship of the nurse with the family is the pivotal factor in any nursing intervention. The nurse must be viewed as a family nurse, concerned about and working toward maximum wellness for the total family. The interaction will probably be channeled through the wife, because of the traditional role assignment for management of health and childrearing. Because of this, methods of including the husband in the interaction may need to be contrived. There may be occasions when he is present in health care settings or in the home at the time of a nursing visit, and needs only to be specifically invited to participate. Men often feel that they are intruding, or modifying their role, by "sticking around" when health or child care is the issue. Their participation, though, can be legitimated on the basis of family responsibility and decision making. Indirect contact can be maintained through the wife, by soliciting his opinion or his sharing in a decision.

Nursing interaction with a woman who is recognized as inadequate for carrying out the mothering role needs to be cautious and creative. Her feelings of inadequacy or dismay with the mother role are in direct conflict with cultural expectations, increasing even more her anxiety and guilt. Her behavior, because of this, will be suspicious and aloof. A suggestion, however indirect, that she is or will be a poor mother will establish an insurmountable barrier.

The relationship with the woman needs to be established as separate and distinct from the nurse's interest in her child, possibly to the extent of ignoring the child during initial contacts. The mother must feel the nurse's interest in her as an individual, with needs and rights outside her mothering role. She also needs to be recognized for the things she *is* doing well; there are always positive elements to be found in any situation. The nurse must be truthful, however, or he will discredit himself as a trustworthy individual.

Because of the probability that the woman has not resolved her own dependency needs (Anthony and Benedek, 1970, p. 536), a minimal dependency on the nurse during stressful situations in family development can prevent panic. With this support, then, she may be able to accept the dependency of her own child on her. This relationship must be considered as long term, as learning will be slow and family stress will predictably continue.

With the nurse's assistance in discussing her activities and concerns, the woman will very likely identify her own difficulty in dealing with her child, or an anticipated child. Such comments as "Children bother me," "They are too much work," or "I don't want to give up my career," may be admissions of the problem, and can be explored further. A woman who is considering pregnancy, but not yet pregnant may be aided in analyzing her own needs relative to the mother role. If the family postpones pregnancy until she is ready to accept its responsibilities, this family has achieved a higher level of organization and an opportunity for success. At this point the mother has involved the child in the picture, and he can now be introduced into the nursing intervention.

Child Care

With the advent of the child into the discourse of the mother and nurse, care needs to be exercised that the mother does not need to compete with her child for the nurse's attention. The mother's problems with child care can be the focus, rather than the child, with the mother and nurse collaborating on working these out. The self-concept of the mother is not diminished by the nurse assuming an authority role, and she is learning to think through her own problems and assume responsibility for making decisions.

Interaction of the mother with the child can be reinforced by pointing out the child's responses to her, however slight these may be. If the mother indicates interest in a specific activity or goal for her child, this can be used to structure interaction. An example of this is the mother who thinks her child should be walking. Whether or not this is developmentally realistic, the nurse can suggest the mother have a "class" with him for 10 minutes each day. He and the mother can develop a plan that is compatible with the child's motor coordination, but more importantly, includes the mother's handling and talking to him. Reinforcement will be needed for the baby's response to the mothering attempts, with care that the mother's expectations of the child not exceed his potential. Nursing intervention with mothers in other areas of child nurturance have been discussed by Rhymes (1966, pp. 1975-1976).

Family Planning

A family's control over its size is a fundamental factor in maintenance of organizational integrity. There is some evidence that the birth of a first child is provoking, even when the pregnancy is planned (Le Masters, 1965, p. 113), as well as when it is unplanned (Dyer, 1963, p. 199). In another limited study, all the failing-to-thrive children had been unwanted (Eckels, 1968, p. 15).

Nursing intervention is appropriate when the family has indicated they do not plan for family expansion within the next 9 months, but are not using reliable contraceptives. The intervention may be limited to giving information regarding contraceptive methods and resources for obtaining them. Usually, though, there are more complex factors when contraceptives are not used and, these must be considered. Concerns that commonly interfere include cultural or group taboos, fear of loss of sexual potency or satisfaction, concern about partner becoming promiscuous, and cancer phobia.

The usual communication and decision-making patterns of the family will affect any behavior change, and need to be considered in planning the intervention. Attempts to have the wife attend a family planning clinic will come to naught if her spouse makes all the decisions and their communication patterns do not allow for discussion of this topic. In such a case, the nurse may need to talk directly to the man, or to involve others relevant to the family in this direction.

Abortion has recently become an acceptable method for controlling family size once impregnation has occurred, and it is being used by many women. Nursing intervention, if abortion is being considered, may begin with suggesting resources. It is possible that further intervention will be indicated by the woman's fear of the procedure, her guilt reaction to it, or increased family strife resulting from it.

Communication Patterns

Although many nurses are not qualified to function formally as a family therapist, most nurses can assist family members in improving basic communication patterns. Successful communication is gratifying, bringing with it a sense of inclusion and security which is essential to family organization. Intervention consists of assisting family members toward an effective feedback system, appropriate verbal and nonverbal messages, efficiency of terminology, and flexibility (Davis, 1966). Families at any level other than highly organized, can improve family interaction through effective communication.

Crisis Intervention

A crisis results from an event that is perceived by the family as stressful, and for which they lack coping resources. Many events occur throughout a family's existence that might precipitate a crisis, such as birth or death, getting sick or getting well, promotions or demotions. It is the defining of the event as a crisis, and the inadequate resources for coping, that differentiate a crisis from simply an event. In working with families who are vulnerable to stress, the nurse can predict that certain events will trigger a crisis and then be available for assistance. This immediate help, whatever the source, is the critical element in crisis resolution. The results have been found to have far greater impact than a remedy for a given problem, and promote increased skill in dealing with subsequent difficulties. If however, the problem and its concommitant anxiety persist, ability to cope with future situations will be lower than the precrisis level (Hill, 1965), and family disorganization may result (Caplan, 1964, pp. 39–41).

General principles have been identified by Cadden which can be applied to intervention at the time of crisis:

1 Help the troubled to confront the crisis by helping him to verbalize and to comprehend the reality of the situation.

2 Help him to confront the crisis in doses which he can manage, being cautious not to overly dampen the impact. The reality of the situation must be kept in the forefront, although some periods of relief from looking at alarming reality are necessary.

3 Help him to find the facts since these are often less awesome than speculations about the situation. Fantasies can be more frightening than reality, however threatening it may be.

4 Help him by not giving false reassurance. Acknowledge the validity of fears and give reassurance that there is faith in his ability to manage.

5 Do not encourage him to blame others, since blaming is a way of avoiding the truth. Blaming may give momentary relief, but will lessen the likelihood of a healthy adaptation.

6 Help him to seek and accept help because he needs it and because, by seeking it, he is acknowledging that trouble exists.

7 Help him accept assistance with his everyday tasks, since a crisis disorganizes and disorients energies due to the excessive amount of energy diverted to the task of resolving the problem (Robischon, 1967, p. 32).

Anticipatory guidance in family development and other family health areas can be useful to many families by providing them with a coping resource (understanding of situation) necessary to avert a crisis in the future.

Nursing Process: Evaluation

The effectiveness of the nursing intervention must be routinely evaluated on the basis of the short-term goals. If these goals have not been met, the reasons for this must be identified and the process reconsidered. Modifications may be necessary at any step.

Achievement of these goals reflects progress of the family toward a higher level of wellness, and subsequent goals can continue to guide the nurse and family efforts toward optimal family health.

COMMUNITY ACTION

Huxley's contention that good mothers make a good society might now be reconsidered. Could he have said as well that good societies make good mothers? Many of the situational factors increasing the family's vulnerability to disorganization are a direct outgrowth of social conditions. Poverty is an obvious example, but basic to this is unequal access to education, occupation, and power related to race or sex.

Health care is not available to all families, even for the acutely ill, and few families have access to services promoting wellness. Very few families will have an opportunity for the nursing intervention discussed above.

Changes in health care will result, not just because a need exists, but because the economics or politics of the situation make change attractive. These realities, once accepted, can be utilized by nurses to promote the community changes necessary for family health. The professional responsibilities of nursing necessitate active involvement at the community level. Nursing intervention is most effective when it results in community wellness, with fewer families that fail to thrive.

THE LUNAS: A FAILING-TO-THRIVE FAMILY

A Working Relationship: The Initiating Event

The Lunas (names are fictional) came to my attention through the personnel of the County Outpatient Clinic. Cynthia had been seen in the clinic for diarrhea, and it was noted that at ten months of age she weighed eight pounds (birth weight, five pounds four ounces) and was developmentally slow. A social service conference with Mr. and Mrs. Luna provided additional information, including Mrs. Luna's limited intellectual capacity and her negative feelings about children. A referral was made to the health department, and I arranged with this agency to assume the nursing supervision of the family.

The nursing process began (initiating event) with my acceptance of the family as a client, but an essential corollary was yet to be decided—would the family accept me? Ordering the limited data available, and relating it to study findings, resulted in the initial inference that this acceptance would not be easily won. Mrs. Luna was undoubtedly conscious of her inadequacies as a mother as well as an individual. Having someone visit her as a result of this could increase her own self-doubts and result in a defensive or hostile reaction. I hoped to have an advantage from the prevailing view among the poor that public health nurses are helpful. The Lunas did not have a phone, but even if they had, I would have chosen to make my first contact in person in order to foster positive personal interaction.

The first goal set was to be accepted to the extent of getting inside the house and agreement for a return visit. Intervention, for the initial visit, was planned as presentation of myself as a public health nurse, a caring and helping person. To be perceived this way by Mrs. Luna, I would need to focus the visit on her rather than on the children. To examine or discuss Cynthia would emphasize the inadequacy of her mothering, and probably establish a barrier between us. The children's welfare, in the long run, was dependent on their mother being able to assume a nurturant mothering role. It was she who had to be the primary client in this failing-to-thrive family.

On my first visit to the Luna household I introduced myself as Ruth Stewart, a public health nurse. I explained that the clinic personnel had said that she had told them she was having problems with the children and they thought she might like to have someone to talk to about this. She replied that they had told her a nurse would be coming (which I had not known), but right now she was moving out of the apartment for a week. The electricity and water had been turned off because of overdue bills, and they were moving in with her husband's family until they had a paycheck. After establishing that they expected to return on Friday, I then asked about returning the subsequent Monday. Mrs Luna agreed to this and we decided on a mutually convenient time. Evaluation of this visit relative to my short term goals indicated satisfactory, though not glowing results. I did not get inside the house, but with an acceptable reason for this. Mrs. Luna received me with minimal suspicion and no hostility, and agreed to a return visit. A nurse-family relationship was begun on the second visit when Mrs. Luna met me at the door and invited me in.

During the next several visits to the Luna home (or rather, homes—they had moved again) I concentrated the nursing process on developing a working relationship with Mrs. Luna. Despite this focus, I learned a great deal about the family through discussion with her and her husband, as well as from observation.

The Family: Data Collection

Alicia and Guadalupe (Lupe) Luna have lived their young lives in this southwestern city noted for its Mexican-American culture and its poverty. The Lunas share in each of these heritages, but hold to the Great American Dream of a home of their own, nicely furnished. Meanwhile, they have moved through a series of small and shabby apartments, with periodic interludes with Mr. Luna's parents, as rent and utility bills got ahead of their pocketbook. They have recently moved to another part of the state in search of a job that might prove more satisfying to Mr. Luna than his night-shift operation of the elevator in a drab mid-town hotel. Perhaps he found use for the bookkeeping he studied cursorily between elevator runs at the hotel.

Mr. Luna was definitely the dominant member of this family, and Mrs. Luna recognized her dependence on him. This husband-father dominance can be expected from study of Mexican-American family patterns but was intensified by personal characteristics in this family. Mr. Luna was slightly built and handsome, and he seemed much younger than his 26 years, possibly because of his boyish gregariousness. He described his high school career as though it was the proving ground for his machismo (the uniquely Latin virility) so that it was not surprising that he did not graduate. His interest in women had not diminished, apparently, as his wife complained about his flirtations with her sister and others. He spent many of his evenings away from home with his male friends, another concern to his wife.

As many of the poor, he considered the daily grind of life rather futile and articulated this dramatically. His hopes for the future, however, belied this apparent anomie. His religion, Catholicism, provided no solace or satisfaction because he "had too much church" when he was a child. His family and his home were a source of pride and he was more actively involved in them than would be expected in Mexican-American, lower-class families. The decor of the apartment was livened by his efforts, one a golden-hued figurehead—a discarded styrofoam wig stand, gilded. He was demonstrably affectionate with both the little girls in the family, one his own child and one a step-child, and helped his wife care for them.

Mrs. Luna was a pretty nineteen-year-old with black eyes and long black hair. She always dressed neatly and attractively, though simply. Her intellectual ability was limited, typified by her being unable to shop without her husband, because she would be short-changed. Communication with her necessitated use of simple, concrete phrases, with continuous evaluation of her understanding. Her husband would take over for her, conversationally, if this was allowed. She accepted her dependence on him as proper. She was an immaculate housekeeper and derived pleasure from this. Her primary sources of enjoyment were shopping trips or movies (particularly horror-type) with her husband. Occasionally, she visited her mother's to watch television because their own set was not working. As her husband, she grew up within the Catholic church, but agreed with his view that she had "too much church" then.

Interaction was limited almost exclusively to the extended family, her own or her husband's. She said she did not have any friends, but that she liked people "who are nice to me." She readily identified her dislike for children and complained about her own making her tired and nervous. Both Mr. and Mrs. Luna wanted to avoid further pregnancies "until we have more money," so she was taking "control pills." Each of her two children had been conceived prior to her marriage, the first occurring when she was sixteen and in the sixth grade. Her mother was "mad" about the pregnancy and insisted that the baby would be placed for adoption. However, when Sally was born she "was so pretty" that her grandmother relented and kept her. Less than a year later, Alicia and Lupe began their courtship, which resulted in her second pregnancy and later, their marriage. Cynthia was born when her mother was eighteen and Sally was twenty months old.

A major theme of any discussion with Mrs. Luna was her reaction to her children. She recognized their dependence on her and used the housework to justify her inattention to them. I never observed her voluntarily initiating verbal or nonverbal interaction with either child. She responded to Sally's active overtures for attention by limited touch or comments, and occasionally would allow Sally to join her in the chair. Cynthia received attention only when she cried, and then primarily through care-taking tasks. Her usual docile inactivity did not provide much stimulus to encourage a response from her mother. During early visits, Mrs. Luna held her stiffly by the arm and at a distance, which reduced body contact between them to a minimum. Mrs. Luna said that her husband would get angry with her because she treated Sally better than she did his baby.

Sally was a bright-eyed, alert 2½ year old, constantly active and demanding attention. She responded with obvious pleasure when she received attention, and especially when this resulted in her being held or sitting close to others (family members or me). She chattered on in a patter that was seldom understandable, even to her mother. She would, on occasion, slow down sufficiently to talk and play with Cynthia, and sometimes tease her. She liked to play with other children, and would dash outside to find some if not watched carefully. Her mother did not approve of this because she got "too dirty."

Cynthia, at ten months, looked like a forlorn, limp doll and reflected many of the characteristics described for the failing-to-thrive syndrome. Her expression was one of "silent despair" and "soberly watchful" most of the time. She showed no interest in her own body, but would respond to items handed to her. She did not have toys because they "mess up the house." Cynthia watched others around her intently and responded to attention from family members (but not from me) by smiling. Other than her plaintive cry, she did not vocalize. Her mother said that she cried "a lot" at night, though this seldom occurred during my visits.

Her physical development was impaired with her weight more affected than her height. She could not sit without support or roll over. She grasped objects held toward her. She remained flaccidly immobile wherever her mother left her—in the playpen or on the couch. She had never rolled off the couch.

Cynthia's failure-to-thrive is only the most dramatic manifestation of the disorganization in the Luna family. The history of the family provides a classical cycle of the problem situations and relationships that trigger further problems.

The Lunas' decision to organize as a family resulted from the circumstance of an unplanned and undesired pregnancy. Another child, also unplanned, is a member of the family by virtue of her stepfather's acceptance. He provided for her as well as his own child and wife on $60 weekly income. The usual stresses of poverty were routine in the family life, and resulted in frequent change of residence. The educational limitations of both spouses and Mrs. Luna's intellectual limitations created additional hazards to family organization.

Mrs. Luna, in discussing her problems within her family, frequently referred to her childhood. Her father had deserted the family when the children were young and he "has nothing to do with us." Her mother remarried, but nothing was mentioned of her stepfather other than he is no longer living. Mrs. Luna always spoke about her mother with anger and described her as "lazy" and "mean." Mrs. Martinez was said to have "kicked out" both Alicia and her brother because they "wouldn't help." She would not allow the Luna family to move in with her when their finances didn't provide the essentials of life, but "she should." Although Mrs. Luna did not feel welcomed by her mother, she talked about her dependence on her. Data are insufficient for definitive inferences, but they suggest a pattern of unresolved dependency needs.

It is the story of Mrs. Luna's life with her mother that offers a clue as to why Sally thrived while Cynthia failed to thrive. At the time of Sally's birth, it was

Grandmother Martinez who responded to her, deciding that she would remain in the family. It is probably that Grandmother also assumed major responsibility for Sally, delegating some to her other daughters, so that Alicia was not burdened with the total dependency of her progeny. Only when Cynthia was born while the Lunas were establishing their own family unit was Alicia expected to bear the full responsibility of motherhood. The family structure could not tolerate this additional—and major—stress, and disorganization resulted.

Goals and Nursing Implementation

Goals, with this family, were established on a long-term basis, with one year chosen as the appropriate interval. Evaluation at the end of the year would indicate the extent to which the goals had been achieved, and provide baseline data for reestablishment of goals and redirection for methods of implementation.

A primary goal, basic to all others, in working with the Lunas was the establishment of trust. In order to evaluate the relationship relative to trust, specific behavioral goals were established. At the end of one year, Mrs. Luna will:

1 continue to agree to nursing visits every two to three weeks;
2 discuss freely the family problems; and
3 talk with the nurse when available about her increased anxiety level, rather than cleaning house.

Mr. Luna's perception of my role was critical to achievement of the goals. Important as this is to the nursing relationship with any family, it was doubly so because of Mr. Luna's dominance in his family. His trust of me would be evaluated through his:

1 continued agreement to nursing visits to his family every two to three weeks; and
2 participation in nursing visits when awake.

Implementation geared towards these goals included planning for home visits every two to three weeks with the family's permission and agreement with the timing. Visits were rescheduled, even though previously arranged, when the situation indicated I was not welcome at the time (i.e., when Mrs. Luna was feverishly cleaning house, probably to reduce her increased anxiety or when Mr. Luna awoke early and wanted to take the family shopping). Permission was requested from Mr. Luna to visit his family, initially through Mrs. Luna and later from him directly. Occasionally, visits were arranged at times at which Mr. Luna could participate. When visits were not specifically scheduled ahead, for various reasons, I would write to Mr. and Mrs. Luna suggesting alternative times, including a postal card for their reply.

The paramount goal was that Mrs. Luna would modify her behavior to provide more adequate mothering for her children. Because her own inadequate self-concept and dependency needs were very likely interfering with this, it was here the implementation had to begin, and not with teaching the tasks of motherhood. It was through the tasks, though, that evaluation could take place, so specific goals were established in relation to the children. Mrs. Luna, at the end of one year will:

4 describe a positive behavior of each child and relate this to her interaction with each;
5 provide toys or toy substitutes for children to play with indoors;
6 allow Sally to play outdoors two to three times weekly;
7 hold Sally, when child initiates this;
8 hold Cynthia three times daily, ten minutes each time; and
9 talk with Cynthia three times daily.

Mrs. Luna's dependency needs were met to a limited extent by my being available on a periodic basis for her discussion of her problems, and for assistance in handling those relative to her children. A positive self-concept was fostered through focus on her and her problems, rather than the children, as well as by avoidance of comments or behaviors that might be interpreted as critical. I also legitimated for Mrs. Luna the reality of the problems of motherhood and housekeeping, and the needs of women beyond these roles. I identified and reinforced the attributes and behaviors that contributed positively to the limited family organization. There was always something positive I could pick up on within the situation and the bounds of truth. An incidental, but important consideration, was my inquiring of Mrs. Luna what she wanted me to call her . . . and her reply was Mrs. Luna.

Data collection was a continuing process, partly because of situational changes, but also because the family's increasing trust in me allowed them to disclose more about themselves and their history. Other data resulted from very specific collection methods [see Client Assessment] that I employed once we were well into a working relationship.

I implemented the client assessment by suggesting to Mrs. Luna that getting more information from her about her own health and the problems she had been discussing would be helpful in our working together to decrease the problems. I explained that I would use a form that nurses used on everybody with whom they work, thus establishing it as a routine procedure, not differentiating her or her problems. She agreed to this readily and a time was arranged for this. Despite the assessment focus on Mrs. Luna, many of the answers involved concern for and problems related to her children. This, then, was used as an approach to suggest doing assessments on the children as well. The same assessment guide was used, in this case, for the children.

The information from the assessments was useful in validating inferences made previously on the basis of limited data and findings from the literature for comparable situations. It was most useful in that it brought the problems Mrs. Luna faced in mothering her young daughters to an operational level. In responding to questions on the guide, Mrs. Luna identified several specific problem areas in the tasks of child rearing. Because of this, additional goals were established as a basis for working together in such areas as controlling Sally and feeding Cynthia. It was Mrs. Luna, though, who initiated the discussion of the problems. At this point, Mrs. Luna and I began working toward her increased interaction with Sally and Cynthia. Unfortunately, it was about this time that Mr. Luna decided to move to an area that appeared more promising economically.

Evaluation

The goals established for the Luna family could not be validly evaluated because the nursing process was interrupted before the evaluation term was completed. However, nursing methodology could be assessed informally relative to family responses.

Contact with the family was maintained until they left the community, with their agreement on the frequency and timing of visits. There were some occasions when they were not home, however, at the time agreed on. Mrs. Luna would later explain, voluntarily, that Lupe had awakened and wanted to go shopping or to visit. Because this was typical of his behavior, it was very probably the reason. My encouragement of Mrs. Luna to do things she enjoyed, as well as maintaining her household roles, may also have contributed to this. I did consider the possibility of avoidance, but the data did not support this.

Mrs. Luna said several times that she liked to have me visit her and contrasted this to the "other nurse" that told her to "feed the kids more."

Correspondence to Mr. and Mrs. Luna suggesting possible visit times was always answered on the enclosed postal card by Mr. Luna. A couple of times he explained that they were to be out of town, but told when they would return. He volunteered that they liked getting these letters.

As the nurse-family relationship continued, Mrs. Luna articulated more specifically and clearly her interpersonal problems, not only with her children but also with her husband and her mother.

After several months, Mrs. Luna identified that she was not as tired as she used to be, and was sleeping better. She attributed this to Cynthia's "getting older." Since, in these few months, Cynthia's needs and behavior had not changed, it suggested a change in her mother's acceptance of her.

Mrs. Luna's mothering behavior modified somewhat during this time. Although she did not hold Cynthia very often, she did begin holding her close to her and in a more relaxed manner. She volunteered that she was "doing more" for the children, although I had never suggested this to her.

The few changes highlighting the eight-month nursing intervention with the Lunas seem woefully insufficient when looking at those problems that remain. Modification to any extent, however, increases the family's capability for coping with the remaining problems, and increases their potential for wellness.

CLIENT ASSESSMENT

Head of Household: Guadalupe Luna
Address: 321 Culebra
Name: Luna, Alicia Sanchez
Name prefers staff to use: Mrs. Luna
Birth Date: 3/24/52
Religion: Catholic (not practicing)
Medical Dx: None
Nursing Dx: Inadequate and insecure mother
Interviewee: Alicia Luna
Interviewer: Ruth Stewart, R.N.
Date: 5/17/71
A   Significant biopsychosocial data related to activities of daily living
  1   Rest and sleep
        Often wakened by children during night and wakes up tired. Likes
        to sleep late in morning. Does not nap.
  2   Elimination
        O.K.
  3   Eating
        Very good appetite, eats three to four times daily if food available
        (financial problems with this). Likes meat particularly.
  4   Breathing
        O.K.
  5   Skin
        O.K.
  6   Senses
        O.K.
  7   Mobility
        O.K.
  8   Recreation
        Shopping with husband, favorite recreation. Likes movies, par-
        ticularly horror. Can only do this if sister will babysit. Goes to
        mother's home occasionally to watch T.V. (None in own home.)
        Does not attend church (too much when a child).
  9   Communication
        Limited because of problems of understanding. Need to use very
        simple concrete statements with her. Husband will take over com-
        munication for her if he's around. She enjoys talking with nurse
        when alone.
  10 Interpersonal relations
        Interaction only with family. No friends. Likes people "who are
        nice to me."
  11 Temperament
        Placid and accepting. Admits nervousness with children, but can't
        get adequate Hx (see A. 9.).

12 Dependence/Independence
    Identifies dependence (extreme) on husband, mother.
13 Education
    6th grade (at 16 years).
14 Work
    Maintains household. Immaculate housekeeper. Does laundry in bathtub.
15 What is important to person
    To remain nonpregnant.
    To have a house and furniture.

B Sociocultural
   See family sociocultural assessment.
C Data related to person's health needs
    1 Patient's and/or family's understanding of condition
       Attributes problems in family to having the children. She does not like children. They make her tired and nervous. Doesn't "have time for them" because of house work.
    2 Patient's and/or family's understanding of condition and events leading up to it
       Expects problems (C.1.) to be reduced because Cynthia is getting older (Sally not mentioned) and if she does not get pregnant.
    3 How condition is managed in home
       Children have been cared for physically, but given little attention or affection by mother. Mr. Luna does assist her with care of children. Generally, situation is just "muddled through."
    4 Previous health care and reaction to this
       Emergency care and prenatal care.
       Now on contraceptive pills—taking O.K.

Nursing Goals: At the end of one year Mrs. Luna will:
    1 Continue to agree to nursing visits every two to three weeks.
    2 Discuss freely the family problems.
    3 Talk with the nurse, when available, about her increased anxiety level, rather than housecleaning.
    4 Describe a positive behavior of each child and relate this to her interaction with each.
    5 Provide toys or toy substitutes for children to play with indoors.
    6 Allow Sally to play outdoors two to three times weekly.
    7 Hold Sally, when child initiates this.
    8 Hold Cynthia three times daily, ten minutes each time.
    9 Talk with Cynthia three times daily.

BIBLIOGRAPHY

Ackerman, N. W.: *The Psychodynamics of Family Life,* New York: Basic Books, Inc., 1958.

Ainsworth, M.: *The Effects of Maternal Deprivation,* Public Health Paper 14, Geneva: World Health Organization, 1962.

Anthony, E. J., and T. Benedek (eds.): *Parenthood,* Boston: Little, Brown and Company, 1970.

Barbero, G. J., and E. Shaheen: "Environmental Failure to Thrive: A Clinical View," *The Journal of Pediatrics,* **71**(5):639-644, 1967.

Bowlby, J.: *Maternal Care and Mental Health,* 2d ed., Monograph Series #2, Geneva: World Health Organization, 1952.

Bregg, E. A.: "Curriculum Conceptual Framework," The University of Texas Clinical Nursing School (System-Wide), October 1971. Mimeographed paper.

Bullard, D. M., H. H. Glaser, M. C. Heagarty, and E. C. Pivchik: "Failure to Thrive in the 'Neglected' Child," *American Journal of Orthopsychiatry,* **37**:660-690, 1967.

Caplan, G.: *Principles of Preventive Psychiatry,* New York: Basic Books, Inc., 1964.

Clarke, A. D. B.: "Learning and Human Development," *British Journal of Psychiatry,* **114**:1061-1077, 1968.

Davis, A. J.: "The Skills of Communication," in D. Mereness (ed.), *Psychiatric Nursing,* Dubuque, Iowa: W. C. Brown Company Publishers, 1966, pp. 44-48.

Dyer, E. D.: "Parenthood and Crisis: A Re-Study," *Marriage and Family Living,* **25**(5):196-201, 1963.

Eckels, J. A.: "Home Follow-up of Mothers and Their Failure-to-thrive Children Using Planned Nursing Intervention," *American Nurses Association Clinical Sessions,* New York: Appleton-Century-Crofts, 1968, pp. 12-19.

Freudenberger, H. J., and A. Overby: "Patients from an Emotionally Deprived Environment," *Psychoanalytic Review,* **56**:299-312, 1969-70.

Hill, R.: "Generic Features of Family under Stress," in H. J. Parad (ed.), *Crisis Intervention,* New York: Family Service Association of America, 1965, pp. 32-54.

LaMarre, C. J.: "Psychological Aspects of the Development of the Young Child," *Medical Services Journal,* **23**:580-586, 1967.

Leaverton, D. R.: "The Pediatrician's Role in Maternal Deprivation," *Clinical Pediatrics,* **7**(6):340-343, 1968.

Legeay, C.: "A Failure to Thrive: A Nursing Problem," *Nursing Forum,* **4**(1):56-71, 1965.

LeMasters, E. E.: "Parenthood as Crisis," in H. J. Parad (ed.), *Crisis Intervention,* New York: Family Service Association of America, 1965, pp. 111-117.

Leonard, M. F.: "The Impact of Maternal Deprivation on Infant Development," *Connecticut Medicine,* **32**(6):466-472, 1968.

Lidz, T.: *The Person,* New York: Basic Books, Inc., 1968.

Lo, W. H.: "Aetiological Factors in Childhood Neurosis," *British Journal of Psychiatry,* **115**:889-894, 1969.

Nye, F. I., and F. M. Berardo: *Emerging Conceptual Frameworks in Family Analysis,* New York: The Macmillan Company, 1966.

Parad, H. J., and G. Caplan: "A Framework for Studying Families in Crisis," in H. J. Parad (ed.), *Crisis Intervention,* New York: Family Service Association of America, 1965, pp. 53-71.

Rapoport, L.: "Working with Families in Crisis," in H. J. Parad (ed.), *Crisis Intervention*, New York: Family Service Association of America, 1965, pp. 129–139.

Rhymes, J. P.: "Working with Mothers and Babies Who Fail to Thrive," *American Journal of Nursing*, **9**:1972–1976, 1966.

Robischon, P.: "The Challenge of Crisis Therapy for Nursing," *Nursing Outlook*, **15**(7):28–32, 1967.

Schaffer, H. R.: "Activity Level as a Constitutional Determinant of Infantile Reaction to Deprivation," *Child Development*, **37**:595–602, 1966.

Spitz, R. A.: "Anaclitic Depression," *Psychoanalytic Study of the Child*, **7**:313–341, 1946.

Taylor, A.: "Deprived Infants: Potential for Affective Adjustment," *American Journal of Orthopsychiatry*, **38**:835–845, 1968.

Wiedenbach, E.: *Clinical Nursing: A Helping Art*, New York: Springer Publishing Co., 1964.

Chapter 26

Early Detection of Child Abuse

Martha Underwood Barnard

"More deaths are attributed to child abuse than are caused by automobile accidents, leukemia, cystic fibrosis, and muscular dystrophy combined" (Hall, 1967, p. 63). Are you contributing to these deaths and many more cases of families with repeated child abuse because of your professional ignorance, denial, and neglect? Chances are you are.

> Three-year-old Tommy is brought into the physician's office for his routine check and immunizations. There is an old cigarette burn on his chest, cat scratches on his arms, and bruises at different stages of healing on his abdomen. The parents tell the doctor that he is a discipline problem. The diagnosis is well child with normal toddler discipline problems. The physician asks the nurse to give the parents a pamphlet on how to discipline their toddler. Two weeks later the parents bring the child in to a local hospital emergency room. The child is dead on arrival.

How can an adult abuse or neglect an innocent child? It is easy for some. It is behavior that has been passed to them from preceding family generations. It has become a way of life. Much to the disbelief of health professionals, child abusers are not all young, minority races, blue-collar workers, or unemployed. It is easy to deny that the problem exists if it can be blamed on some other "type." The fact is that it exists in all races, classes, and occupations.

The problem centers on the preventive aspects of child abuse. Since this tends to occur in different generations of the same family, there must be early detection to stop this continuous cycle. The purpose of this chapter is to provide the nurse or appropriate health professionals with a means of identifying suspected child abuse cases or of identifying families with the potential for child abuse. If health professionals are made aware of the characteristics of these families, then prediction of the possibility of neglect or child abuse can take place. Only through prediction can early prevention and intervention be initiated to help inhibit the familial cycle of neglect and abuse.

BACKGROUND KNOWLEDGE

Statistics show that there are an estimated 10,000 to 15,000 diagnosed child abuse cases per year in the United States. What is more alarming is that there are many cases that are never diagnosed because they are not obvious. It has only been in the past decade that the "obvious" child abuse cases were included in the differential diagnosis of the physician. Before (and still in many cases today) the diagnosis of failure to thrive, rickets, scurvy, or accidental subdural hematoma is made instead of child abuse.

The first reported case of child abuse was in April 1874 in New York. It involved a nine-year-old girl who had been discovered as having been seriously physically abused. A nurse reported the case to the American Society for Prevention of Cruelty to Animals. Three years later, in 1877, the American Humane Association was organized and from this the Children's Division was formed. In their motto they state:

> The Children's Division of the American Humane Association is dedicated to promotion of more and better child protective services to the end that all children may be protected from neglect, abuse, rejection, or exploitation; and their right to a normal and secure childhood may be safeguarded (American Humane Association, 1969, p. 3).

It was not until August 1946 that any further literature was written on the possible abuse to children. At that time Dr. John Caffey wrote an article entitled "Multiple Fractures in the Long Bones of Infants Suffering from Chronic Subdural Hematoma." In this article he reported six case studies of patients who "exhibited 23 fractures and 4 contusions of the long bones. In not a single case was there a history of injury to which the skeletal lesions could reasonably be attributed and in no case was there clinical or Roentgen evidence of generalized or localized skeletal disease which would predispose to pathological fractures" (p. 163). The public and the professionals still denied the abuse. In 1961 the term *battered child syndrome* was coined by Dr. C. Henry Kempe in an address he delivered at an Academy of Pediatrics' convention in Chicago. It was used to characterize a "clinical condition in young children who have received serious physical abuse, generally from a parent or foster parent" (1962, p. 17). The public started becoming aware, and their cry for legislation was heard. In 1963, California, Colorado, Florida, Idaho, Minnesota, Ohio, Oregon, Pennsylvania, South Dakota, Wisconsin, and Wyoming enacted laws concerning the reporting of child abuse. Today all states have laws requiring physicians, registered nurses, and other people involved in child care to report diagnosed cases of child abuse, and many states require the reporting of any suspected case of child abuse.

In all these cases, whether they are mottos or laws, they are only as good as the person who abides by them and they are as harmful as the person who fails to abide by them. These reports should not be used to punish the parents but should be used to make it possible for early therapy to be initiated with those families that have child abuse existing in their home environments. Equally as important it is hoped that the nurse and other health professionals will not have to continuously act under the laws but rather be able to identify characteristics that would predict the potential for families abusing their children; therefore they would be able to intervene and prevent the actual event from occurring.

For the purpose of this chapter, child abuse will be defined as any physical and mental assault against a child by an older individual and/or the failure to protect the child from obvious danger in his environment (Elmer, 1963, p. 180). Within the framework of this definition the following subjects will be discussed: familial characteristics, types of abuse, identification of the potential for abuse, and nursing intervention.

It is of the utmost importance for health professionals to use collected data on families that have abused their children. An awareness of these facts will enable the nurse to make a systematic evaluation of individuals in a family or of the entire family. Characteristics that have been found in past studies of these families can be used to identify similar characteristics in other families, thus making it possible to be aware of the existing potential for abuse or neglect.

Studies have shown that these parents come from all income levels and job types, including the professional group. These people come from all religions. Some live in immaculate homes, while others live in a filthy, cluttered environment.

On the other hand the parents have common problems that should alert the nurse to the possibility of abuse. Some basic characteristics of parents have been illustrated in several studies. Young (1964) summarizes these characteristics in the following manner:

> As a group the abusive parents seemed to see other people as victims, resources, or enemies. They made contacts rather than friends. They trusted no one. They did not often visit other people, and they invited few into their houses. They rarely joined groups or organizations and most of them did not participate in religious groups. As they frighten others, so they themselves responded chiefly to fear (1964, p. 68).

She found through her studies that "unlike neglecting parents, those who abuse their children tend to be possessive of them" (1964, p. 64). She found that most of the parents had alcoholism as an acute problem, and separation was more common than divorce (1964, pp. 72–73).

Fulk (1964) cites a study that classified these parents into three types. One type involved the parent with "continual hostility." The second type shows the parent as being very "rigid, compulsive, and lacking warmth." The third type shows the parent with "strong feelings of passivity and dependency and is found competing with their children for the love of their spouse" (1964, p. 11). Wheelock states that in all the parents studied there was "the urge to release aggression against a helpless object" (1966, p. 95). Many times these parents expect their children "to perform like adults" (Hopkins, 1970, p. 590).

Similarly, Kempe is quoted as stating:

> Often parents are described as psychopathic or sociopathic characters. Alcoholism, sexual promiscuity, unstable marriages, and minor criminal activities are reportedly common amongst them. They are immature, impulsive, self-centered, hypersensitive, and quick to react with poorly controlled agression. Data in some cases indicate that such attacking parents had themselves been subject to some degree of attack from their parents in their own childhood (1962, p. 18).

It must be emphasized that all these characteristics do not have to be linked with all parents. They may come in any combination. On the other hand they may not be prevalent only among those parents who abuse their children. In essence, they must be regarded as those characteristics that will warn the health professional to be extra sensitive to the possibilities of future problems within the family unit. Indeed it is only a more sophisticated means of anticipating problems and providing anticipatory guidance.

Certainly there are two sides to this story. The child is one that usually has caused some type of hardship in the home. Possibly the child was conceived illegitimately or at a time when it created a financial burden. If the child was premature or had some neonatal problems, he may have caused an additional financial burden.

The mother, on the other hand, may have some resentment toward the child if she had any type of problems (emotional and/or physical) during her pregnancy. At the same time the father may have some real feelings about his wife being pregnant. He may feel left out of this part of her life, or he may have some jealous feelings toward the child because he does not get the same amount of attention he received before his wife became pregnant.

> In one case the mother stated to the author that her husband had lost his job about 2 weeks before she had gotten pregnant. "I had to give him an extra amount of attention in order to keep him from being mad all the time. Any time I started feeling tired or getting sick to my stomach after I got pregnant, it made him mad. He would get mad and say that no damn pregnancy was going to get in his way." After the birth of the baby he still did not have a job. "He'd sit around the house wanting to have sex relations. Either the baby would start crying before or during the time we were having relations. He'd get up and start whipping him until he'd knock him out!" Later the mother found that any time the baby would cry she would get up and stick a bottle in his mouth or lock him in his room and turn the music up in order that her husband could not hear him cry.

In other cases infants that are born with a low birth weight would suggest the possibility of abuse. Klein states in his study that "multiple factors may be operating to select the low birth weight infant for battering, i.e., preexisting mental retardation, maternal deprivation, and isolation from mother in the newborn period. Not only may low birth weight predispose to battering but certain social characteristics of the mother may predispose to delivery of low weight infants. Specifically, the increased incidence of low birth weight infants among women from deprived backgrounds where prenatal care is either not available or not utilized is well known" (Klein and Stern, 1971, p. 17). Low birth weight should also alert the nurse to the possibility of the mother's feeling guilty for not carrying a full-term infant or not providing the infant with the proper nutrients during the gestational period of his life. This guilt is only compounded by the mother's not being able to fondle the infant and develop the mother-child relationship because of the infant being placed in the high-risk nursery. The mother's frustration and the increased financial costs may result in a good environmental media for abuse.

Other parents may experience frustration as the child goes through certain developmental stages. For example, the newborn being brought home for the first time will most likely cause some tension in the home environment. In many cases, if the neonate tends to cry a lot, the parents may take this as a personal attack. They may feel inadequate as parents, or they may feel the child does not appreciate what they are doing for him. The more anxious the parents become, the more anxious the child becomes, thus again leading to a very highly emotional relationship. Another stage of development that may bring out the jealousy or the inadequacies of the parents is the toddler state when toilet training is started; and the child has now discovered that his world must be explored. He does this through climbing and destroying things in the home environment. When told not to do these things, he usually responds with a "no."

Other parents see their child in the oedipal stage as one who is competing for the love of their spouse. This may be the breaking point for an impulsive parent. At this time they see this child as "a competitor, as someone taking and getting what belongs to him. The child is an unconscious symbol of someone or something that once caused him pain" (Wasserman, 1967, p. 177).

Other characteristics of children that should lead the nurse to be aware of abuse are symptoms of brain damage, a tendency to be accident prone, and assaultiveness in the child's nature. The child who tends to whine and cry a lot or be quite hyperactive will also produce hostile feelings in his parents or the people caring for him.

EVIDENCE OF ABUSE

The nurse should be aware of the variety of abuses for which the child should be observed or examined. This can be done during the admission of a child to a ward or during the physical examination the nurse does during the clinic or home visit. Abuse ranges from severe burns, caused by hot water, cigarettes, radiators, etc., to more minor chronic types of physical findings, such as cuts at different stages of healing. In addition, forms of beating or throwing the child from heights will cause severe internal damage, such as hemorrhage, broken bones, or subdural hematomas. On the other hand, the child may have only a few bruises at different stages of healing.

Young (1964, pp. 55, 60) stresses that physical abuse is not the only type of abuse. Mental abuse also plays an important part in these children's lives. Just the mental abuse alone is enough to cause severe permanent personality damage. In one case presented by Young, the child's head was shaved by his parents, and then they continually called him a criminal.

Another form of abuse may be lack of environmental stimulation. These children may plot low on their growth grids. Evidence has shown that the weight is affected more than height; however, they can both be affected. In some cases, children start to gain weight after appropriate environmental changes such as foster homes, hospitalization, or volunteers visiting the homes.

The important point is that the nurse must be aware of the wide range of types of abuse and be prepared to identify characteristics of the child and his family that would indicate initiating immediate supportive nursing intervention or referring this child for further medical evaluation.

Last but not least, child abuse or neglect should be suspected at any time the child is found to have a subdural hematoma, multiple unexplained fractures, skin lesions and bruises at different stages of healing, and soft tissue swelling on any part of the body. In addition, a high degree of suspicion should be present in the case of a child who deviates below the 25 percentile on the growth grid and does not perform up to his age ability on a developmental test. (Denver Developmental Screening Test is recommended for use.)

THE NURSING ROLE

The nurse will be involved in either making or assisting in making the diagnosis of child abuse. It is at that time he will be responsible for referring the family to the appropriate health professionals and legal authorities. In order that this is done correctly all health team members must have a thorough understanding of the causes, familial characteristics, legal implications, and health professional obligations of child abuse. In most cases, no matter how severe, the nurse and other health team members must keep in mind that their obligation is to salvage the family, not to punish it. If the nurse does not feel capable of doing this, then he should find a professional that he can refer the family to for proper care.

The nurse will be able to make a more complete evaluation of a child and his family if he is able to do it in a systematic manner. Knowledge and skill of assessment, physical examination, and evaluation are necessary to make such a systematic appraisal. In addition the nurse should identify his own assessment guideline to suit him in this appraisal. In all guidelines the following information should be included:

1 Chief complaint (if present)
2 Prenatal history
   a Was this an expected pregnancy?
   b Were the mother and father married at the time that pregancy was diagnosed?
   c If they were not married, did they get married after the diagnosis was made?
   d During what month of gestation did prenatal care begin?
   e Did the mother follow the recommendations of her obstetrician?
   f Was there any illness during pregnancy, e.g., nausea, vomiting, weight gain?

g   Was the mother hospitalized for this illness?
h   Were any drugs taken by either parents during pregnancy? (Should include alcohol, marijuana, hard drugs, tranquilizers, and aspirin.)
i   Why were these drugs used?
j   At what point during pregnancy did the mother take the drugs?
k   Did the parents attend any prenatal or infant care classes?

3   Labor history
a   How long was labor?
b   What did labor mean to the mother, e.g., painful, pleasant, etc.?
c   Was there someone besides the medical personnel to support the mother during labor and delivery?
d   If so—who?

4   Delivery history
a   How long?
b   What type?
c   What type of anesthesia?
d   Apgar of the baby

5   When did the mother first see her baby?
6   When did the father first see his baby?
7   Did baby go home when the mother did?
8   Did the family have insurance covering hospitalization expenses for the mother and her infant?
9   Is mother on birth control now?

10 Family history should include:
a   Height
b   Weight
c   Age
d   History of any diseases
e   Education background
f   Occupation
g   How did each individual adjust to the infant?

11 Genetic history of family members:
a   Congenital defects
b   History of mental retardation

12 What size family did the parents come from?
13 What size family is the infant a member of?
14 Were the parents expected children?
15 How were the parents disciplined as children?
16 How does the husband treat the wife when he gets mad? (Mothers are much freer to talk about how their spouse reacts to them when he is mad as opposed to how he reacts toward the children.)
17 Are there extended family members living in the same home environment? If so, who?

18 Nutrition habits:
a   What?
b   How much?
c   Is the infant on a demand feeding schedule?

    d Does the baby require a lot of burping?
    e Does the infant vomit frequently?
19 Elimination habits:
    a How many times?
    b Type of care?
20 Sleep:
    a Where?
    b How often?
    c Through the night?
    d Does he nap?
21 Crying patterns:
    a Why does he cry?
22 Growth and development:
    a Measurements (height, weight, and head circumference) should be plotted on growth grids. Watch for deviations (anything below 25 percentile should be questioned). Should be done in home environment if possible and/or repeated if a deviation is present.
    b Developmental tests.
23 Systematic physical appraisal (again include any deviations from the normal as well as the personal hygiene of the child).
    a General appearance
        1 Skin
        2 Nails
        3 Hair
    b Head
    c Eyes
    d Ears
    e Nose
    f Throat
    g Mouth
    h Neck
    i Chest
    j Heart
    k Abdomen
    l Extremities
    m Spine
    n Genitourinary
    o Rectum
    p Anus
    q Neurological exam

Before taking a history, it is of the utmost importance that the nurse takes time to develop rapport with the family. While taking the family history and performing the child's physical, the nurse will want to observe for specific signs that will cause him to suspect child abuse. For example, he should be suspicious when the adult or parent bringing the child to the clinic or hospital (or on a home visit) does not volunteer information concerning the child. In the cases where some type of injury (minor or major) is apparent on the child's body, the nurse should be aware if the parents (or caretaker for the child) become irritable when being asked about how the injury occurred. Parents may get their stories mixed up (either between each other, or they may give a history that varies several times in a period of an hour or varies from day to day). Be aware of the parents that blame the injuries on the child's siblings or the child himself.

If the child is admitted to the hospital for evaluation of nonaccidental injuries, there are certain things to observe about the parents and the child. In addition to the history and chief complaint varying from the physical findings, the nurse will also find that as the hospital stay continues, the parents seldom, if at all, ask about their child's prognosis or as to when he will be discharged.

In addition, he will want to observe the child who tends to withdraw from his parents or adults in general. Specifically he will want to note if the child tends to withdraw from men or women, or if he tends to withdraw from his parents and not other adults.

Further, the nurse should be aware of the child's response to painful stimuli. For example, during a treatment that would normally be painful for the patient, the nurse should observe to see if the patient reacts to the painful stimulus. In many cases the child is so used to having pain inflicted that he appears to have become somewhat conditioned to it, if it is really possible to do so.

According to Morris (1963), the nurse should be aware of children who seem less fearful of hospitalization than other children. Abused children also become apprehensive when adults approach other crying children. Further, at the time of discharge they announce that they do not want to go home, or they become very depressed at the thought of going home.

INTERVENTION

Intervention must be initiated immediately if child abuse or neglect is suspected. In the case of families that have characteristics that would indicate the potential for abuse, much anticipatory guidance must be initiated.

Professional contact must be continued with these families, especially during the early years of childrearing. Support and guidance must be given to these parents to help them over certain hurdles of development.

On the other hand, in the cases where there is a diagnosis of abuse, it must be kept in mind that if the parents have brought their child for medical attention then this is their way of asking for help.

In *no* case should a parent be blamed for the child's injuries. In all cases the parent should be considered as much of a patient as the child. It should be emphasized to these families that the professional team is there to help the entire family, not punish them. These adults (either ones with the potential for abuse or ones that have abused their child) have been punished enough in their lifetime. They now need much guidance and support. They need to be accepted for once, even with all their negative characteristics.

Initially, the nurse will have or should gather the data that have been described previously. All baseline data should be entered very specifically in the patient's chart. In the case where the abuse patient and his family have been identified by another health professional, the nurse still has the obligation to collect data, work with the parents, and work closely with the health team. All these nursing situations require very skilled observations and charting of nursing histories. There is never room for any subjective thoughts. Specific statements, interactions, and physical findings should be charted by all health team members.

The nurse should work closely with the physician, social worker, juvenile officer, and any other professional dealing with these families. Plans should be made together for assessment of the family situation, home environment, and recommendations for future health team and legal involvement.

In the cases where the abused child is kept in the home, a nurse should make a home visit. This is for evaluation of the home environment as well as being a means for developing a better rapport with the family. The family taking the child home needs frequent visits in the home during the period immediately following discharge. This can be done by the nurse or social worker. In ideal cases both should be making these home visits. In the cases where there are no nurses or social workers to make these visits, volunteers trained by health professionals can offer much support to these families on a daily basis. The number of required visits cannot be predetermined. These must be determined after frequent evaluations of the home situation are made by the professionals of the team working with these families.

On the other hand, in the cases where the potential for child abuse and/or neglect is identified, the nurse is the appropriate health professional to support the parents and give anticipatory guidance in relation to childrearing and accident prevention. Again, in the cases where there are not enough nurses to do such things, trained volunteers with close professional supervision will be helpful.

In all cases, it is of the utmost importance that the health team professionals work closely together. Any nurse questioning or suspecting abuse should refer to the appropriate physician for further evaluation. In the case where the nurse (or any professional) is more sure of the case being abuse, he is then obligated to refer to the appropriate authorities. This will vary according to the institution, county, and state in which he works.

Once the communication breaks down between members of the team working with these families, then the families get different messages. Thus the support and guidance becomes disintegrated, confusing the adults and child once again. The confusion leads to frustration. The frustration produces the potential for further child abuse.

Most important teamwork, early detection, and continuous evaluation of the intervention are required to guide these parents through their crisis.

CONCLUSION

In conclusion, the nurse and other health team professionals must make themselves aware of the characteristics of these children and their families. This knowledge then leads to the possibility for early detection of the potential or suspected case of child abuse. Once the step of detection has occurred, the entire health team should work together on the assessment, the intervention, and the continuous evaluation of these cases. Together, they should make recommendations for the care delivered to these families.

The aftermath is not the time to intervene nor is it the time to make the diagnosis of child abuse. It's too late, way too late. Have you been too late?

BIBLIOGRAPHY

American Humane Association: *Children's Protective Services,* Denver, Colorado, 1969, p. 3.

Caffey, J.: "Multiple Fractures in the Long Bones of Infants Suffering from Chronic Subdural Hematoma," *American Journal of Roentgenology,* **56**:163-173, 1946.

Elmer, E.: "Identification of Abused Children," *Children,* **10**:180-184, 1963.

Fulk, D. L.: "The Battered Child," *Nursing Forum,* **3**:10-26, 1964.

Hall, M.: "The Right to Live," *Nursing Outlook,* **15**:65-67, 1967.

Hopkins, J.: "The Nurse and the Abused Child," *The Nursing Clinics of North America,* **5**:589-598, 1970.

Kempe, C. H., et al.: "The Battered Child Syndrome," *Journal of American Medical Association,* **181**:17-24, 1962.

Klein, M., and L. Stern: "Low Birth Weight, Battered Child Syndrome Linked," *American Journal of Diseases of Children,* **122**:15-18, 1971.

Morris, M., and R. W. Gould: "Role Reversal: A Necessary Concept in Dealing with the Battered Child Syndrome," *American Journal of Orthopsychiatry,* **33**:298-299, 1963.

Wasserman, S.: "The Abused Parent of the Abused Child," *Children,* **14**:175-179, 1967.

Wheelock, S. E.: "The Abused Child Syndrome," *Hospital Topics,* **154**:95-96, 1966.

Young, L.: *Wednesday's Children,* New York: McGraw-Hill Book Company, 1964.

Chapter 27

The Woman and Her Family Facing Therapeutic Abortion

Barbara J. Clancy

The purpose of this chapter is to explore possible feelings and needs patients and their families may experience while facing the crisis of a therapeutic abortion, and how nursing personnel can meet their needs at this time.

OUR CHANGING TIMES

In the past few years several states have liberalized their abortion laws, and in the past year there have been drastic and rapid changes made in an attempt to meet the needs of our changing society. One need is related to the fast-growing population, and the emphasis placed on this facet of ecology (Hellman, 1971).

There is no doubt that family planning and sound contraceptive advice are far superior to population control by means of abortion; however, our country does not seem to be able to stabilize its population by means of contraception alone (Peck, 1968). Many young women experience contraception failure due to either lack of use or lack of understanding of the means of contraception. In addition many unwed girls become pregnant because they doubt their fertility; and once pregnant, they are unhappy (Krantz, 1971). Others may seek pregnancy as a means of displaying independence, but find they feel dependent during the pregnant state (Young, 1954). The middle-aged woman who has raised her family may find another pregnancy intolerable.

There are varied individual reasons why women seek an abortion. The reality of the situation is that abortion will become a means of population control for an increasing number of families. Therefore, what one's feelings for or against abortion are is not the question. As nurses we have to face this reality and deal with it in a positive and professional manner.

Many lay persons are beginning to examine their views on abortion; and a large majority, including some Roman Catholics, agree that under certain circumstances such as rape, incest, a deformed fetus, or threat of death to the mother an abortion should be permitted (Harain, 1968; Peck, 1968). The Catholic church officially continues to take the stand of "no abortions"; however, there seems to be a trend toward some relaxation of views (Peck, 1968).

Some authors feel that psychiatrists should not become involved in the web of abortion (Corcoran, 1969; Whittington, 1970). It is difficult to judge if a person will have a long-term psychiatric sequela because of a refusal for an abortion (Whittington, 1970). Usually a stable person can handle an abortion with relative ease, whereas an unstable person (the person who can obtain an abortion easily) may be more apt to have long-term effects (Simon, 1967). There is a normal period of depression after an abortion; however, most studies show the long-term effects are more positive than negative (Marder, 1970). In Scandinavia, there have been long-range research studies comparing children of mothers who have been refused abortions with children of mothers who had not requested abortions. The children who had mothers who were refused abortion had an increased number of psychiatric problems, more arrests, increased school dropout rates, and earlier marriages (Forssman and Thuwe, 1966).

Planned parenthood associations, public health departments, women's liberation groups, and medical centers in any locality are a few of the agencies where information may be obtained.

If a nurse, due to moral or religious convictions, cannot give preabortive advice and counseling, then a referral should be made to someone who can help this patient. If this is neglected, then the professional obligation to the patient has not been fulfilled.

TYPES OF FAMILIES SEEKING ABORTION

While working with the patient experiencing an abortion, personnel must realize that each situation is unique and requires an individual approach.

The young unwed adolescent may have become pregnant for the variety of reasons mentioned previously (Krantz, 1971). This patient may be hostile to personnel and family and is acting out feelings that life has dealt a cruel blow. She really is expressing anger at herself that is displayed in many ways (Young, 1954). If the personnel can understand the reason for this behavior, they can help the patient work through these feelings.

Often the pregnant, unwed adolescents are trying to cope with the crisis of abortion completely alone, without family or friends, at a time when love and understanding are needed. Often their families are hurt or angry and are punishing the girls by making them go through the procedure alone. They may have denied the reality of their pregnancy and therefore sought medical assistance late in their pregnancy, which may increase the physical and psychological danger. These are the patients who have been described as "spoiled" or "unappreciative" or "hostile." The patients who are able to "act up" often are able to work through their feelings. The quiet, uncommunicative, or "good" patients may be the persons who need the most help.

The young girl who has the support of her family and possibly a boyfriend is not only the fortunate person but the exception. In most states if the patient is younger than twenty-one, the parents or guardian must sign the operation permit and therefore know about the abortion.

The author has talked with several parents of girls having an abortion. They seem to be appreciative of the fact that personnel are interested in them as well as their daughters. A statement such as, "You go and eat supper while I stay with your daughter," can show acceptance. One father sent his daughter roses and upon a comment about the flowers said, "My little girl needs to know that Dad loves her."

Another mother could not understand why her daughter did not confide in her about the sexual involvement with her boyfriend because of the close mother-daughter relationship. One physician explained to this mother that young girls often attempt to avoid disappointing their parents and therefore will be silent about their sexual experience. It has nothing to do with lack of love or respect for one another (Rockwell, 1971).

There is no doubt that an abortion affects not only the young girl but her family. It may be difficult not to place blame, but the goal of the family should be to avoid dwelling on the past and to stress the positive approach of returning to a normal pattern of life as soon as possible.

The young adult over twenty-one does not need parental permission for an abortion. Therefore, whether family and friends are to be involved is the patient's decision. If the physician or nurse informs the family of the situation on his own, this is a breech of confidence.

If a young woman decides to withhold information about the abortion from her family, she will experience this crisis alone. The young adult may have chosen to withhold knowledge because of fear of hurting the family and/or fear of rejection. Whatever the reason, the patient needs the support and acceptance of the personnel.

The attitudes and feelings of married women seeking an abortion may be quite different than those of the unwed person. The married woman who becomes pregnant may desire to postpone having a family until she and her husband are financially and psychologically "ready" for the role of parenthood.

Another couple may decide that their present number of children is the ideal family and, with another pregnancy, seek an abortion. One mother stated that she dearly loved her three preschool children, but the thought of another one in diapers "was intolerable." Another mother whose youngest child was of beginning school age sought an abortion because she had wanted to resume her teaching career. She stated, "I love my four children, but I need more in life than babies and diapers. I find I'm a better mother when I can be satisfied by working." This woman and her husband requested permanent sterilization after the abortion procedure.

Women going through menopause may become pregnant. Some persons may be able to cope with this situation, others may not. If this patient seeks an abortion, she and her husband may also wish permanent sterilization.

No matter what the family situation, there are normal guilt feelings after an abortion. The amount of support obtained from family and medical and nursing personnel may be a determining factor in the woman's ability to cope with these feelings in a positive way. Everyone has a philosophical versus a real-life view of how they would work through a crisis situation. Sometimes the two views do not coincide. The most important factor is what the patient allows the abortion to do to her, and finally the patient must forgive herself (Rockwell, 1971).

FEELINGS OF PERSONS INVOLVED IN ABORTION

Many patients about to have an abortion have fears about the procedure itself, the doctor performing the abortion, the hospital routine, and what people will think (Beck, Newman, Lewitt, 1969).

If the patient is to have the dilatation and curettage procedure, the aspect of general anesthesia may be an additional fear. Patients going to surgery may fear death from anesthesia.

Often, patients have been so involved with gaining approval for an abortion that they have no idea what will happen to them prior to, during, or after the procedure (Peck, 1968). Patients may be so anxious about their situation that they may not have heard the explanation that was given. For most patients this is a deep emotional experience, and it is difficult to imagine their true feelings.

There seems to be a group cohesiveness when patients undergoing an abortion are in the same room. They seem to sense their common problem and can give support to one another. There may be some patients who want to be alone; and, if hospital facilities are conducive to fulfilling the patient's desire for privacy, this should be arranged.

For many young patients the hospitalization for an abortion may be their first hospital admission. This experience, even under the best circumstances, is frightening. The adolescents are really not adults, yet because of the adult situation of being pregnant, often are treated as adults.

The patients often express their concern about what people will think of them. The unwed adolescents and young adults are usually withdrawn and quiet, but often will begin to talk when one demonstrates sincere concern for them. In the author's experience it seems as if married women need to explain their reason for the abortion by initiating this topic. In general the married women seem to display less guilt; however whether or not this is true is hard to ascertain.

It is imperative to focus on the feelings and needs of the medical and nursing personnel as well as the need of the patients and their families. If we are involved, committed persons, we cannot condemn. The right amount of empathy, compassion, and commitment are the necessary aspects for working with the patient having an abortion.

For as long as obstetrics and maternity nursing have been practiced, goals have been directed toward bringing new life into the world. Those persons who enter this specialty of medicine and nursing have specific reasons for choosing this field. Therefore we cannot condemn the personnel for having problems adapting to the rapid changes occurring in the maternity area.

Due to the rapid change in the laws concerning abortion, some hospital facilities were not large enough to cope with the influx of patients. Some nurses complained that the time normally spent with the maternity patient was now spent with the abortion patient (Zahourek, 1971). It is evident that extensive adaptation and flexibility on the part of the medical and nursing staff are necessary. Possibly it is an error to place the patient having an abortion on the maternity unit.

How can the personnel be helped to work through problems of adaptation? Some hospitals have tried group sessions for all professional and non-professional personnel (Goldman, 1971; Leroux, et al., 1970). Expressing feelings both for and against abortion, with the guidance of obstetricians, psychologists, and psychiatrists, is a positive approach to the problem.

Feelings will be expressed in some way, and patients have told of being treated punitively by hospital staff. Patients stated they did not expect open acceptance, but neither did they expect hostility (Goldman, 1971). Others have said they had feelings of guilt and depression that may have been attributed to treatment by the personnel (Marder, 1970).

Hostility demonstrated by personnel toward a patient should not be tolerated. Hostility may be demonstrated in a verbal and nonverbal manner or shown by what one does not say. Unless the staff is able to give the patient the support and acceptance needed, they should not work with the patient having an abortion.

Although one can understand the feelings of the staff, these patients should not be treated in a condemning manner. As nurses we have no right to pass judgment or to set standards for other persons. These patients should be treated as any other patient being admitted to the hospital. They have problems and concerns similar to many patients, and should be given the same considerations (Krantz, 1971).

In the author's experience nursing students have been able to support the patient and family experiencing abortion. They have expressed the desire to care for these patients and have on occasion helped the staff understand their own negative feelings. The students of today generally are liberal and broad-minded in their views, and several have stated that although they may not approve of abortion themselves, life styles are changing and a nurse must be flexible in the approach to nursing care.

METHODS OF THERAPEUTIC ABORTION AND NURSING CARE INVOLVED

Nurses need to be informed of the various methods of performing therapeutic abortions and the specific nursing care involved.

The method preferred and used most often by physicians because of the relative safety is the suction dilatation and curettage. This method is used prior to the fourteenth week of gestation. If this technique is used after the first trimester, the danger of uterine perforation and hemorrhage may be increased because of the thinning uterine wall and the additional blood supply to the pelvic organs (Beck, 1969). In this method the patient is given a general anesthetic, the cervix is dilated, and the endometrial lining is cur-etted and suctioned from the uterus. The patient may be hospitalized for 24 hours or less, depending on the policies and the facilities of the institution. The patient is dismissed when the vaginal bleeding is minimal or has ceased.

Many patients and their families are confused about hospital policies and the abortion procedure. Therefore explanations should be repeated a second or a third time prior to the beginning of any procedure, so that misconceptions can be clarified.

While preparing the patient for the dilatation and curettage procedure, the usual preoperative safety precautions are performed. The patient may be given either a general or a spinal anesthetic and anticipatory teaching should be given. A preoperative medication may be given depending on the anxiety level of the patient and the orders of the anesthetist. The abortion procedure itself is over rapidly; but the patient will remain in the recovery room until the vital signs are stable, the bleeding is minimal, and she is completely conscious. How long the patient will remain under medical supervision usually depends on the specific needs of the patient. This can vary from a few hours to 24 hours. Although the physical care is minimal, how the nurse ministers this care is most important.

An amniocentesis may be performed and amniotic fluid is withdrawn from the uterine cavity by means of a needle inserted through the abdominal wall or the vagina. The amniotic fluid is replaced by an equal amount of a hypertonic saline solution. This causes death of the fetus probably due to chemical changes; however, the physiology of the process is not completely understood (Cameron, 1970; Manabe, 1969b). An oxytoxin intravenous infusion is started to enhance contractions. The patient experiences labor discomfort in the process of expelling the dead fetus. This method may cause complications and therefore is used only if dilatation and curettage is contraindicated. Grave, but rare, complications reported in the literature include cardiovascular shock, hypertension and apneic episodes, acute pulmonary edema, extensive hemolysis, kidney necrosis, central nervous system disorders, as well as maternal death (Manabe, 1969b). A dilatation and curettage is performed after the fetus is expelled to decrease the chance of hemorrhage and infection.

The patient should have an explanation of the amniocentesis prior to and during the procedure. The patient should know when she can expect to experience uterine contractions and how the contractions will feel. Many patients are unaware that the process involves labor in order to deliver the fetus.

Since circulatory complications may occur from the saline instillation, the patient's vital signs, urinary output, and response level should be watched closely and reported to the responsible physician.

Once the patient begins to experience uterine cramping, an oxytocic drug is given by intravenous infusion. The patient is usually on bed rest and becomes increasingly uncomfortable as the contractions increase in intensity and frequency. Demerol or another analgesic is usually given early in labor since this does not seem to stop contractions as in labor at term (Krantz, 1971). The patient needs all the physical care of the normal laboring patient, such as vital signs, need to void, clean and dry bed linen, sacral pressure to ease discomfort, oral hygiene, help with breathing and relaxing techniques, and an explanation about her progress.

When delivery of the fetus is imminent, the patient *should not be left alone.* When the amniotic fluid ruptures, the fetus is usually delivered soon. Being alone can be horrifying to patients and has been expressed as, "The worst thing that ever happened to me." Others have said, "Thank you for not leaving me *then!*" There should be enough nursing personnel assigned to these patients so they will not be alone. Often the body of the fetus is expelled before the after-coming head since the head is the largest part of the fetus and requires further cervical dilatation. The patient may become panicky that the head will not be delivered unless this is explained as a normal occurrence (Rockwell, 1971). The patient is observed for several hours and then dismissed if all signs are normal.

A hysterotomy is an incision into the uterus in order to remove the fetus and placenta. If the woman is at the period in her life when additional children are undesirable or hazardous to her health, a tubal ligation or a sterilization procedure may be done at this time.

The nursing care following this procedure is the same as for other minor surgery. The patient may be hospitalized for 2 or 3 days if no complications arise.

A hysterectomy, or removal of the uterus, is a major surgical procedure involving a hospital stay of approximately a week. Older patients who have had several children or cases when the uterus is diseased may select this procedure.

The nursing care involved is the same as for any major surgery: preventing respiratory complications, maintaining fluid and electrolyte balance, promoting bowel and bladder elimination, building physical strength, teaching rehabilitative aspects, and maintaining positive self-image and emotional health.

Prostaglandins are chemically identified as hydroxy fatty acids which effect contractility of smooth muscle. Prostaglandins have been used to induce labor and more recently to terminate pregnancy after the fifteenth week of gestation (Embrey, 1970; Filshie, 1970). These drugs have few complications and seem to simulate normal labor in a more satisfactory manner than other oxytocins (Embrey, 1970). Although prostaglandins are not presently being used in this country, their use may become prevalent in the future as a means of affecting abortion.

Although there are specific nursing measures involved depending on the type of abortion procedure, there are also general nursing measures that are important for all patients. Obviously the patient is the prime focus rather than the abortion procedure itself. The nursing care given during an abortion can be viewed as a positive rather than a negative experience (Malo-Juvera, 1971). The abortion process and care received may affect the way a patient's life will go (Rockwell, 1971). If the patient is to have a positive experience with a later pregnancy, she needs support, preferably from a member of her family and from medical and nursing personnel.

A patient can easily sense if she is being judged or condemned. Disapproval can be shown by gestures, by avoidance, or by overt verbal comments made in the halls or supposedly out of the range of the patient's and family's hearing. Nurses should work toward understanding patients and displaying this acceptance of them as individuals, by their actions.

Having an abortion is a crisis time for this patient and her family. It is feasible to apply crisis theory to the nursing care of a patient having an abortion, as has been done in other crisis situations. For example, a patient in crisis has decreased defenses and at this time is often willing or able to accept an alternative action not previously accepted. Also, a patient in crisis may become very angry after the shock of the situation. When the patient is angry, she may find an inner strength to help in the coping mechanism (Robischon, 1967).

Emotional support is very important for these patients. We have no right to moralize or even talk about their situation unless they obviously want to talk about it. We must use psychiatric nursing principles, which also include knowing when to be silent and let the patient take the lead. One cannot assume that all patients will feel better by talking about their problem. Physical presence, by someone who really cares, is often the best emotional support.

If the patient is under twenty-one, the family or guardian will know about the abortion. If the patient is over twenty-one, she will make the choice of informing or not informing her family. We have no right to try to change her mind according to what we might do. It may be wise to keep in mind that the patient has more facts about the situation than we do.

If family members or the man responsible for the unwanted pregnancy are present, they should be able to be with the patient if this is what the patient desires. If the family is supported, they may in turn be able to give support to the patient. If their presence is harmful, they should be asked to leave; however an explanation for this action, given in a firm but professional manner, is needed.

The patient may decline to inform close friends about the abortion. This may be wise since the fewer persons who know about the experience the easier the rehabilitative process may be (Rockwell, 1971).

NURSING CARE FOLLOWING THE ABORTION

The emotional reaction immediately following an abortion varies with each patient. Some patients seem euphoric, others withdrawn, or some will cry because of guilt or from relief that the procedure is over. They may wish to be alone or desire the presence of a supportive person. The nurse should be alert to the specific needs and follow through accordingly.

Nurses in the recovery room have stated that many patients who have had an abortion by means of dilatation and curettage often cry and become very active, often thrashing, while recovering from anesthesia. This behavior may be indicative of guilt and concern as to whether the proper decision was made (Rockwell, 1971). The normal grief period following abortion is from 2 to 3 months; and if the depressed state persists, the patient should seek professional help (Rockwell, 1971; Simon, 1967). Support for the patient in the recovery room is most important, since this may decrease later feelings of guilt.

Follow-up care for these patients may be impossible if they are from out of state and/or they wish to remain anonymous. The patient is advised to see a physician for a pelvic examination in 4 weeks to rule out the possibility of infection and to ascertain if the pelvic organs have returned to the prepregnant state. She should understand the importance of this examination and be given a return appointment if she lives in the immediate vicinity.

A public health nursing referral may be indicated for some patients who exhibit specific problems; however, a referral for all patients is impractical as well as impossible. Since patients do exhibit a normal depression, they should be told to expect these feelings. They should be given a phone number to call in their respective cities if they wish to talk with someone familiar with psychiatric counseling. Various hospitals performing abortions should have a list of phone numbers of helping agencies in the key cities so that a patient will know where to turn for help if needed. Follow-up care should be available but *never* forced.

Contraceptive advice should be given to all patients following an abortion. The chance of a need for a second abortion should be avoided if possible. It has been demonstrated that those having one unwanted pregnancy are in a high-risk group for a second unwanted pregnancy (Leroux et al., 1970). Other studies show that many young girls seeking an abortion are unaware of the types of contraceptives or how they could be made available to them ("Nurses' Feelings," 1971). Some persons feel that legalized abortion will decrease contraception use; however, the contrary has been demonstrated in the past (Peck, 1968).

Most states have laws against giving contraceptive advice to patients who are under legal age, except on permission from the parents. When permission for the abortion is obtained, it may be feasible to obtain contraceptive permission.

Contraceptive advice should be given freely and in terminology based on the patient's level of understanding. This advice can be given in a positive rather than a negative manner and will be more acceptable. For example, "Planning for children shows that you are a responsible person," rather than "You don't want to have another abortion, do you?" The latter statement is condemning in the approach and may be ineffective.

CURRICULUM DEVELOPMENT

If additional states continue to liberalize the abortion laws, it may be important for schools of nursing to include essential content to meet this specific need. Some schools are beginning to see the need for the inclusion of course content on abortion, contraception, and sexuality (Goldman, 1971; Malo-Juvera, 1971).

There may also be a need to develop continuing educational workshops to help the practicing nurses and physicians gain background knowledge, practical experience, and understanding of the patient seeking an abortion.

CONCLUSION

Unwanted pregnancy is one of the greatest social problems facing our country today and affects families on all income levels. Society pays dearly, and for many years, for the consequences of the unwanted child ("Abortion," 1970).

In the future nurses will be called upon to be involved in helping a patient seek an abortion. Studies have shown that illegal abortion has not decreased appreciably except in areas where the "red tape" has been cut extensively (Harain, 1968; Peck, 1968). Women resent having a board of persons dictate what they can and cannot do with their lives. For this reason, it seems feasible to say that when "abortion on demand" is a reality or when a woman and her physician are able to decide on an abortion, then illegal abortions will diminish appreciably.

Nurses should be knowledgeable about the types of abortions and how and where to refer a patient through legal channels. Not only public health nurses, but all nurses may be approached for this information. If patients are not referred through proper channels, they may be directed to commercial agencies which may take advantage of this vulnerable patient. Legal action has been taken against some of these agencies that have been making large profits from the increased number of abortions (*American Medical News,* 1971).

BIBLIOGRAPHY

"Abortion: The Lonely Problem," *RN,* **33**:34–39, 1970.

American Medical News: American Medical Association, Chicago, **14**:1, June 7, 1971.

Beck, M. B., S. H. Newman, and S. Lewitt: "Abortion: A National Public and Mental Health Problem—Past, Present, and Proposed Research," *American Journal of Public Health,* **59**:2131–2143, 1969.

Cameron, W.: "Techniques of Abortion," *The Journal of the Kansas Medical Society,* **71**:375, 1970.

Corcoran, C. J.: "Abortion: A Catholic View," *Illinois Medical Journal,* **135**:300–302, 1969.

Embrey, M. P.: "Effect of Prostaglandins on Human Uterus in Pregnancy," *Journal of Reproductive Fertility,* **23**:372–373, 1970.

Filshie, G. M.: "Therapeutic Abortion Using Prostaglandin E$_2$," *Journal of Reproductive Fertility,* **23**:371–372, 1970.

Forssman, H., and I. Thuwe: "120 Children Born after Application for Therapeutic Abortion Refused," *Acta Psychiatrica Scandinavica,* **42**:71, 1966.

Goldman, A.: "Learning Abortion Care," *Nursing Outlook,* **19**:350–352, 1971.

Harain, G.: "Abortion or Compulsory Pregnancy," *Journal of Marriage and Family,* **30**:246–251, 1968.

Hellman, L. M.: "Family Planning Comes of Age," *American Journal of Obstetrics and Gynecology,* **109**:214–224, 1971.

Krantz, K. M.: Personal Communication, 1971.

——— and J. Semmens: *The Adolescent Experience: A Counseling Guide to Social and Sexual Behavior,* New York: The Macmillan Company, 1970.

Leroux, R., et al.: "Abortion," *American Journal of Nursing,* **70**:1919–1925, 1970.

Malo-Juvera, D.: "Preparing Students for Abortion Care," *Nursing Outlook,* **19**:347–349, 1971.

Manabe, Y.: "Abortion in Mid-pregnancy by Extraovular Instillation of Rivanol Solution Correlated with Placental Function," *American Journal of Obstetrics and Gynecology,* **103**:232–237, 1969*a*.

———: "Danger of Hypertonic-Saline Induced Abortion," *Journal of the American Medical Association,* **210**:2091, 1969*b*.

Marder, L.: "Psychological Experiment with a Liberalized Therapeutic Abortion Law," *American Journal of Psychiatry,* **126**:1230–1236, 1970.

"Moonlighting Medics: Liberal Abortion Law Proves to Be a Bonanza for New York Doctors," *New York Times,* **51**:1, 1971.

"Nurses' Feelings: A Problem under New Abortion Law," *American Journal of Nursing,* **71**:350–353, 1971.

Peck, A.: "Therapeutic Abortion: Patients, Doctors, and Society," *American Journal of Psychiatry,* **125**:797–803, 1968.

Robischon, P.: "The Challenge of Crisis Theory for Nursing," *Nursing Outlook,* **15**:28–32, 1967.

Rockwell, W. L.: Personal Communication, 1971.

Simon, N. M.: "Psychiatric Illness Following Therapeutic Abortion," *American Journal of Psychiatry,* **124**:59-65, 1967.

"The R.N. Panel of 500 Tells What Nurses Think about Abortion," *RN,* **33**:40, 1970.

Walker, E.: "Study of Sexuality in the Nursing Curriculum," *Nursing Forum,* **10**:18-30, 1971.

Whittington, H. G.: "Evaluation of Therapeutic Abortion as an Element of Preventive Psychiatry," *American Journal of Psychiatry,* **126**:1224-1229, 1970.

Young, L.: *Out of Wedlock,* New York: McGraw-Hill Book Company, 1954.

Zahourek, R.: "Therapeutic Abortion and Cultural Shock," *Nursing Forum,* **10**:8-17, 1971.

Chapter 28

Family Rehabilitation: An Adult with a Myocardial Infarction

Jean A. Yokes

The family as the basic structural unit in Western society reacts to illness in a variety of ways. An acute myocardial infarction in a family member may be lethal or catastrophic both medically and socioeconomically. It has especially profound consequences for the family, being not only detrimental to the patient, but also to this fundamental unit. This chapter intends to examine these consequences from the point of view of nurse-patient-family therapeutic relationships. It intends to propose mechanisms of professional interaction which will optimize the potential for maximum normalization of postillness health status.

To have an understanding of the family structure, awareness of the typical behavioral characteristics of the coronary-prone individual may be of value ("Psychological and Social Factors," 1964; Ostfeld, 1967; Jenkins, 1971; Rosenman et al., 1964). These characteristics may affect the family structure. Behavioral patterns have been reported in the literature. The typical picture of the coronary prone is an individual who lives in an industrialized society; has enhanced drive; is ambitious, competitive, and has an excessive sense of urgency of time. He is dedicated to work and is unable to relax. The restless, competitive attitude of attempting to squeeze as many actions and events in as small a space of time as possible is behaviorally manifested by hurried speech, rapid gestures, and a harried facial expression. The burden of overinvolvement creates stresses which are associated with metabolic changes such as altered serum lipids and cholesterol and altered blood coagulability.

The Western Collaborative Group, a group of individual investigators interested in prevention of coronary artery disease, was formed on the West Coast. They have presented longitudinal prospective studies of import relevant to this point (Rosenman, et al., 1966). Their studies characterize the coronary-prone individual as one who has suffered extreme disappointment, frustrations, anger, and sadness; and has been subjected to geographical relocations. He uses denial and controls his emotions, keeping them hidden from himself and others. Physiologically this individual has increased serum lipids, augmented postprandial hypertriglyceridemia, an accelerated coagulation, enhanced daytime excretion of catecholamines, and an elevated diastolic blood pressure. As a result of a particular psychosomatic mode of an individual's adaptation to stressors there may be a pathogenetic relationship between the central nervous system responses, including the neurohormonal component, and resultant strain manifested as coronary artery disease (Rosenman et al., 1970). Hans Selye (1956) has described stress as functional and structural changes which occur due to the organism's physiochemical adaptation responses to maintain homeostasis. The stressor may be of a physiologic nature such as a coronary occlusion or a psychologic nature such as fear of death.

Psychologic and physiologic stressors are a part of an individual's everyday life. In nursing these are seen in the patient as a sequela of illness and hospitalization. A stressor of psychologic origin is hospitalization and isolation of the individual from familiar surroundings, familiar possessions, and familiar people. An example of a physiologic stressor is that of chest pain from a heart attack.

A conceptual framework of stress, operationalized to provide definitive measures for a therapeutic plan of nursing intervention to alleviate stressors, is warranted. Clinical nursing studies conducted to determine effective modes of intervention may provide a direction toward formulation of nursing theory and scientific nursing therapy. At the ANA clinical sessions, Rhetaugh Dumas (1966) discussed stress and its utilization as a therapeutic nursing measure. She stated that nursing activities might be conceived in relation to stress: those which facilitate prevention, mitigation, or alleviation of stress; or those that sustain an individual through the stressful period and promote restoration of optimum functioning and well-being.

The family experiences a crisis when a member has an acute myocardial infarction. Nursing is in need of a systematic assessment for crisis intervention and methods for alleviation of stressors experienced by family members when changes in life's activities due to illness occur. An examination of general stressors created by our culture may lead to a better understanding of the family's response to crisis.

In order to gain a perspective of the cultural stressors and an individual's adaptive responses, books like Toffler's *Future Shock* (1970) and Reich's *The Greening of America* (1970) make vivid the impact which "Americanism" is having on the individual and family in our society. Reich believes that individuals are living with preindustrial modes of adaptation in an age when technology controls our lives. Religious and philosophical views, values, and laws have not changed in keeping with the economic, political, and social changes in society. Individuals are structured by Madison Avenue advertising, mass education, and mass production of goods, the molding of dress, and the molding of behavior and thoughts by bureaucracy. Real experiences are substituted by simulated ones so that power, money, and status in a bureaucracy create a climate for competition, subjugation, and subordination. Sensory overstimulation may occur due to rapid transportation, communication, and transience of the community and an abundant supply in choices of consumer products. Families must make frequent adjustments to new communities when the breadwinner is promoted and transferred to a new job in the company. Inability to cope and exhaustion of the individual may result. Family cohesiveness may be strained.

A discussion of the family cannot exclude the individual children, their roles in the family, personality characteristics, and interpersonal relationships. If it is true that a cultural lag exists, certain effects must be experienced by the children and certain adaptations made by them. One could hypothesize that due to lack of close family ties, children of these characteristic families may become hippies, college dropouts, drug addicts or may try to please the family member to the exclusion of developing their own interests and potential.

On a daily basis the absence of fulfillment of human needs such as recognition and self-actualization in the coronary-prone individual may lead to resultant stress and perhaps to an increased risk for coronary artery disease. The family of the coronary patient must cope with the cultural stressors as well as the stressors of the crisis created by illness.

The medical literature has described the coronary-prone individual, but little mention has been made of how family members have adapted their life styles to the behavior of the coronary-prone individual. The male character in the novel *Hurricane Years* (Hawley, 1968) exhibits the personality profile described in the medical literature. He had a high level of ambition and experienced many frustrations at work. Sadness and disappointment were experienced during childhood. The relationship between husband and wife lacked closeness, lacked a sharing of feelings, lacked goals, and lacked freedom of expression. His wife developed interests apart from his so that at the time of her husband's heart attack, there was little to sustain them through the crisis. In the novel, the physician and nurse contributed to the husband's and wife's readjustment in life style: a beginning toward the establishment of a sharing relationship, the husband's change in attitude toward his job, and the resolution of the fear of a future heart attack.

Inclusion of the family in the nursing care plan facilitates the goal of optimum rehabilitation of the patient. The literature is lacking in depth analysis of the family of an acute coronary patient, their emotional responses, coping mechanisms, and adaptive behaviors. An attempt is made to describe observations of how families cope with hospitalization, death, or return to the community during the crisis of an acute myocardial infarction in a family member. An assessment tool of the family situation and therapeutic intervention is suggested so as to promote optimum family adjustment during the crisis and subsequent rehabilitation.

IMMEDIATE CRISIS

The person suffering severe chest pain will usually deny its significance and on the average will arrive in the emergency room 6 to 8 hours after the pain begins, unless prompted by others to seek immediate care. An individual who is being treated for coronary artery disease and does not obtain relief from coronary vasoldilators will generally seek medical assistance immediately. If the strickened individual collapses in a state of shock, hopefully help is available to provide emergency measures until he is placed in an intensive care unit.

SUDDEN DEATH

Outside the environs of the intensive care unit staffed with highly trained nurses, sudden death from electrical heart failure is a well-known, but as yet a barely preventable, complication of acute myocardial infarction. Even if all persons were trained in resuscitative procedures, a striking example of an unpreventable death is that of a husband who, without waking his wife, is aroused in the middle of the night with pain he attributes to indigestion. Thinking a glass of milk will ease his discomfort, he goes to the kitchen. The next morning his wife finds him dead on the kitchen floor. The wife, due to lack of knowledge of her husband's situation, is unable to resuscitate and possibly prevent death. When chest pain occurs, denial by the individual, family, or others present, may also prevent immediate transfer to the hospital and access to life supporting services.

Unexpected death of one's spouse would seem, if measurable, to produce a greater degree of emotional shock to the family than death which occurred following the hospitalization of the victim. The family would not have had time to deal with and begin to develop coping mechanisms in the former situation.

The following is an example of the coping mechanism displayed in the case of sudden death. The wife, who was in her early thirties, lived near her small home town. Following the sudden death of her husband, she resigned from her job. Being basically of a relatively dependent nature and having close family ties nearby, she looked to her parents for emotional support. Following the busy plans of a funeral, grieving followed the typical pattern of regression to a more dependent mode of behavior. Withdrawal and depression occurred while the wife stabilized herself and adapted to a new pattern of living, that of total responsibility for the care of her son of junior high school age. In this instance, finances were not a worry as the husband left a sizable inheritance.

When the widow's energy became once more outwardly directed, the home was sold. The widow and son moved in with her divorced sister several states away. The summer months were spent in an environment of continual partying, poor eating habits, and irregular sleeping patterns which resulted in the widow's 20-pound weight gain.

In the interim, the son, being without the disciplinary love of a father and having a frequently absent mother, experienced loneliness and began having difficulty in school. In the fall the widow decided to occupy some of her time with a job. Continued preoccupation with adjustment to the change in life style and frequent attendance at parties interfered with effectiveness at work. Many times, extended lunch hours were taken during which no one knew of her whereabouts. The following spring the widow seemed more relaxed, an apartment was obtained, and shortly thereafter she met a man with three children and was soon married.

Pathological responses to widowhood may take the form of extended withdrawal from the environment with self as the center of concern. Most likely this would occur in a situation where the widow or widower had greatly depended on the spouse and did not have close family ties or friendships. In this instance a health worker cognizant of the situation could begin to develop a relationship providing emotional support to draw out feelings, help identify them, and help the survivor begin the process of coping and adaptation. Socialization may occur at a slow rate. Feelings may consist of hostility, anger, denial, and an irreplaceable loss. The latter may be accentuated if the couple was older, was married a long time, had a close relationship, and the widowed had a dependent personality, and felt greatly insecure without the spouse. Anxiety and extreme weight loss may be the manifested physiological and psychological responses to the stress of change in accustomed life style. The goal of care would be one of support, respecting the wishes of the survivor spouse and suggesting to the survivor that he remain in the same environment during the initial adjustment phase. Support should be given in the development of friendships with gradual addition of activities outside the home. If of a working age, a job could help provide responsibility and diversion for the widowed.

It has been the writer's experience that families differ in their need of intervention and support during a crisis. Those families who have close ties within the primary family, with relatives and with members of the local community, seem to have a cushion of absorption of the emotional and sometimes financial shock experienced when a family member has an acute myocardial infarction. This same support remains present during the later stages of rehabilitation. Given this situation there appears to be a lesser degree of need for intervention and support by the nurse and other health workers.

Another observed phenomenon which seems to have an effect on the degree of intervention and support needed is that of the family's environment and their manner of adaptation to the environment. The writer has found that families living in predominately agricultural areas exhibit less need for intervention and support by a nurse. The author's speculation has resulted in the concept that those individuals who depend on nature's whims of sun, rain, hail, snows, and tornados for their livelihood, such as farming and husbandry, develop a philosophy of life (agrarian) and an ability to more effectively cope with a crisis than do those individuals who live in an urban area and have their lives affected by business and social organizational demands.

Those people from agricultural areas appear less anxious and seem to be less disturbed by the dependency role and interruption in the familiar daily activities which illness and hospitalization demands. They seem to have more acceptance of events which they have no control over than do those individuals who are competing for status and income in metropolitan areas of high family mobility. The agrarian community, in most instances, appears to provide adequate support during bereavement in the case of death of a community member. The bereaved is kept active with visits by friends and the sustenance of gifts of food.

HOSPITALIZATION

In the last few years the communication media has informed the public of intensive coronary care technology. Even so, when the family arrives in the intensive care unit they may be overwhelmed with the monitoring equipment at the bedside and the newly acquired dependency of their family member. Before the family enters the room, the nurse should briefly explain the condition of the patient and the use of the equipment, and be receptive to the fears and anxieties expressed by the family. This family may need help in canceling previously made commitments. Visitor policies may be mentioned when appropriate. Later, at a feasible time, when the patient's condition is stabilized, the nurse may elicit information from the family which would aid in assessment and intervention in the nursing care of the patient. This manner of planning care would hopefully diminish feelings of isolation and loneliness felt by the family as well as provide a better rationale for rehabilitation goals for the patient. When appropriate, the patient should also be involved in providing information. The following is an assessment tool which may be a useful guide to obtaining a nursing history.

Pattern of daily living
    Eating habits
    Sleeping habits
    Personal hygiene habits
    Bowel habits
    Drug use
    Smoking habits
    Drinking habits
    Exercise habits
    Relaxation measures
    Pleasurable activities and avocation
    Vocation and working habits
Languages spoken
Religion
Description of residence
Handicaps and protheses
Marital status
    Children, their ages, sex, roles and interpersonal relationships; closest relationship; and significant others
Visitors
    Their relationship, their support to and interaction with the patient
Unusual stresses preceding the heart attack
Previous illnesses and hospitalization including attitude toward hospitalization
Hospitalization insurance and financial status
Other health agencies involved with the family
Patient's and family's current understanding of the illness
Patient's and family's current effective and ineffective coping mechanisms and adaptive behaviors
Patient's and family's previous history of coping with stress and change
Family unit's characteristic life style and daily interactions

The assessment of the patient and family is an ongoing process. Short-, intermediate-, and long-term goals for rehabilitation should be defined. Problems should be identified. Priorities should be established. Strengths and weaknesses exhibited by the patient and his family should be sought, and the strengths mobilized and supported. Methods of diminishing inhibiting factors should be sought.

Following formulation and institution of interventive techniques, evaluation and modification of the nursing care plan should occur when appropriate. This information should be recorded so that when the patient is transferred, those responsible for his care have guidelines for continuity. Privacy of information elicited should be maintained. Judgment must be made by the nurse of what questions to ask and when. A combination of direct and indirect methods of interviewing may be warranted. This will vary according to the quality of rapport which the nurse establishes as well as the wishes of the patient and family to reveal and share information. If the family exhibits adequate adaptive behavior, the nurse's role may be one of giving support when needed and answering questions.

The nurse may not be in the best position to elicit information and initiate interventive measures that will help the family with coping with the crisis of an acute myocardial infarction. After consultation with the physician, the referral of complex cases to a social worker, psychiatrist, psychologist and/or pastor may be indicated. Pertinent information helpful in providing nursing care may be elicited from these other team members.

The family should be made to feel as wanted guests in the hospital. The nurse, because of his continual presence, is probably in the best position to act as host. Ideally a visitor's waiting room with an outside phone is made available for family use. The nurse should introduce the family members to the other visitors present and help them feel as comfortable as possible. If a coffee machine is available, possibly the visitors would find some comfort from a cup of coffee. Directions to local lodging, restaurants, and places of relaxation should be given.

From observations of interactions among the families in the waiting room, it would seem that since they share in a common crisis situation this stimulates rapport between members of families. They attempt to be supportive to one another. If one person leaves the room for a while, the remaining visitors know where he can be reached. If a phone call comes in for a visitor who is temporarily absent, the visitor answering the phone locates the person who is being called. Crisis seems to have the advantage of removing the stereotyped pleasantries that often impede immediate development of a relationship. However, these relationships usually are situational and terminate once the stress of the crisis has diminished.

One could speculate that with the occurrence of an acute myocardial infarction, the family members experience many kinds of feelings. They may relive many past events and experience feelings of guilt, sadness, anxiety, and melancholy. Frustration may be experienced due to their inability to have control of the crisis situation—that control being allocated to the health team personnel providing patient care. Helplessness may result in situations when communication attempts are thwarted. In observations of the wives of male patients, some seem to experience a need to be needed. In their interactions with their husbands, they may exhibit "take charge" behavior. Formerly, in this kind of situation, the wife ventilated her feelings more than her husband. Inclusion of the family in the progress of the patient and in his care may help relieve some of the feelings of helplessness and frustration. If one family member appears to have a good rapport with the patient, this family member may be guided to contribute to alleviation of the patient's anxiety and fear. An example of this is a patient whose native language is not English and, in the regression caused by illness, resorts to his native tongue to communicate needs. A family member can help bridge the communication barrier and in so doing help alleviate some of the fear and frustration experienced by the patient.

Preparation of the family for the patient's transfer to an intermediary unit and/or to the general medical unit should begin as soon as is feasible and the patient's condition appears stabilized. This should be approached with a manner indicating progress of the patient, who will no longer need intensive observation and care. For many patients and families this move may be a threatening experience for them as many of them feel the security of the coronary care unit and fear that if a complication occurs outside the unit, immediate help will not be available. This is a realistic concern which most hospital care systems have not been able to alleviate as yet.

Following discharge from the coronary care unit the patient usually goes through a depression. This is likely due to previous denial of the infarct and its life-threatening meaning, energy lost through mobilization of forces to maintain oneself during the immediate crisis, and subsequent realization once the patient has left the cornary care unit of the meaning of the infarct and change in life style that may result. Fear of another heart attack may be incapacitating. Previous personal and social factors may influence the degree of depression. With gradual acceptance, activity will be directed outward to the environment and effective behavior modification manifested in order to adapt to the new life style. The family should be included in the therapeutic plan during this stage of resolution of illness. Possibly telemetry and a better prepared general nursing staff may help provide security in case of complications after discharge from the coronary care unit.

Dependence on others is a normal sequence of illness. Trust of the health team members may take time to establish but is quickly destroyed. Once the health team is committed to providing service, they assume responsibility for maintaining trust as well as progression of patient and family to independence and self-determination. Denial, anger, and depression are normal processes one goes through when illness occurs. They allow a drawing inward from the environment while effective coping and adaptive measures are sought. The family should be helped to understand and cope with this depression in the hospitalized family member. The family may also experience the same psychological responses. They will need a chance to verbalize their feelings and problems in adaptation.

Withdrawal and listlessness from the environment may indicate severe depression and may be a warning of maladaptation and need for concerted external intervention to prevent suicidal sudden death. Ideally, a mental health worker is available for intervention. Ginsparg and Statten (1970) suggest these steps in health crisis intervention:

Adjustment to the illness

a Help the individual to accept the fact that he [or the family member] has suffered damage to a vital body organ
b Help him to become aware of the psychological meaning his damage has for him
c Familiarize him with the reality factors of his illness, such as extent of damage, degree of recovery and the limitations which are necessary as opposed to those which are unnecessary

Adjustment to the life situation

a Explore with the individual his current life situation and his priorities in life, his satisfactions, commitments, etc.
b Help the individual identify the stress situations which create difficulty for him
c Help the individual to deal better with these situations, either by eliminating them from his life, or developing different ways of handling them

Since the family will experience changes in daily life style and emotional stress, the steps suggested by Ginsparg and Statten may be utilized by the nurse and other team members in helping the family cope and move toward reconciliation. One change in routine is daily trips to the hospital. In the early hospitalization phase, if the spouse is not working, he may spend most of his time in the waiting room. This is a total change in daily routine. At this time changes in the home are experienced by the absence of this family member. In the case of the husband who had been hospitalized, the wife and children must assume or redirect those daily responsibilities in family life which he fulfilled. If the wife is hospitalized, help may need to be brought into the home if young children are present.

The nurse's role is one of recognizing maladaptations and assuming responsibility for the proper referral. The nurse should be aware of and minimize family dependency. He should have knowledge of community resources and assume responsibility for mobilizing them so that the family can begin the process toward autonomy.

PREPARATION FOR DISCHARGE

According to Hahn and Dolan (1970) the impact of illness is too overwhelming to begin teaching while the patient is in the coronary care unit but following discharge from the coronary care unit, the nurse's clarification of the physician's instructions was found helpful in patient adjustment. They found that the nurse's evaluation of the home situation, job, and customary activities helped the patient in his application of information. Hahn and Dolan assessed the reaction of the patient to his diet, drugs, and therapies in preparation for helping the patient assume responsibility for his own health care during rehabilitation. Inclusion of the patient's family in the teaching program was found helpful. In this study the patient's readiness for teaching was evaluated by the physician, and the teaching was conducted in individual, frequent short sessions. Four areas were covered: (1) disease process, (2) medications, (3) activity, and (4) diet. The patients were quizzed before discharge by the nurse and misunderstandings clarified. The day of discharge, instructions given by the physician to the patient and family were reinforced and clarified. Staff conferences regarding teaching and nursing care were held periodically.

Separate patient and family group therapy discussions after discharge from the hospital would provide further opportunity for clarification and would mobilize group support and an opportunity to ventilate and share in problems experienced and their effective solutions. Other health team members would be valuable at these group discussions if they were also included as team members during the patient's hospitalization. These sessions would provide for continuity, follow-up, and, hopefully, optimum rehabilitation.

RETURN TO COMMUNITY

According to statistics, about 60 to 70 percent of patients who experience a myocardial infarction can resume fulltime activity (Ostfeld, 1967). Optimum adaptation and rehabilitation has been shown to occur when the patient has adequate hospitalization insurance and a job to which to return.

According to Thomas (1966), the family is the most important primary group in the handicapped person's life. It has the greatest influence on how the patient views himself and whether his social functioning is appropriate to his disability. The family members may be a positive factor in rehabilitation. Or the family may be a negative factor contributing to the stressors experienced by the coronary victim. The wife whose husband has had a coronary experiences fear of a recurrant heart attack and ever-present sudden death. The health team should help the wife ventilate fears and develop a workable means of handling these fears. This may be an important topic for group therapy discussions posthospitalization. The family may have more difficulty making adjustments than the patient. Interpersonal relationships may suffer as many families do not want to talk with the patient about the heart attack. Group therapy may be of value in bridging these communication gaps.

Reasons for imposed disability are family overprotectiveness, expectations of the family that pose hardships on the handicapped, excessive patient dependency, severe anxiety, past history of psychological illness or depression, instability of work history, ethnic background, multiple diseases, dietary restrictions, and use of anticoagulants.

An iatrogenic factor may be introduced inadvertently by the physician who does not use treadmill testing of activity level tolerance of the patient. An aid to rehabilitation is work evaluation units whereby the treadmill is utilized, reconditioning exercises prescribed, and a prescription for daily activities formulated with the patient and family. In the case of severe physical limitation of the patient, a community-based nurse may need to evaluate the physical environment in the home and suggest alterations of the environment.

Socioeconomic obstructions to rehabilitation are time spent in litigation for workmen's compensation, fear of the employer to hire a person who has had a coronary or to assign him a job he can do, lack of job retraining, higher income on pension or from disability insurance, and society's attitudes.

Glasser and Glasser (1970, p. 7) have identified three main factors which can be utilized to determine whether a given event becomes a crisis for the family:

1   Hardships created by the change or event itself

2   Family resources: role structure, lack of rigidity and previous experiences with crisis situations

3   Whether the family perceives the event as a threat to their status, goals and objectives

Those families which seem best able to adequately respond to a crisis seem to exhibit a commitment and participation in family involvement; they have interdependence in instrumental and socioeconomic roles and are flexible in adapting to changes within the family as well as to external situations in the community. A suggested assessment tool for determining the family's ability to adequately cope with change and need for intervention is (Glasser and Glasser, 1970, p. 158):

    1 Solidarity in family structure (Amount of intimacy, social integration, emotional integration, togetherness, understanding, companionship)
    2 Sexuality
    3 External relationships in the community (Friends, school, local grocer, barber, or beautician)
    4 Internal instrumentality (The division of work)
    5 Division of responsibility in previous four categories

According to Thomas (1966), negative influencing factors are role discontinuity, role conflict, role strain, and nonfacilitative interdependence (marital strain). One role of the health worker is mobilizing the individual's internal resources for coping and adaptation.

The unique emotional components of a cardiac ailment are unknown but may be related to change in body image and the individual physical and emotional attachments to the heart. There is, of course, the emotional, poetic attachment to the heart, as well as knowledge of the amount of physical reserve of the heart which may or may not be hindered by information from the physician and others. The family's views of the change in body image may contribute to the family's emotional response to the patient. The children may have difficulty with the possible role changes, role identities, and responsibilities. In case of depression, hostility, irritability, or paranoid reactions created by the heart disability, the appropriate health worker may be invaluable.

The nurse and others involved in rehabilitation can use the crisis situation which makes individuals more susceptible and less resistive to outside help to explore with the family means of changing life styles, bringing the family closer together, and finding more satisfying relationships. Two books written for the layman may be suggested reading for the patient and family: List's *A Psychological Approach to Heart Disease* (1967) and Brenton's *Sex and Your Heart* (1968). Also of value in adjustment may be local clubs such as "Cardiacs Anonymous."

In the case of one follow-up of a patient postdischarge, the major concerns seemed to be loss of dominance in family relationships and in family business matters, change of diet, and not knowing the level of optimum physical activity. The profile of the individual was a male in his early fifties, widowed, who owned his own business in which his two sons worked. With the help of several home visits by a nurse, the man's anxiety seemed to diminish as evidenced by decreased pulse rate, increased physical activity, and a development toward acceptance of relinquishing total responsibility for the family business to the sons who had some different opinions regarding the business management.

Systematic data collection on previous life styles of families who have a family member with a myocardial infarction, knowledge of their adaptive behavior characteristics, as well as experimental effective therapeutic intervention are needed. This knowledge could be invaluable to primary prevention as well as identifying content for inclusion in nursing and health delivery education curricula.

BIBLIOGRAPHY

Andreoli, K. G., et al.: *Comprehensive Cardiac Care,* 2d ed, St. Louis: C. V. Mosby Company, 1971.

Aquilera, C., M. Messick, and M. Farrell: *Crisis Intervention: Theory and Methodology,* St. Louis: C. V. Mosby Company, 1970.

Bogdonoff, D.: "Psychological Impact of Coronary Care Unit," *Advanced Cardiac Nursing,* Philadelphia: Charles Press, 1970, pp. 176-183.

Brenton, M.: *Sex and Your Heart,* New York: Coward-McCann, Inc., 1968.

Caplan, G.: *An Approach to Community Mental Health,* New York: Grune & Stratton, Inc., 1961.

Dumas, R.: "Utilization of Stress as a Therapeutic Nursing Measure," *ANA Clinical Sessions,* New York: Appleton-Century-Crofts, 1966, pp. 193-212.

Ezra, R.: *Social and Economic Effects on Families of Patients with Myocardial Infarctions,* Denver, Colo: The Graduate School of Social Work, University of Denver, 1961.

Ginsparg, L., and E. Statten: "Psychiatric Aspects of Rehabilitation in Coronary Artery Disease," *Proceedings of the 78th Annual Convention,* American Psychiatric Association, 1970.

Glasser, P., and L. Glasser (eds.): *Families in Crisis,* New York: Harper & Row, Publishers, Incorporated, 1970.

Gorton, V.: *Behavioral Components of Patient Care,* London: The Macmillan Company, 1970.

Hahn, H., and N. Dolan: "After a Coronary—Then What?," *American Journal of Nursing,* **70**:2350-2352, 1970.

Hawley, C.: *Hurricane Years,* New York: Fawcett World Library, 1968.

Hellerstein, K.: "Rehabilitation in Coronary Artery Disease," *Advanced Cardiac Nursing,* Philadelphia: Charles Press, 1970, pp. 184-196.

Jacobson, G. F., et al.: "Generic and Individual Approaches to Crisis Intervention," *American Journal of Public Health,* **58**:339-342, 1968.

Jenkins, C.: "Psychologic and Social Precursors of Coronary Disease," *New England Journal of Medicine,* Part 1, pp. 244-255, Feb. 4, 1971; Part II, pp. 284-317, Feb. 11, 1971.

Jezer, A.: "The Workshop in the Coronary Spectrum," *Journal of Rehabilitation,* **32**:68-71, 1966.

List, S.: *A Psychological Approach to Heart Disease,* New York: Institute of Applied Psychology, Inc., 1967.

Miller, M. G., and J. Brewer: "Factors Influencing the Rehabilitation of the Patient with Ischemic Heart Disease," *The Medical Journal of Australia,* 1:410–416, 1969.

National Nursing Conference: *Post-hospital Care of Coronary Patients,* Richmond, Va., Feb. 25–26, 1970.

Ostfeld, M.: "The Interaction of Biological and Social Variables in Cardiovascular Disease," *Milbank Memorial Fund Quarterly,* 45:13–18, 1967.

"Psychological and Social Factors in Cardiovascular Disease," *The Heart and Circulation,* 2d National Conference on Cardiovascular Diseases, Washington, D.C., 1964, pp. 241–242.

Reich, C. A.: *The Greening of America,* New York: Random House, 1970.

Rosenman, R. H., et al.: "Coronary Heart Disease in the Western Collaborative Group Study," *Journal of the American Medical Association,* 195:130–136, 1966.

————: "Coronary Heart Disease in the Western Collaborative Group," *Journal of Chronic Diseases,* 23:173–190, 1970.

————: "A Predictive Study of Coronary Heart Disease," *Journal of American Medical Association,* 189:15–22, 1964.

———— and M. Friedman: "Behavior Patterns, Blood Lipids, and Coronary Heart Disease," *Journal of the American Medical Association,* 184:934–938, 1963.

Schiller, E., and G. Morris: "A Practical Rating Scale for Early Identification of the Problem Case," *Medical Journal of Australia,* 1:889–892, 1971.

"The Patient with a Myocardial Infarction," Supplement, *American Journal of Nursing,* 64:C-1–C-32, 1964.

Thomas, J.: "Problems of Disability from the Perspective of Role Theory," *Journal of Health and Human Behavior,* 7:2–13, 1966.

Toffler, A.: *Future Shock,* New York: Bantam Books, Inc., 1970.

Chapter 29

The Family with a Mentally Retarded Child

Raeone S. Zelle

In 1966, members of the International League of Societies for the Mentally Handicapped from thirty-three countries convened in Paris to attend the Third International Congress. For three days many experts discussed stress on families of the mentally handicapped. In his introductory address, Dr. Hutchison (1967) from Great Britain stated:

> It is only in recent years that it has come to be generally accepted that the presence of a mentally retarded person in the family causes stresses to that family, not only to the parents but to the other members, and it is only in recent years that some attempt has been made to alleviate these stresses, thus ensuring that the family enjoys, as far as possible, a normal family life.

Nurses are in an unique position to help the family cope with the stress caused by the definition of one of the members as mentally retarded. They provide service in varied settings including the home over an extended period, and their professional role is viewed as a helpful and acceptable part of the cultural pattern of our society (Ehlers, 1966; Freidson, 1959; Wolfensberger, 1967). However, a holistic approach seems to be a generalized ideal rather than a reality. What seems to be lacking is a conceptual frame of reference for family assessment and intervention. As Farber (1960a) pointed out, common sense or vague generalities do not specify the variables which can be important determinants of the severity of the stress nor the necessary steps to be taken by family members in counteracting the stress.

The author (1969) found that public health nurses in a large, urban health department relied solely on their generalized professional frame of reference to assess the effect of a retarded child on family relations and life. They were not sensitized to observe all the important dimensions which have been found to be affected, and they did not utilize a uniform system for classifying and recording observations. The most comprehensive assessment was made by the nurse who had visited the family frequently over the longest period of time when the father was at home. The least comprehensive assessment was made by the nurse who had visited the family for the shortest period of time and had never seen the father. The above results raise questions regarding the handicapping effect of the lack of a conceptual guide for family assessment, the corresponding lack of uniformity especially in light of the ever-present problem of personnel turnover and family mobility, and the traditional working day which often precludes involving the father.

The intent of this chapter is to draw upon the theoretical explorations and formalized investigations of family stress and crisis which have been conducted in recent years to develop a frame of reference for family assessment and intervention. Hill (1965), Parad (1965), Caplan (1964), and Farber (1964) are but a few of the members of various disciplines who have made important contributions to the better understanding of family interaction and stress. Farber has related much of his research to the family in which one of the members is mentally retarded, and the author feels that his conceptual model provides a workable framework for nursing.

CONCEPTUAL FRAMEWORK

Farber views the family as a set of mutually contingent careers. A career is defined as a progression of roles which unfold in a patterned sequence in a life cycle. A man and woman marry and have children, and the children progress through various stages: infancy, school age, adolescence, and adulthood. The parents retire and eventually die, ending the life cycle of one family unit. Movement in the cycle from one stage to the next is stimulated by a change in the roles of the children which in turn causes a shift in the roles of the parents and redefinition of values and obligations in accordance with conventional norms.

In families with a retarded child, the course of the child's life is different from his brothers and sisters. Regardless of his birth order, he eventually becomes the youngest, slows down the movement of the family life cycle, and prevents development of later stages (Farber, 1964). (A mildly retarded child's career may not be perceived as arrested if he becomes an independent member of the community.) The family members are faced with a set of circumstances which differ from conventional norms, and there is no tradition or broad group experience to guide them in coping with the deviant child and the disruptions which evolve. Doubt and disagreement can arise, reflected in tension in the system of family roles and changes in the value system of one or both parents. Members must reorient their lives with respect to the child's peculiar career, and sharpening differences can arise between the family and the community of normal families (Farber, 1959; 1960a).

It would seem evident that the retarded child could be termed a threat to homeostasis in accordance with Caplan's definition of crisis. However, a crisis involving the concept of equilibrium is viewed as time-limited, and a new steady state can be achieved within a relatively short period (Caplan, 1964, p. 53). Clinical observations and research findings would seem to support Farber's contention that a crisis evoked by a handicapped child can be enduring in nature (1964, p. 407). He defined a crisis as an induction of a new distortive process in family life "which is counter to the ordinary organization of the norms and values of the family members" (1964, p. 392). A process approach permits a more adequate analysis of the coping mechanisms which must be employed to counteract the distortive effect. Farber recognized certain regularities in the process and developed a framework of phases which was applied to the family with a mentally retarded member as follows:

1 During the first phase, the family attempts to handle the deviance within the existing arrangement and system of norms and values. As long as the family can maintain a fiction of normality, no family crisis exists. The problem may be explained away as an easily remedied illness, slow maturation, or a lesser handicap.

2 Distortions in family relationships finally force the family to define the child as deviant. Members can no longer explain away his special needs and demands or handle them within the existing system of roles and values. The initial impact of the crisis process marks the second phase.

3 Distorted relationships within the family precipitate revisions in extrafamily relationships, and this marks the third phase of the crisis. Extrafamily activities may have to be restricted because of the special needs of the child or altered because of the unsupportive attitude of certain individuals and groups. New extrafamily coalitions must be formed which provide help and support in handling the problem.

4   A continuation of family life is sustained through a rearrangement of age and sex roles to adjust to the arrested career of the retardate. The rearrangement is the fourth phase. Members must develop strategies to cope with the deviancy in the family organization and life cycle.

5   If strategies cannot be employed to minimize the disorganization to a tolerable level, the fifth phase of the crisis evolves. The deviant child is eliminated by permanently placing him outside the home. Farber (1964, p. 430) terms this the *freezing out* phase.

IMPLICATIONS FOR NURSING ASSESSMENT AND INTERVENTION

Of course, in reality a family does not conform to a generic classification and proceed from one phase to another in an orderly, precise manner. There is an intertwining of phases and even regression at times in response to a new or renewed source of stress. However, it is important for the nurse to assess the approximate phase of adjustment, the severity of the crisis as perceived by the family in relation to important variables which will be discussed later, and the type and effectiveness of coping strategies which are employed. The assessment can be used as a baseline for planning appropriate intervention and establishing priorities of service.

First Phase of the Crisis

If the family is in the first phase, their primary need is a warm, permissive, and nonjudgmental relationship with a professional person who allows them to absorb the painful reality at their own pace. Olshansky (1962, p. 191) pleads with professionals to not rush the process of acceptance. "In most cases one can ask what will be lost if the parent is unable for several years to view his child as mentally defective." Professional persons sometimes become impatient with the family's so-called lack of acceptance and tendency to shop for various diagnoses which may be a reflection of their own lack of acceptance of mental retardation or seeming helplessness in the situation. Mandelbaum (1960) contends that the reaction should be viewed as a normal attempt to offset the tremendous blow to the self-concept of the parents which can be understood and justified if we examine the following symbolic meanings of a child:

1   The parent views the child as a physical and psychological extension of himself, and a defective child is seen as a reflection of his own inadequacies and imperfections.

2   The child is a means of vicarious satisfaction to the parent, and he feels frustrated when he realizes that his child cannot fulfill his hopes and aspirations (Cummings and Stock, 1962, p. 744).

3 The child is a means by which the parents can transcend death and derive some degree of immortality. The birth of a defective child may precipitate existential conflicts regarding the meaning of life and the relative insignificance and helplessness of man (Roos, 1963, p. 347).

4 The child is viewed as a personalized love object, and parents are expected to love a defective child who may be aesthetically unacceptable to them (Dalton and Epstein, 1963, p. 525).

The author (1969) interviewed mothers and fathers of severely mentally retarded children, and her impressions corroborated the reports of other writers (Begab, 1963; Oberman, 1963; Yates and Lederer, 1961), that fathers have a more difficult time adjusting to the reality. As the instrumental leader or head of the house, he is concerned with the continued maintenance of the family name and place in the community, and some of the above areas of meaning would be more crucial to him. In the American society, the man is expected to maintain a masculine, controlled image. All the wives stated that they had no problem communicating with their husbands, but most of the husbands stated that they kept their worries and concerns to themselves. The following excerpts of taped interviews illustrate the constraint of expression.* The fathers were responding to the question, "How did you feel at first?"

Father A: (long pause) "Oh, it's kind of hard to explain I guess. (pause) It's just that a (pause) just so he's going to turn out to be a special child I guess."

Father B: "Well, it's really hard to say exactly how I felt. It is just hard to explain how you feel about something like that I suppose."

Father C: "I didn't believe it, and I still don't. All I think is she is just slow and coming along. . . . I still think she is all right."

Because of his working hours, the father cannot always attend diagnostic evaluations and follow-up conferences or be at home when the public health nurse visits; and he, therefore, is not exposed to as much professional help and support as his wife. Professionals (Quast, 1968; Schild, 1971; Wolfensberger, 1967) are beginning to emphasize the importance of involving both parents to promote communication, mutual understanding, and collaborative problem solving. If the burden of decision making and responsibility is placed upon one parent, this can lead to disassociation and marital friction. Hopefully, the nurse will begin to challenge the traditional schedule in both his own place of employment and other agencies which restrict or negate involvement with the father. He may be the first professional person to detect the child's

---

* Separate taped interviews with fathers and mothers served as raw data for the author's master's thesis (1969). Identifying information has been changed. Subsequent excerpts are from the same source.

delayed development and may be accepted in a counseling role when other professional persons would be rejected because of the unthreatening connotation attached to both his title and involvement with the family.

Some professional persons still cling to the old adage that parents must work through their feelings before they will respond to help with the special needs of the child. The author has found that this is not true in most cases. Too often, parents are left to struggle on their own, especially during the initial period of infancy which can be stormy. If it takes 1½ hours to feed the baby because of a weak suck and lethargy, the parents will be responsive to suggestions regarding the most effective nipple and the stimulative value of taste and temperature, even if they explain the problem away by rationalizing that some babies "just do not feed well." There is no reason why the nurse cannot go along with their definition of the problem initially, especially in view of the fact that a threatening contradiction may close the door to further intervention. Concrete, practical help often opens the door to a trusting relationship which catalyzes expression of concerns.

Second Phase of the Crisis

The need for professional help is no doubt even more acute in the second phase of the crisis when the fiction of normality begins to crumble. Investigators have described a gamut of emotions which pours forth during the painful definition process—anger, disappointment, shame, guilt, depression, frustration, etc. (Auerbach, 1961; Dalton and Epstein, 1963; Kramm, 1963; Mandelbaum and Wheeler, 1960; Roos, 1963). Positive feelings of love and nuturance also come forth, developing a state of ambivalence (Schild, 1971). Again, the trend is toward viewing these reactions as normal rather than neurotic responses to a tragic event. Professional persons are also beginning to recognize that some of the stress may stem from "inept, inaccurate, and ill-timed" professional intervention (Murray, 1969; Matheny and Vernick, 1969; Wolfensberger, 1967). Many parents know absolutely nothing about mental retardation, and the last thing they need is involvement with a professional person who also knows nothing. Unfortunately, intervention which centers on a rehashing of feelings may be a cover up for a sense of inadequacy in dealing with questions and practical management problems. Wolfensberger admonishes professional persons to seriously assess their limitations and assume responsibility for developing competence. The professional affiliation or degree is really irrelevant; the person must possess the following qualifications to function as an intervener: (1) competency in communication and interviewing skills, (2) background knowledge and clinical experience in the area of mental retardation, (3) an orientation to community resources and management trends, (4) positive attitude toward mental retardation, and (5) sensitivity to the practical, situational needs of families (Wolfensberger, 1967, p. 355).

There is a beginning recognition of the need for a reality rather than a therapy-oriented approach and long-term counseling preferably by one primary intervener (Wolfensberger, 1967). Parents need frequent opportunities to regurgitate and recapitulate in order to finally assimilate information and work through feelings (Wolfensberger, 1967, p. 356). The public health nurse's intervention has historically met the above criteria, and this may explain why parents have viewed him as the most helpful professional person (Ehlers, 1966; Freidson, 1959; Logan, 1962). The family may have established a close relationship with him even before the birth of the retarded child because of other health needs. Too, since he routinely provides service in the home setting, he can observe practical problems firsthand; and he no doubt deals with these problems more than members of any other professional discipline.

However, nurses cannot develop a false sense of security because of the bouquets which have been thrown their way. The author has come in contact with many nurses who feel very inadequate and inexperienced in the field of mental retardation. It is imperative that nursing education and service realize the trend toward community-based care and prepare nurses to function as intelligent members of the team. Because of the multifaceted nature of mental retardation, one individual cannot possibly develop the breadth and depth of expertise required to deal with all the needs of the family. The nurse must learn to seek and utilize consultative help from specialized persons in his own profession and to develop a collaborative working relationship with members of other disciplines which involves a sharing of responsibility and expertise. There is a need for a primary intervener to promote continuity, and it is important that this person either be present or be fully informed of contacts with other professional persons to prevent bewildering the family with contradictory opinions and recommendations.

The severity of the impact of the definition process has been related to a number of variables by researchers. The sample in many of the studies consisted of middle- or upper-class white parents (mothers primarily) of severely retarded children which restricts generalization. Also, very few of the studies were experimental in design. However, it is felt that a brief discussion of the findings will sensitize the nurse to the importance of defining predictive variables which will identify high-risk families and critical periods.

Farber (1960b) reported a relationship between socioeconomic level and perception of stress. In families of relatively high socioeconomic status, the diagnosis precipitates a "tragic crisis" in which anticipated life careers are frustrated and plans are demolished. The reaction is more immediate and emotional in nature. In families of relatively low-socioeconomic status, the diagnosis does not precipitate an immediate abstract reaction. They are more vulnerable to an evolving "role organization" crisis precipitated by an inability to cope with the burden of the child's needs superimposed on other family demands. The reaction is to the here-and-now, and the mother is more apt to complain of physical strain. Other investigators have reported that lower-class families are less traumatized by the definition of the child as retarded (Ehlers, 1966; Giannini and Goodman, 1963; Kramm, 1963; Michaels and Schucman, 1962). The relationship between religious beliefs regarding the meaning of tragedy, absolution of guilt, and the value of children and the parental reaction has also been studied. Farber (1959), Zuk et al. (1961), and Kramm (1963) found that Catholic parents were more accepting of the diagnosis; however, other uncontrolled variables may have also been relevant. Farber (1959) found that the personal adjustment of the parents prior to the birth of the child is an important variable in determining vulnerability to stress.

The degree of handicap, sex, and birth order have also been identified as important variables. Hall (1961) and Auerbach (1961) reported a linear relationship between the severity of the handicap and the degree of stress. However, Cook (1963) and Denhoff (1960) reported that a diagnosis of mild retardation can have a greater impact on the parents. Farber et al. (1960) found that the initial stress is sex-linked, with the mother experiencing greater trauma if the retarded child is a girl and the father experiencing a markedly greater impact if the retarded child is a boy. These reactions were felt to relate to a need to live through a child and other identification factors. However, Farber (1959) found that the effect shifts later, and the marital integration of the parents is more adversely affected by a mentally retarded son. The disruption increases with age especially in lower-class families which was felt to infer that there is a greater perceived arrest in his anticipated career. Parents become increasingly disappointed with his failure to meet societal expectations. Kramm (1963) reported that the impact is more intense when the child is the firstborn, which may be related to greater expectations and hopes being invested with the first birth. Conversely, Quast (1968) noted that there seems to be less of an impact if the retarded child is the youngest. Dreams have been fulfilled by the other siblings, and the parents have acquired childrearing skills. Farber (1959) found that the younger the retarded child and the higher the degree of dependency, the greater was the effect on the adjustment of the normal siblings. Both Farber (1959) and Fowle (1968) found that the normal sister experienced greater role tension than the normal brother which was attributed to the fact that greater domestic demands were placed on her. Conversely, they found that the normal brother experienced greater role tension when the retarded child was institutionalized. Farber concluded that heretofore he had been expected to stay out of his mother's way, and now he was exposed to increased demands to conform to family routines. Other investigators reported that the siblings experience no adverse effect from the definition of a brother or sister as retarded (Caldwell and Guze, 1960; Graliker et al., 1962).

In the last few years, two studies have been published which involve a minority sample. Budner et al. (1969) found that Puerto Rican parents identify a developmental lag later and are less traumatized by a diagnosis of mental retardation than Caucasian parents. However, they have more difficulty coping with realistic management problems, which is congruent with the "role organization" crisis model. Both Budner et al. (1969) and Andrew (1968) found that minority families do not receive as much help, and they receive help later. Dager (1964) reported studies of families without a father which have possible implications. It was found that mothers tend to be more overprotective of their children, and the sons especially manifested dependent and infantile behavior. Assuming that this effect may also hold true if there is a retarded child in a one-parent family, the increased dependency would be superimposed on the retardation and intensify the management burden.

Third Phase of the Crisis

The establishment of priorities and the nature of nursing intervention must also be based on an assessment of adjustments which family members are forced to make in extrafamily relationships which Farber defined as the third phase of the crisis. The nurse needs to look at the degree of support and help the family is receiving from relatives, neighbors, friends, religious groups, other parents of retarded children, etc. Individuals and organizations in the community can serve as very valuable resources if they reinforce the reorientations which the family has to make and if they help relieve day-to-day burdens and demands. Some of the parents who have participated in group counseling sessions at Alta California Regional Center (a state-supported, community-based, multidisciplinary service for the mentally retarded) have become quite knowledgeable in relation to basic information about mental retardation, the "feeling work" involved with the definition process, and practical management approaches; and they have effectively served as counselors to other parents.

Unfortunately, the above persons and groups can be unsupportive if they base their intervention on conventional norms and values which are incongruous with the new script which family members have to develop (Farber, 1959). If they fail to understand the difference in the demands and expectations of a retarded child and a normal child of the same chronological age or have many misconceptions, their advice and comments can generate doubt and anxiety at a time when the parents are struggling to come to grips with their new role as illustrated in the following excerpt:

> You explain it to them and they sit there in a big. . . . You know they don't even understand anyway; and then when Paul does do something wrong they say why don't you do this.

An unsupportive attitude permeated all the extrafamily relationships of this family including the relatives:

> Like my mother-in-law, he'll grow out of it; now that's her attitude. He'll grow out of it. There's nothing wrong with him. He'll grow out of it whatever it is, but he's not mentally retarded. But yet she won't take him, you know. . . . That's a different story. Whatever it is he'll grow out of it, but she isn't going to have anything to do with it in the meantime.

The following excerpt illustrates that professional intervention can also be unsupportive:

> The minute he examined Betty he said, "We suggest you put her in an institution, and the sooner you do it the better." And it was so against my way of thinking and every time I would go he would start going at it again, and I would come home in tears everytime. And so finally John said, "You're just not ever going back to that doctor again. . . ."

Some parents may actively continue associations which are based on conventional norms and values as a means of escaping the problems and responsibilities of having a mentally retarded child. They may become overly involved with organizations, neighbors, or friends to avoid facing the task of developing new coping mechanisms. On the other hand, the family may become so overwhelmed and bogged down with the care of the child or the stigmatic connotation that they withdraw from community involvement and the potential supportive rewards.

Because of the multifaceted nature of mental retardation, individuals and groups in the community can seldom deal with all the needs. The family may find themselves thrust into a dependency on professional resources. This forced dependency may be in sharp contrast to a proud pattern of independence and self-sufficiency; and parents may need help in adjusting to the changed role and the interminable frustrations of frequent medical visits, agency policies, and possibly incompetent professionals. As the two studies indicate, minority groups have difficulty locating resources. There is a need for more vigorous casefinding among these groups to help families secure needed medical services and to also provide early, practical help which may prevent evolvement to a "role organization crisis." However, the intervention may have to be intensive in nature to effectively relieve the burden of family roles and promote the functionality of the child. Unfortunately, in many areas there is a paucity of services which meet these criteria. Even nurses are finding themselves bogged down with large caseloads because of the elimination of staff in response to economic pressures. Although middle- and upper-class parents are more sophisticated in locating and utilizing resources, they too are confronted with gaps in service. In addition to the need for assistance with medical and management problems, they especially may feel a need for intensive professional counseling to work through the "tragic crisis." Because of the greater emphasis on conventional norms in the middle- and upper-class social system, they possibly are more often exposed to unsupportive community relationships which feed into emotional reactions.

Nurses must assume a more active role as social and health planners to catalyze the upgrading of existing resources and the development of new resources. They are in an unique position to identify needs, but they frequently are not represented among professional disciplines at the planning level. To qualify for a more active role, they must become more cognizant of the political and bureaucratic mechanisms involved in decision making (Noble, 1970, p. 199). Nurses must also utilize their creativity on both a large and a small scale to expand the beginning trend toward the development of lay and paraprofessional resources, especially in view of the rising cost of service (Arnold and Goodman, 1966; Standifer, 1964).

Fourth Phase of the Crisis

Whether members can learn to take on the role of a "family-with-a-mentally-retarded-child" is to a large extent dependent on the strategies which they develop to adjust to his arrested career. This marks the fourth phase of the crisis. His inability to perform his age-sex roles stimulates a revision of heretofore rather taken-for-granted role relationships of family members and forces the family to consciously assume new modes of behavior. Unfortunately, there is no cookbook which defines what the new roles or related expectations should be (Perlman, 1963).

It is the author's impression that the mother experiences the greatest stress during this shifting and adjustment process. She is considered the primary caretaker in most families and more acutely feels the tug and pull of the needs of family members. Both Fowle (1968) and the author (1969) found that the wife was perceived as manifesting greater role tension than the husband. The following excerpt illustrates the pressures which she may experience (family had just institutionalized retarded child):

I don't know it's a funny thing because it's been so long since the kids all sat at
one table and ate you know together. . . . But I just did things as I had the time
for them. That's what I did so things got a little bit different and disrupted here
you know . . . I couldn't keep up with everything . . . I used to push the kids aside
at least I think I did when—a lot of times I did when I could have been helpful
to them.

The father can sometimes feel like a displaced member of the family, and
his companionship needs are left unmet as expressed in the following excerpts
in response to the question, "Do you ever feel left out?"

Father A: "Why sure because my wife is always doing for her you know."

Father B: "Yeah sometimes, sometimes it bothers me because she's
always got to be looking after John you know. I kinda feel left out once in a
while."

As mentioned earlier, all the normal children have to assume an older
child role regardless of their chronological age. Normal sisters may especially
be exposed to increased domestic demands beyond that which their chronological age would warrant (Farber, 1959; Fowle, 1968). Parents may also
place increased pressure on the normal siblings to excel to compensate for the
arrested career of their retarded brother or sister (Farber et al., 1960). Their
socialization needs may suffer because of the restrictive demands of the
retardate's management. Parents may be very hesitant to let friends visit
because of the child's susceptibility to infections, and involvement in organizations may have to be forfeited because of the lack of transportation and/or
surrogate responsibilities.

The nurse can assume a therapeutic role in helping families develop
coping strategies. A holistic approach is essential in developing an equilibrium between the needs of all family members. Many new approaches have
been developed to promote maximum functionality of the retardate which
can in turn lighten the burden of care. However, this goal is self-defeating if
it involves a program which dominates the energy and time especially of the
mother. The needs of other family members are neglected, and the retarded
child becomes accustomed to a self-centered existence which may be shat-
tered later when he enrolls in a community program or he is placed outside
the home (Morgan, 1967).

Quast (1968) suggested that the role and responsibility of the father be
expanded to minimize the burden of the mother's role and interdependency
between her and the child. The father generally becomes more actively involved with the children as they evolve in their career from the dependent
infancy stage; and he balances the mother's protectiveness with a more
future-oriented emphasis on independence and adaptability. However, the
sustained infantilism and dependency of the retarded child's arrested career

often inhibits or delays the formation of this relationship (Miller, 1969, p. 79). The author makes a special point of identifying ways the father can become involved with the management needs of the infant during group counseling sessions (conducted at Alta California Regional Center). Gross motor activities initially appeal to his masculine orientation especially when he is convinced that the infant will not break. Interest and involvement progresses to all areas of management, and he proudly reports developmental growth. The author has also found that siblings will eagerly assume responsibility for stimulative games and activities if their involvement is appropriately restricted.

The author has observed another coping strategy which is effective, and her impressions corroborate Farber's (1960a) findings. It seems that when parents can agree on a common goal or orientation, there is less disintegration and disorganization in family life, and the needs of the retarded child are more apt to be placed in proper perspective. In some families, the parents are very traditionally oriented, and goals and values revolve around the children and the continuance of the family name and status in the community. Both parents accept a sharp division of labor with the husband focusing on economic needs and the wife on domestic needs. For some families, a happy, congenial home may be the primary focus; and satisfaction is derived from close interpersonal relationships rather than social mobility or community status. For other families, the emphasis may be placed on climbing the middle-class ladder of success. Both parents place high value on career involvement, and the needs of the children are adjusted to social and employment demands.

If the family has developed an effective, solidifying family orientation, the nurse should relate to their value system instead of imposing his own. One of the important strengths is a healthy marital relationship which is the primary cohesive force in any family unit. The nurse should not insist upon the father's involvement with the daily domestic-oriented needs of the child if both parents accept sharply defined roles. On the other hand, he should realize that a home-oriented father may very definitely want to be involved in all facets of care. He must not react with scorn if career-oriented parents delegate the care of the child to a babysitter or withdraw him from a good program because the father is promoted and transferred. The effectiveness of coping strategies must be assessed from a holistic point of view. The retarded child's development is not a reliable criterion in and of itself. He may be progressing beautifully at the expense of the needs of the other family members.

Unfortunately, many parents do not attain the above degree of perfection. The nurse will come in contact with families who are so fatigued from emotional and/or physical stress that they have no energy for constructive planning or problem solving. Professional persons have to painfully admit at times that some families are beyond help (Hersh, 1961) or are not amenable to help. The saving grace for some of these families is coping strategies which alter the arrested career of the retarded child to a certain extent or relieve the burden of the roles of family members. Enrollment of the child in a developmental or special education program shifts the burden of his care during the day and often promotes functionality. Homemaking and babysitting services can alleviate the pressures placed on especially the role of the mother and siblings (Adams, 1968). Also, short-term respite in an institution or local community facility may prevent a complete breakdown and may free the parents to redirect their energy and develop appropriate strategies which will permit reentrance of the retarded child to the home. As discussed in the previous section, hopefully some of these strategies can be employed earlier on a preventative basis.

Fifth Phase of the Crisis

If the family cannot develop strategies to minimize the disruption to a tolerable level, the only alternative may be to evolve to the fifth phase of the crisis and permanently remove the child from the home—freeze him out. As illustrated by an earlier interview excerpt, some families are pressured by the physician to evolve to this phase at the moment of birth, and the advice may be supported by other professional persons. Wolfensberger (1967) points out the serious social, ethical, and moral implications involved. He argues that persons in a counseling role have a responsibility to help the family base the decision on carefully thought-out issues relating to the welfare and needs of the child and other family members, the value system of the family, and the feasibility of other coping strategies.

Researchers have identified variables which may influence evolvement to this crisis phase. However, again the studies have shortcomings which restrict generalization, and some of the findings are contradictory. Tizard and Grad (1961), Saenger (1960), and Graliker et al. (1965) found that the greater the degree of physical and mental handicap, the higher the probability that the family will be forced to choose this alternative. In congruence with the "role organization" and "tragic" crisis conceptualization, Farber et al. (1960) and Downey (1963) found that families at a high socioeconomic level place the child because of abstract reasons involving interference with the goals and aspirations of other family members and community opinion. The tendency is to place the child early and forget about him. Families at a lower socioeconomic level place the child because of present-oriented situational demands and pressures, and they delay placement longer and tend to remain in contact with the child. Saenger (1960), Wortis (1967), and Budner et al. (1969) report that the lower the socioeconomic level, the higher the likelihood of institution-alization. However, Graliker et al. (1965) found no socioeconomic difference between parents who placed or kept their child at home.

Hopefully, professional persons in the community and facilities will become more future-oriented in their thinking. Admission priorities have often been based on the degree of family breakdown. Placement may be the only strategy which will preserve the integrity of certain families, and the retardate should be accepted for admission before the deterioration has become a reality and has progressed to an emergency status. Too, the author feels that all parents should have the privilege of spending the retirement years alone without a dependent child to care for. A girl afflicted with cerebral palsy who was suddenly placed in a residential facility after her mother's death contends that:

> It is better to gently untie the apron strings which hold the family together, than to have them suddenly severed by the sharp knife of death . . . Now I see that if I had gone into a "home" before my mother's death . . . she could have given the attendants hints on my personal care. Still more important, I would have had the assurance of her love and understanding as I ventured into the unknown (Morgan, 1967, pp. 10-11).

Hersh (1970) identified a pattern of reactions to the stress involved with relinquishing the role of primary caretaker. There is an initial sense of loss followed by a sense of relief from the burden which is accompanied by a feeling of guilt and ambivalence. The nurse can be very helpful during this stressful period and especially if he has been involved with the family over a period of time and has developed a trusting relationship. He can support their decision and provide ego strength while they work through their reaction to the loss. He can also help the institutional staff develop a family-centered approach to the care of the retarded child, especially in view of the trend toward community placement. If the parents feel left out and disengaged, their ties with the child are more likely to continue in name only.

CONCLUSIONS

The crisis framework sensitizes the nurse to the dimensions of family life which can be affected and the coping tasks which have to be accomplished. Except possibly in the case of the retardate who has a mild mental impairment, the child's arrested career precipitates a lifelong adjustment. Olshansky (1962) defines this as a state of "chronic sorrow" which varies in relation to time, situations, and families. There is a need for an "open-door" accessibility to supportive professional help as the family moves through the phases of adjustment or regresses in response to increased stress which may be related to maturational and developmental indices. When the child reaches school age, the contrast in the progress and development of the subnormal child and the children of friends and relatives is brought into sharper focus and may precipitate the first feelings of anxiety about the future. When the child reaches adolescence, new fears will arise regarding delinquency, sexual exploitation, and the right of sexuality. When the child reaches adulthood, the burden of dependency is a source of stress for both the parents and the normal siblings (Hutchison, 1967).

Whether the retarded child is at home, hospitalized for an illness, enrolled in a school program, or placed in a residential facility, a nurse may be involved with his care. Hopefully, incompetence, judgmental impatience, and prejudice will not prevent nurses from addressing themselves to the stress which the family may be experiencing and reality-oriented needs. Hopefully, rigid traditional working hours will not prevent them from incorporating the whole of the family in intervention. Also, hopefully, professional defensiveness or jealousy will not prevent them from sharing responsibility and information with each other and with other team members to provide continuity of service and focus. The following quotations vividly portray the chronic burden which the childrearing needs of the retarded child can impose on the family and the inability of the family to shoulder the burden alone:

Family A (mother): "We went to Ohio last year for two weeks and Peter stayed at Institution X. And it was—I think I had quite a traumatic experience coming home. I was quite depressed because after two weeks of this freedom of doing what I wanted to do weekends and everything, going out where I wanted to go and having no problem leaving the children for a couple hours with friends or relatives without having to sit down for 45 minutes explaining exactly what they should do in case Peter fell, uh had a convulsion, or anything else. And it was such a change coming back to this routine again of planning and preparing and always being on the alert, that I was about really fed up."

Family B (father): "I guess as long as we can keep getting some sort of help from somebody you know we can work it out. If it wasn't for the help. I may sound like I am on a bandwagon, but I think that's a good thing. It's helped us and it's helped probably other people. Without it, you know, (pause) it would have been a disaster."

BIBLIOGRAPHY

Adams, M. E.: "Problems in Management of Mentally Retarded Children with Cerebral Palsy," *The Cerebral Palsy Journal,* **29**:3-7, 1968.

Andrew, G.: "Determinants of Negro Family Decisions in Management of Retardation," *Journal of Marriage and the Family,* **30**:612-617, 1968.

Arnold, I., and L. Goodman: "Homemaker Services to Families with Young Retarded Children," *Children,* **13**:149-152, 1966.

Auerbach, A. B.: "Group Education for Parents of the Handicapped," *Children,* **8**:135-140, 1961.

Begab, M. J.: *The Mentally Retarded Child: A Guide to Services of Social Agencies,* Washington, D.C.: U.S. Government Printing Office, 1963.

Budner, S., L. Goodman, and R. Aponte: "The Minority Retardate: A Paradox and a Problem in Definition," *Social Service Review,* **43**:174-183, 1969.

Caldwell, B. M., and S. B. Guze: "A Study of the Adjustment of Parents and Siblings of Institutionalized and Noninstitutionalized Retarded Children," *American Journal of Mental Deficiency,* **64**:845-861, 1960.

Caplan, G.: *Principles of Preventative Psychiatry,* New York: Basic Books, Inc., 1964.

Cook, J. J.: "Dimensional Analysis of Child-rearing Attitudes of Parents of Handicapped Children," *American Journal of Mental Deficiency,* **68**:354-361, 1963.

Cummings, S. T., and D. Stock: "Brief Group Therapy of Mothers of Retarded Children outside of the Specialty Clinic Setting," *American Journal of Mental Deficiency,* **66**:739-748, 1962.

Dager, E. Z.: "Socialization and Personality Development in the Child," in H. T. Christensen (ed.), *Handbook of Marriage and the Family,* Chicago: Rand McNally and Company, 1964.

Dalton, J., and H. Epstein: "Counseling Parents of Mildly Retarded Children," *Social Casework,* **44**:523-530, 1963.

Denhoff, E.: "The Impact of Parents on the Growth of Exceptional Children," *Exceptional Children,* **26**:271-274, 1960.

Downey, K. J.: "Parental Interest in the Institutionalized, Severely Mentally Retarded Child," *Social Problems,* **11**:186-193, 1963.

Ehlers, W. H.: *Mothers of Retarded Children,* Springfield, Ill.: Charles C Thomas, Publisher, 1966.

Farber, B.: "Effects of a Severely Mentally Retarded Child on Family Integration," *Monographs of the Society for Research in Child Development,* vol. 24, no. 2, serial no. 71, 1959.

————: "Family Organization and Crisis: Maintenance of Integration in Families with a Severely Mentally Retarded Child," *Monographs of the Society for Research in Child Development,* vol. 25, no. 1, serial no. 75, 1960a.

————: *Family Organization and Interaction,* San Francisco: Chandler Publishing Company, 1964.

————: "Perceptions of Crisis and Related Variables in the Impact of a Retarded Child on the Mother," *Journal of Health and Human Behavior,* **1**:108-118, 1960b.

————, W. C. Jenne, and R. Toigo: "Family Crisis and the Decision to Institutionalize the Retarded Child," *Council for Exceptional Children, NEA Research Monograph Series,* series A, no. 1, 1960.

Fowle, C. M.: "The Effect of the Severely Mentally Retarded Child on His Family," *American Journal of Mental Deficiency,* **73**:468-473, 1968.

Freidson, E.: "Specialties without Roots: The Utilization of New Services," *Human Organization,* **18**:112-116, 1959.

Giannini, M. J., and L. Goodman: "Counseling Families during the Crisis Reaction to Mongolism," *American Journal of Mental Deficiency,* **67**:740-747, 1963.

Graliker, B. V., K. Fishler, and R. Koch: "Teenage Reaction to a Mentally Retarded Sibling," *American Journal of Mental Deficiency,* **66**:838–843, 1962.

———, R. Koch, and R. A. Henderson: "The Study of Factors Influencing Placement of Retarded Children in a State Residential Institution," *American Journal of Mental Deficiency,* **69**:553–559, 1965.

Hall, W. T.: "Family Disorganization as Associated with Severity of Handicap (by Cerebral Palsy) of a Minor Child," unpublished doctoral dissertation, Minneapolis: University of Minnesota, 1961.

Hersh, A.: "Case Work with Parents of Retarded Children," *Social Work,* **6**:61–66, 1961.

———: "Changes in Family Functioning Following Placement of a Retarded Child," *Social Casework,* **15**:93–102, 1970.

Hill, R.: "Generic Features of Families under Stress," in H. J. Parad (ed.), *Crisis Intervention: Selected Readings,* New York: Family Service Association of America, 1965.

Hutchison, A.: "Stress on Families of the Mentally Handicapped," *Stress on Families of the Mentally Handicapped,* Belgium: International League of Societies for the Mentally Handicapped, 1967.

Kramm, E. R.: *Families of Mongoloid Children,* Washington, D.C.: U.S. Government Printing Office, 1963.

Logan, H.: "My Child Is Mentally Retarded," *Nursing Outlook,* **10**:445–448, 1962.

Mandelbaum, A., and M. E. Wheeler: "The Meaning of a Defective Child to Parents," *Social Casework,* **41**:360–367, 1960.

Matheny, A. P., Jr., and J. Vernick: "Parents of the Mentally Retarded Child: Emotionally Overwhelmed or Informationally Deprived?" *The Journal of Pediatrics,* **74**:953–959, 1969.

Michaels, J., and H. Schucman: "Observations on the Psychodynamics of Parents of Retarded Children," *American Journal of Mental Deficiency,* **66**:568–573, 1962.

Miller, L. G.: "The Seven Stages in the Life Cycle of a Family with a Mentally Retarded Child," State of Washington Department of Institutions, Division of Research, Research Report, vol. 2, no. 2, 1969.

Morgan, I. M.: "Untie the Apron Strings," *Cerebral Palsy Journal,* **28**:10–11, 1967.

Murray, M. A.: *Needs of Parents of Mentally Retarded Children,* Arlington, Tex.: National Association for Retarded Children, 1969.

Noble, M. A.: "Nursing's Concern for the Mentally Retarded Is Overdue," *Nursing Forum,* **9**:192–201, 1970.

Oberman, J. W.: "The Physician and Parents of the Retarded Child," *Children,* **10**:109–113, 1963.

Olshansky, S.: "Chronic Sorrow: A Response to Having a Mentally Defective Child," *Social Casework,* **43**:190–193, 1962.

Parad, H. J., and G. Caplan: "A Framework for Studying Families in Crisis," in H. J. Parad (ed.), *Crisis Intervention: Selected Readings,* New York: Family Service Association of America, 1965.

Perlman, H. H.: "Social Diagnosis Leading to Social Treatment," *Social Work in*

Child Health Projects for Mentally Retarded Children: Selected Papers, District of Columbia, Department of Public Health, 1963.

Quast, W.: "The Role of Interpretive Parent Interview in Diagnoses of Children," in J. L. Khanna, (ed.), *Brain Damage and Mental Retardation: A Psychological Evaluation,* Springfield, Ill.: Charles C Thomas, 1968.

Roos, P.: "Psychological Counseling with Parents of Retarded Children," *Mental Retardation,* **1**:345–350, 1963.

Saenger, G.: *Factors Influencing the Institutionalization of Mentally Retarded Individuals in New York City,* New York: New York State Interdepartmental Resources Board, 1960.

Schild, S.: "Counseling Services," in R. Koch and J. C. Dobson (eds.), *The Mentally Retarded Child and His Family,* New York: Brunner/Mazel, Publishers, 1971.

Standifer, F. R.: "Pilot Parent Program: Parents Helping Parents," *Mental Retardation,* **2**:304–307, 1964.

Tizard, J., and J. C. Grad: *The Mentally Handicapped and Their Families,* New York: Oxford University Press, 1961.

Wolfensberger, W.: "Counseling the Parents of the Retarded," in A. A. Baumeister (ed.), *Mental Retardation Appraisal, Education and Rehabilitation,* Chicago: Aldine Publishing, 1967.

Wortis, J.: "Successful Family Life for the Retarded Child," *Stress on Families of the Mentally Handicapped,* Belgium: International League of Societies for the Mentally Handicapped, 1967.

Yates, M. L., and R. Lederer: "Small, Short-term Group Meetings with Parents of Children with Mongolism," *American Journal of Mental Deficiency,* **65**:467–472, 1961.

Zelle, R.: "A Study to Determine the Need for a Conceptual Guide to Assess the Effect of a Retarded Child on Family Relations and Life," unpublished master's thesis, Seattle, Wash.: University of Washington, 1969.

Zuk, G. H., et al.: "Maternal Acceptance of Retarded Children: A Questionnaire Study of Attitudes and Religious Background," *Child Development,* **32**:525–540, 1961.

Chapter 30

Suicide as a
Family Nursing
Problem
Martha L. Mitchell

"Are suicidal behaviors apt to present themselves to me as a nurse in the context of my practice?" Assume that this deserving question evokes affirmative responses from an overwhelming percentage of nurses in virtually all areas of nursing practice. Assume too that the number and distribution of nurses answering yes not only reflect the magnitude of the suicide problem in our society, but also mirror its appearance within our health care institutions. These tentative yet potentially realistic assumptions suggest another important inquiry which is central to this chapter: What significance does the individual nurse's awareness of threatened, attempted, or committed suicide hold for his ability to render family-centered nursing care?

Most nurses recognize that the distance is great indeed between the mere acknowledgment that "yes, the suicide problem does crop up in my practice" and the ability to give skilled nursing care, once aware of the problem. When this distance is measured in terms of the nurse's objective of family-centered nursing care, a major factor is the way the nurse conceptualizes the problem of intentional self-destructive acts. Suicide, to a unique degree among health-illness problems, evokes characteristic subjective responses which tend to force attention onto the suicidal act and actor. Thus, in dealing with suicide, the overwhelming tendency is to turn toward the singular, discrete, and concrete aspects of the problem and away from its more abstract and complex relationship aspects. Because of these tendencies, the issue of the nurse's conceptual framework becomes especially important in order that the family perspective not become totally lost in the anxious shuffle of "saving the suicidal actor from himself."

One major purpose of this chapter is to examine some factors which pose difficulties for the nurse who attempts to relate the immediate problem of self-destructive behavior to the larger context of family-centered nursing. A second major purpose is to evaluate the need for a conceptual framework which integrates the threefold elements of suicide, family, and the nurse's role. The first and second sections of the present chapter correspond to these two major purposes. The third and final portion suggests one theoretical frame of reference, that of interpersonal communications, to illustrate its application to the problem of suicide. Through its fundamental appeal to the inevitability of communication in human relationships, communication theory provides a particularly useful means for understanding and responding to suicide as a family nursing problem. It will be seen that this theory suggests that neither self-destructive acts nor others' responses to this problem can be adequately understood without considering the communicational context in which they occur. Ultimately the discussion proceeds toward the conclusion that skilled nursing care relating to suicide necessarily focuses on the matrix of interpersonal relationships surrounding the patient, the most salient of which is frequently the actor's family.

FACTORS AFFECTING RESPONSES TO SUICIDE

The contemporary literature on the subject of suicide has proliferated rapidly, this topic having become fair game for theorizing, investigations, and speculations among a wide range of fields that do not ordinarily share common concerns. Closer scrutiny of the suicide literature discloses that a continuum of self-destructiveness has been proposed as conceptually valid. Thus suicide, when defined in the conventional sense of death directly resulting from a victim's intentional act of self-destruction, is said to belong to the same class of events as threatened suicide, attempted but unsuccessful suicide, and other diverse forms of self-destruction. The latter group, for example, refers to those persons who die or suffer from excessive intake of alcohol or other toxic agents, to the "accident prone," and to the patient with serious chronic illness who blatantly and repeatedly defies the rules of his regimen.

The overwhelming emphasis among the different scholars of self-destruction is on explaining suicide. That is, the overriding concern is the question, *Why?* What are the causes? What motivates persons to act in a way that will obviously bring about premature death? In contrast to this concern, less attention has been directed to prevention, and far less still to the whole area of others' perceptions of and reactions to self-destructive behavior.

To explain adequately the direction which scholarly interest in suicide has and has not taken is difficult. From a pragmatic standpoint, the prevailing preoccupation with "solving" suicide carries with it at least an implicit assumption that elucidation of causes will ultimately permit preventive control over this social problem. However, the comparatively small effort made to identify patterns of interpersonal response to suicidal behaviors deserves particular notice, especially by nurses. Greater insight into characteristic reactions evoked by suicide can illuminate some crucial elements of suicide itself. It can also assist the nurse to understand ways in which personal reactions to self-destruction interfere with motivation to maintain a family nursing perspective. There are two factors in particular which influence the nurse's responses and require understanding: first, the nurse's social and professional values; and second, the issue of the nurse's therapeutic responsibility for suicide.

Values

At the level of societies in general, evaluations of suicide have covered the spectrum, from best to worst; and in no period, including our own, has there been unanimity in such evaluations (Diggory, 1968, p. 3). The preponderant view of suicide in Western cultures has been that it is wrong, or at least undesirable. Analysis of the particular reasons expressed for condemning suicide are especially revealing of the fact that social evaluations of this act are very bound up with larger prevailing values and beliefs about man's nature, about the purpose or ends of life, and about man's relationship with his fellow man. Examples of different value judgment statements illustrating this point are: (1) "Self-murder is a sin." (2) "Suicide evades a social responsibility (to the state, the family, etc.)." (3) "The suicide is a quitter and a cop-out." A fourth example of a stigmatizing value judgment substitutes the conclusion of "madness" for "badness." The significant shift here is that malevolent motives are, in effect, canceled by appeal to the insanity hypothesis. Thus, some persons say unequivocally that the suicidal act is overdetermined by unconscious and uncontrollable motives, wishes, or desires. Other persons put essentially the same judgment in more everyday language. As one observer noted: "In England, you must not commit suicide on the pain of being regarded a criminal if you fail and a lunatic if you succeed, (and) the same can be said of reactions to suicide in many sectors of this country" (Rome, 1965, p. 32).

Society's members, including its health professionals, typically pass value judgments on persons whose acts violate its standards of normalcy or decency. This realization has its manifestation in the mandate so frequently encountered that "the nurse should be nonjudgmental toward patients." Perhaps more realistic counsel would take into account the now well-known fallacy of absolute scientific neutrality and recommend instead that the nurse make a conscious effort to identify and allow for those values which preform judgments. In this regard, then, it is especially noteworthy that society's evaluation of suicide typically stresses that causative factors reside *within* the individual—sinfulness, insanity, moral weakness, and the like. An unintended consequence of these individual, idiosyncratic explanations has been to de-emphasize the environmental, interpersonal conditions which generate or reinforce self-destructive acts. The nurse's objectivity about his own tendency to share in the larger society's overriding views of suicide is a helpful precursor to taking a family perspective in relation to nursing care.

Secondly, the suicidal actor's behavior challenges that whole constellation of values cultivated during the professional nursing socialization process which extol the nurse's commitment to preserving and enhancing life. During basic nursing education, the nurse develops the self-expectation that he will labor even to heroic lengths to save life, promote health, and prevent illness and injury. Life is valued highly as well as his own personal efforts to enhance and protect it. An understandable conflict can thus arise when the nurse is face-to-face with a person who has explicitly communicated his wish to die by his own hand. On the surface of things is the tricky incongruity of working to save the life of one who is willfully determined to end it. Or, to phrase the nurse's personal dilemma in another way: How can I be helpful to a person whose action says that he wants to die?

The foregoing question may or may not be a conscious thought to the nurse. Nonetheless it is often operating and deserves special commentary. On the one hand, the question maximizes the lethal intent aspect of the attempter's behavior and minimizes the marked feelings of ambivalence toward life and death which typically characterize the actor. On the other hand, the question implies a definition of both persons, nurse and patient, which emphasizes the difference between them. The implied definition is based, in part, on the fact that the nurse perceives that an important aspect of self (i.e., the wish to see oneself and to be seen as a helpful person) is being threatened by the patient. The suicidal behavior represents and symbolizes this threat to his professional self-image and predictably centers attention on the act. When this happens, the nurse experiences less obvious need to identify how many feelings he may share in common with the patient and his family. Paradoxically, it is oftentimes less threatening to focus almost exclusively on the suicidal act than to take into account and relate to other behaviors of the patient and family which communicate their feelings of helplessness and despair. For example, the actor's depression or his avoidance of interactions with the staff, the family members' expressions of guilt or indifference to the actor—these may also threaten the nurse's own feelings but be more difficult to deal with than the life-threatening act itself.

In suicide, then, it is the self-destructive *act* which is viewed as the double-edged threat. Practically speaking, it jeopardizes the actor's life or well-being; symbolically, it threatens the nurse's highly valued image of himself as helpful. The combination provides ample reason for anxiety and, consequently, for the issue of control over the act to become the immediate, pressing concern of the health team. There are two common manifestations of this excessive preoccupation with control which are contradictory on their surfaces, yet each shares anxiety as its common source. The first is the counterphobic attitude in which the potential helper rationalizes the necessity to place complete and final responsibility for all acts on the actor (Yochelson, 1965, p. 3). An example of the form this attitude assumes is the carte blanche statement: "Well, if a person wants to kill himself, that's his business. . . . You can't stop him anyway." The second manifestation goes to the opposite extreme and consists of a whole battery of ritualistic observational checks, "sharp searches," and the like. The latter routines are oftentimes indiscriminately, automatically implemented by nurses with the manifest aim of saving the actor from killing himself. One can legitimately question whether these rituals derive from the patient's and family's needs. Or do they primarily serve the latent function of allaying the nurse's anxiety over what else, if anything, he can do that will prove helpful? So much energy can be expended in the rigid execution of these controls that there is little left for understanding the communicational effects of these behaviors on the actor and his family. Indeed, one might speculate whether nurses' absorption with the issue of control over the act and actor is in inverse proportion to their planning family-centered nursing care.

The Issue of Therapeutic Responsibility

Practices and attitudes prevailing within the health care system in relation to suicide powerfully influence the nurse's perceptions and the ways he defines his nursing role when relating to the problem. The specific, observable patterns of behavioral responses to suicide which operate in any one setting are an outgrowth of many complex, interrelated variables. In all instances, these behavioral practices provide an immediate context of informational clues telling the nurse how he is expected to view his therapeutic relationship with the suicidal actor and his family. In the experience of the writer, there is a marked disinclination on the part of nurses, especially in nonpsychiatric areas of nursing practice, to relate in any direct or systematic fashion to the actor and his family around the issue of self-destruction. An important source of these avoidance tendencies can be located in the institutional practices which surround the nurse. Certainly, nurses working in psychiatric settings are not immune to their own avoidance maneuvers when dealing with suicide. But a significant difference in role expectations operates on psychiatric services, due in large part to the fact that suicidal risk is often the explicit reason for hospitalization and a formalized aspect of the treatment program.

There are two conflicting sets of expectations which foster an ambiguous picture of the nurse's therapeutic responsibility in suicide. The first set conveys a positive expectation and stems fundamentally from the nurse's knowledge that suicide *is* regarded as a health problem in this country. The literature variously describes suicide as a public health problem, as a mental health problem, and as one which is the rightful responsibility of health professionals of all kinds. Nurses basically know this well. Implicitly the nurse is also aware that suicide is much more complicated than either physical or mental health. It is a universal, uniquely human problem having many parameters. As Porterfield puts it: "The problem of suicide is octagonal. Its angles are: (1) semantic, (2) statistical, (3) historical, (4) religious, (5) philosophical, (6) psychological, (7) sociological, and (8) action-related" (1968, p. 31). The long-standing debate about whether a person has the right to kill himself or has the obligation to continue with the business of living obscures the obvious: some 22,000 persons are known to intentionally kill themselves each year in this country. A majority of these victims met the customary standards of normalcy before their demise. And there remain, of course, the families of these victims, together with the countless others who agonize over the same decision of whether to kill themselves as the expression of their ambivalence about continuing with the pain of living.

As seemingly obvious as the first positive expectation level may be, a second set of expectations simultaneously operates which offsets the first and throws the nurse's appropriate therapeutic responsibility into a more negative light. Even though the nurse is cognizant that therapeutic intervention in suicide is not identical with the performance of those physical care activities required for the bodily harm the actor may have inflicted on himself, he often experiences little support for initiating the more abstract therapeutic functions. Powerful incentives or restraints for assuming psychotherapeutic role activities are part and parcel of the reward system which surrounds the nurse's employment. The system of rewards most commonly prevailing within our health care institutions favors technical and instrumental nursing functions, efficiency in role performance, and physical care activities. If the nurse intends to expand his therapeutic responsibilities beyond these valued behaviors, it is important that he identify messages from peers, the nursing supervisor, or the physician which may distinctly warn him to avoid getting involved with the patient and his family.

A common practice which may subtly but negatively effect the nurse's sense of therapeutic responsibility derives from the expectation that the psychiatrist will be summoned for consultation or treatment. There are realistic and sound reasons behind this recommended practice of referral. The involvement of the psychiatrist may evoke a wide range of attitudes among nurses. Where a predisposition to avoid the suicide issue already exists, the referral practice may reinforce the nurse's avoidance and foster a "hands off" impression. Frequently underlying this "hands off" stance is the false assumption that if the nurse wishes to avoid interference with the psychiatrist's work, he should also avoid the suicidal actor's and family's problems.

Some major factors which affect the nurse's responses can be summarized as follows. The nurse has a learned self-expectation to make a therapeutic contribution when relating to the suicidal actor and his family. He also recognizes that appropriate nursing responses transcend the physical safety of the actor, or even the actor himself. However, prevailing social and professional values, as well as institutional practices, commonly militate against a family nursing perspective. Rather they favor interventions which center on the immediate, concrete task of controlling the act and actor. It seems obvious, therefore, that if the nurse strives for a more holistic, family-centered approach to the problem, it will be no mere accident. Understanding factors internal and external to himself which act as barriers to a family-centered response to suicide is one important step. A second pivotal task in integrating suicide within the framework of family-centered nursing rests in identifying the theoretical perspective which the nurse employs.

THEORIES OF SUICIDE IN RELATION TO FAMILY-CENTERED NURSING

The nurse who is motivated to gear nursing care to the whole family's needs is simultaneously attempting to reconcile three variables: (1) suicide which is an individual act, (2) the family which is a social system, and (3) nursing care. This point warrants explicit recognition when one turns to the dominant theories of suicide. While these theories can facilitate understanding of the first variable, they do not obviously or easily extend understanding of the other two.

There are two dominant but contending theoretical explanations of suicidal phenomena which appear in the literature. The first is the psychological approach, the prototype of which is the psychoanalytic theory of suicide. This perspective concentrates on internal, individual motives and psychodynamics in order to explain self-destructive behaviors. The second major approach is the sociological, which is concerned with forces in society which cause the individual to commit suicide. These dual approaches will be briefly reviewed to illustrate their implications for family-oriented nursing care.

The most enduring, pervasive psychological theory of suicide is the psychoanalytic, originally advanced by Sigmund Freud and later elaborated and refined by Karl Menninger. The classical psychoanalytic formulation of suicide stemmed from Freud's theory of depression and, later on, his postulation of a death instinct. In short, the psychoanalytic theory says that depression can be understood as aggression turned inward on the self, rather than externally directed. By the same token, suicide is hostility directed inward toward the introjected love object. Shneidman has aptly summarized this explanation of suicide as "murder in the 180th degree" (1970, p. 7). Throughout the psychoanalytic approach, ambivalent feelings of love and hate, the wish to kill and be killed, figure heavily as explanatory factors. External events in the patient's current life situation are viewed as mere precipitants of depression and suicide but are not completely ignored.

Use of the psychoanalytic theory to achieve understanding of an individual case of suicide entails a retrospective, longitudinal analysis aimed at elucidation of the internal, unconscious, dynamic forces which determined the act. Practically speaking, nurses often experience difficulty in employing and relating the highly abstract concepts of psychoanalysis to their work. Moreover, it can be seen from the foregoing comments that the psychological view of the suicidal individual is essentially a monadic one. That is, the unit of concern is the individual patient. The monadic view leaves little room to study either the effects of the actor's behavior on other persons (e.g., on his spouse) or the series of interactions which formed the context for the occurrence of the act (Watzlawick, 1967, p. 21). Recognition of this almost exclusive concern with the individual actor's state of mind is very salient for the nurse who seeks to conceptualize care in terms of a family system.

The sociological study of suicide became established at the turn of this century by Durkheim's (1951) famous work, Le Suicide. Most of the ensuing research investigations into the sociology of suicide bear the stamp of his model. Characteristically, these studies aim at generalizations about the ways suicide rates depend upon and reflect certain conditions in a society. For example, Durkheim postulated three types of suicide (egoistic, altruistic, and anomic) and said these would be predictably related to (1) a given society's regulation of its members' aspirations, and/or (2) whether persons were excessively or weakly integrated within their social group.

The sociological approach has been criticized on some of the following counts. On the negative side, some critics observe that the theory is not sufficient to explain many actual cases of suicide, such as those stemming from idiosyncratic, personal motives or those which are responses to unique cultural situations of interpersonal disharmony (De Vos, 1968, p. 112). Second, it has been said that the theory inadequately differentiates between social conditions which favor successful as opposed to attempted suicide (Shneidman and Farberow, 1970, p. 200). On the positive side, the sociological approach has demonstrated that certain factors are highly and consistently correlated with suicide, such as: physical illness; mental illness; excessive drinking; unemployment; broken homes; and more general factors of race, age, and sex. Knowledge of these and other statistical correlates is of great value to the nurse in predicting high-risk suicidal situations.

That the sociological approach has generated these useful, predictive data brings out another characteristic of the theory which warrants final commentary. Namely, this theory focuses upon the questions of what environmental, social factors "produce" suicide and how to predict its occurrence. The theory is therefore concerned with suicide as an outcome. It does not attempt to study the converse question: What effects or what outcomes does suicide bring about in the social environment? The latter question has more than just theoretical merit. Clinicians dealing with suicidal patients and families have long been aware that not only are marked social responses to self-destructive acts predictable, but the actor's anticipation of these responses also comprises an important part of his suicidal motive. In other words, these recurrent clinical findings suggest the need to conceptualize suicide as more than a terminal outcome, even if the act proves fatal. A framework is needed for placing suicide within the actor's here-and-now relationships with significant others.

In an evaluation of both the sociological and the psychoanalytic approaches and combinations of these two, Gibbs comments: "Indeed, the theories are so diverse that they share only one thing in common—none of them provide truly adequate explanations of suicide" (1968, p. 29). Meanwhile the quest for a general theory of the cause(s) of suicide goes on. As it does, the nurse may very profitably use the insights contained in the sociological and intrapsychic approaches, also recognizing that neither theory expressly attempts to understand individual self-destruction in terms of the actor's present interactions with his family. Indeed, the very effort within both approaches to identify the possible or hypothetical *causes* of suicide is a central issue in relation to the nurse's objective of conceptualizing and relating to the family as a system of closely related persons. Theories which postulate cause-effect relationships tend to be unidirectional and linear in nature, rather than analyzing phenomena as circular and interdependent behavioral events (Watzlawick, 1967, p. 31). The very notion of a social system (e.g., the family) involves a different conceptual model than a cause-and-effect one; it studies the reciprocal effects of behaviors upon the persons who interact and comprise the system. These points again raise the need for a conceptual framework which supports the nurse's ability to locate self-destructive acts and therapeutic interventions within the broader context of human communication.

A COMMUNICATIONAL APPROACH

In the terms of communication theory, the family is a closed information system in which variations in a member's behaviors are fed back into the family system in order to correct the system's response (Jackson, 1957, p. 80). Implicitly contained within the latter conception is the principle that any individual's behavior invariably carries some information (feedback) to the other(s) with whom he interacts about their relationships with one another. The word *communication* is used synonymously with behavior. Thus, behavior of all kinds inevitably carries some message(s) to the participants in the interactional system, whether the form of the communication be verbal, nonverbal, symptoms, silences, or self-destructive actions. The sender of a message (such as the suicide attempt) may or may not achieve the effect (feedback) he desires in the receiver, but some effect is unavoidable. Each person in a relationship cannot *not* communicate and the meanings each attributes to their respective communications depend upon and in some way effect their relationship with one another (Watzlawick, 1967, p. 51).

Satir (1970-1971, p. 245) describes the systems and communication approach to therapy in this way:

> [It] treats the apparent dysfunctional behavior in any one individual as the inevitable outcome of the kind of system and the means and style of communication currently operating in the family. Therefore, the system and the communication are seen as affecting all members with one person showing the evidence, as in the iceberg, or another way of putting it, by becoming the target or the scapegoat of that family system. The healing or the change in this instance comes about through changing the family communication and the system that supports it.

What implications do these theoretical points have for the nursing care of families with a suicidal member? The answer involves two aspects. First, the nurse understands and views suicide as one symptomatic act, information-bearing in nature, within the interpersonal system of the family. Dramatic and life-threatening though the suicidal act may be and/or overtly disturbed though the suicidal actor may appear upon observation, the nurse's focus shifts away from exclusive attention on the individual actor's behavior and onto the context in which the act occurs. That is, the unit of study becomes the patterns of family interaction which precede and follow the self-destructive behavior. The underlying assumption is that a self-destructive action is a manifestation of a family problem which has reached crisis proportions.

Second, the nurse understands his own therapeutic potential in interacting with one, several, or all members of the family in a new light. This new view is based on the fundamental premise that his own behavior always communicates. Whether or not he intends any message to occur at all, the nurse inevitably communicates whether the problem is viewed exclusively as an individual one or as a manifestation of a breakdown in family relationships. How the problem is viewed will, of course, influence what nursing responses are forthcoming. Thus, the nurse's behaviors "show" the family from the outset how the nursing problem is being viewed and how the nurse views his ability to be helpful to them. The nurse's behavioral inputs will in some measure influence the family's relationships with one another.

One could legitimately argue that these dual implications also pertain for a wide range of health-illness problems which confront the nurse. That this contention is a valid one rests in the fact that the potential for applying communication theory to family nursing problems extends far beyond the problem of suicide. It therefore seems relevant to examine further the special communicational value of suicide. The issue at hand may be condensed into a single question: If one views a suicidal act to be a dramatic form of feedback within a system which as a whole is functioning badly, does it make any special difference that the content of the actor's message is self-destruction?

The foregoing question suggests that all the various types of self-destructive behavior share a similar element, even though there are different degrees of lethal intent associated with threatened, attempted, or committed suicide. The element common to all is that the actor communicates his willingness to risk severance of his interpersonal relationships through death. One plausible interpretation of suicide is that the suicidal person has perceived within his life situation that his relationships with other persons have deteriorated or will change in ways that are intolerable to him (Gibbs, 1968, p. 17). The potentially suicidal individual thus is defined and defines himself in such a way that his own self-destruction becomes, *for him,* a logical alternative. Inherently contained in every suicidal threat or attempt is the potential for a fatal termination of relationships; when the actor succeeds, the severance of relationship becomes total and complete. As seemingly obvious as this point may be, it points up the crux of suicidal behaviors; that is, the content and relationship aspects of suicide are virtually inseparable.

Precisely because of the profoundly communicative nature of suicide, it becomes crucial to consider the *effects* which the suicidal behavior has on others. In other words, what changes in the actor's relationships ensue? The wish to evoke specific responses may not always be consciously intended by him, but some effect is inevitable. Even a silence or lack of response by the significant others in the actor's life communicates. Indeed, can there be a more stinging rejoinder to a suicidal attempt than no response at all?

Several studies are revealing of families' responses. Robins et al. (1959, p. 733) report that of 134 consecutive suicides, over two-thirds (69 percent) had communicated suicidal ideas to family, close associates, and helping persons such as ministers and physicians; 41 percent had specifically stated the intent to commit suicide. In the majority of instances, the suicidal communications were of recent onset (months), repeatedly verbalized, and expressed to many persons. Persons close to the suicidal victims seemed unable to know how or even whether or not to respond to the suicidal communications, a finding which was interpreted by the authors in terms of fear arousal. Kobler and Stotland's (1969, p. 268) study examines the question of whether the nature of the social response to suicide attempts increases the likelihood that suicide will eventually occur. Their findings clearly affirm both the question and their contention that "if the response to the plea [for help] is hopeless and helpless, suicide is more likely to occur.... An implicit or explicit fear or expectation of suicide is most often communicated by a hopeless, helpless response, and this communication is important in facilitating suicide" (Kobler and Stotland, 1969, p. 264).

Stengel (1969, p. 77) describes the effect of suicidal acts on persons close to the actor-victim. In fatal outcomes, the effects are in common with bereavement but more intense than typical grief reactions. There is an upsurge of posthumous love associated with guilt feelings and self-reproach for not having cared and loved enough. Nonfatal acts usually call forth more complex yet helpful responses which transform the individual's life situation, if only temporarily. Stengel summarizes the matter of communication in suicide this way:

> It is important therefore in every suicidal attempt to ask what change it has achieved. That is why a purely intrapsychic appraisal is not enough. It ignores the communicative function of the suicidal act. If it is fatal, it is a final message; if it is not fatal, it is part of a dialogue. And you cannot understand a dialogue if you take notice of one participant only (Stengel, 1969, p. 79).

Reports of the predictable problems confronting families during suicidal crises are rarely found within the literature, and usually the family's problems are only alluded to in a hintful fashion. By the same token, there is a virtual omission of family-oriented practices within the health care institutions which come into contact with these families. To cite one glaring example: What nonpsychiatric or psychiatric facility regularly holds a conference for the whole family after a suicidal episode to help the family deal with the strong feelings and confusions that suicide generates? There is good reason to believe that helpful, caring responses by those close to the suicidal person constitute crucial feedback to the desperate attempter after his act, serving as a deterrent to a future repetition. Mobilizing the family's helpful responses before or after a suicidal crisis is a need to which nurses could readily address themselves, for the benefit of the whole family unit.

The paucity of family data and family-centered care practices in relation to suicide reflects one important premise underlying this chapter: Potent forces operate in favor of suicide being studied and related to as an individual problem, not as a family one. The Nurse's awareness and understanding of these individual-oriented forces is believed important to his ability to provide family nursing care in suicide. With some therapeutic initiative, there is a wide open opportunity for nurses to expand customary suicidal health care practices to include the family dimension. Through direct interactions with families and through systematic observation of and gathering data about the problems which families encounter, nurses can make an immediate contribution to this virtually ignored *family* health problem area.

BIBLIOGRAPHY

Bosselman, B. C.: *Self-destruction: A Study of the Suicidal Impulse,* Springfield, Ill.: Charles C Thomas, 1970.

De Vos, G. A.: "Suicide in Cross-cultural Perspective," in H. L. P. Resnik (ed.), *Suicidal Behaviors: Diagnosis and Management,* Boston: Little, Brown and Company, 1968.

Diggory, J. C.: "Suicide and Value," in H. L. P. Resnik (ed.), *Suicidal Behaviors: Diagnosis and Management,* Boston: Little, Brown and Company, 1968.

Dublin, L. I.: *Suicide: A Sociological and Statistical Study,* New York: Ronald Press, 1963.

Durkheim, E.: *Suicide,* trans. by J. A. Spaulding and G. Simpson, Glencoe: The Free Press, 1951.

Freud, S.: "Mourning and Melancholia (1917)," *Collected Papers,* **4**:152-170, London: Hogarth Press, 1949.

Gibbs, J. P. (ed.): *Suicide,* New York: Harper & Row, 1968.

Hendin, H.: *Suicide and Scandanavia,* New York: Grune & Stratton, 1964.

Jackson, D. D.: "The Question of Family Homeostasis," *Psychiatric Quarterly Supplement,* **31**, Part 1:79-90, 1957.

Kobler, A. L., and E. Stotland: "Suicide Attempts and the Social Response," in W. A. Rushing (ed.), *Deviant Behavior and Social Process,* Chicago: Rand McNally, 1969.

Menninger, K. A.: *Man against Himself,* New York: Harcourt, Brace, 1938.

Porterfield, A. L.: "The Problem of Suicide," in J. P. Gibbs (ed.), *Suicide,* New York: Harper & Row, 1968.

Robins, E., et al.: "The Communication of Suicidal Intent: A Study of 134 Consecutive Cases of Successful (Completed) Suicide," *American Journal of Psychiatry,* **115**:724-733, 1959.

Rome, H. P.: "Changing Attitudes toward Suicide," in L. Yochelson (ed.), *Symposium on Suicide,* Washington: The George Washington University School of Medicine, 1965.

Satir, V. M.: "A Humanistic Approach," *International Journal of Psychiatry,* **9**:245-246, 1970-1971.

Shneidman, E. S.: "Orientations toward Death: A Vital Aspect of the Study of Lives," in E. S. Shneidman, N. L. Farberow, and R. L. Litman, *The Psychology of Suicide,* New York: Science House, 1970.

——— and N. L. Farberow: "Attempted and Committed Suicides," in E. S. Shneidman, N. L. Farberow, and R. L. Litman, *The Psychology of Suicide,* New York: Science House, 1970.

——— and ——— (eds.): *Clues to Suicide,* New York: McGraw-Hill Book Company, 1957.

Stengel, E.: "A Matter of Communication," in E. S. Shneidman (ed.), *The Nature of Suicide,* San Francisco: Jossey-Bass, 1969.

——— and N. G. Cook: *Attempted Suicide: Its Social Significance and Effects,* London: Chapman-Hall, 1958.

Watzlawick, P., J. H. Beavin, and D. D. Jackson: *Pragmatics of Human Communication,* New York: W. W. Norton, 1967.

Wolff, K. (ed.): *Patterns of Self-Destruction: Depression and Suicide,* Springfield, Ill.: Charles C Thomas, Publishers, 1970.

Yochelson, L. (ed.): *Symposium on Suicide,* Washington, D.C.: The George Washington University School of Medicine, 1965.

Chapter 31

The Family with a Terminally Ill Child

Jo-Eileen Gyulay and Margaret Shandor Miles

One of the greatest crises any family can experience is that of having a child diagnosed with a terminal illness. The child is an integral part of his family; thus the threat of losing him through death, creates stress on the entire family. Their response to him and his illness affects the way he copes with his disease. Strengthening the ability of his parents and entire family to handle the crisis is an important focus of any team caring for the terminally ill child. Nurses, members of the team, are in a unique position to help the child and his family as they face the many stresses involved.

In the past, the time between the diagnosis and actual death of the child was a short, stormy period, and most of the nursing and medical care focused on the acute needs of the hospitalized child. Gradually, the parents, particularly mothers, were included in the care plans. Nurses knew the child only as a very sick patient in the hospital. If he did go home, in a remission, the nursing staff did not see him or his family again until he was readmitted in another acute state.

Today, however, the medical care of children with such formerly fatal diseases as leukemia, tumors, and Hodgkins disease has changed drastically. New drugs and other modes of therapy have considerably altered the prognosis until they can now be considered chronic diseases which may eventually be fatal. Much of the care is given on an outpatient basis so that he can stay in his home and live as normal a life as possible. Admissions to the hospital during acute exacerbations or complications may be many months or years apart, particularly during the early course of the illness.

This change in the course and treatment of such terminal diseases in children requires a change in the nursing role and focus. Nurses must begin to expand their role from that of giving acute episodic care to that of giving care that focuses on the child and family throughout the course of his illness, in whatever setting he is found: clinic, school, community, or family. The nursing process should begin at the time of diagnosis and extend until weeks or months after the child's death. Continuity of care by the same nurse may be possible in some settings, but it is also important that nurses from a variety of settings begin to work together as a team providing care, sharing experiences and observations, and planning together.

Since the children are seen most frequently in the outpatient setting, the role of the nurse in this setting is vital. They must begin to establish themselves as members of the hematology/oncology team who see the patient at each visit. Their role in assessing, counseling, and teaching families can be invaluable to them. The clinic nurse can also be the key person to establish communication with community and hospital nurses, since he may be closest to the medical team caring for the child. Ideally, this role should be flexible enough to allow opportunities to visit the child and family when they are admitted to the hospital and to discuss their needs with the hospital nurses. They also need time to make home and school visits, to make phone calls, and to write letters to the family and community nurses who are involved in the care.

School and community nurses can be important assets in helping the family when they return to their community as they face the many adjustments the disease will bring. These nurses can also assess the response of the community to the child's illness. Ironically, in a large city, the family may be isolated and given no support from the community. In a small town, the entire community is affected and usually wants to help. However, they may need guidance in understanding the illness and in giving appropriate help. The school community (pupils and teachers) will also need guidance in understanding the illness and knowing how they can help the child when he returns to school. Some crises he will face will include: long absences, being different (loss of hair, weight gain or loss, and bruising), fatigue, and having other children tell him that he's going to die. Working with the community should only be done with and through the parents, not without their consent and assistance.

Hospital nurses must learn more about understanding and helping a family in acute crisis, since most admissions are for an acute exacerbation or the terminal phase. They must increase their skills of assessing families during these times. A plan can be developed whereby the entire nursing staff, on all shifts, is working toward helping the child and family. Too often, with the lack of understanding and an organized plan regarding an individual child and family, the staff ends up working against each other, keeping their feelings (of hostility, anger, pity, helplessness) to themselves, and frustrating the family in many ways. Ideally, the child should be admitted to the same ward each time, so that the family can develop trust in their nursing staff, and the staff can become familiar with the individual needs of the child and his family.

The authors, based on their experiences as nurse clinicians who are part of a pediatric hematology/oncology team at a large university medical center, would like to share with the readers their ideas about family-centered care for these children and their families. Discussion will focus on the importance of assessment as the cornerstone of the nursing process, and on nursing interventions important to help the families as they face the stresses experienced during various phases of the illness—diagnosis, remissions, exacerbations, terminal phase, and postdeath. Because it is the most common terminal illness of childhood, the authors will use acute leukemia as a prototype for discussion. However, the principles discussed would apply to any long-term fatal disease of childhood.

ASSESSMENT

In any setting, it is important for the nurses involved with the family to know the individual family and child, their life styles and needs, and their particular ways of coping with this stressful situation. No two families are alike, and no two families will react to the diagnosis the same way. Reactions depend on many things, including previous experiences with illness and death, modes of coping with crisis, and the special meaning this child has to the family (Chodoff, 1964, pp. 743–744; Friedman, 1967, p. 498).

It is important from the time of diagnosis to begin assessing the child and family. One of the most efficient ways of beginning to collect these data is by doing a nursing history soon after the child is diagnosed. The parents and the child can be interviewed together and separately. The nursing history also helps the family know the staff is truly interested in them as individuals, thus helping to establish a trust relationship. Assessment, however, does not end with the interview but is a continual process throughout the child's illness.

The authors have found the following outline, adapted from Dorothy Smith's "A Clinical Nursing Tool" (1968) to be helpful in beginning to collect data and assess the families:

I Information about the family
  A Parents—age, educational level, occupation, health history, emotional makeup (temperament), brief marital history, hobbies and activities, roles in the family
  B Siblings—age, educational level, health history, role in the family
  C Extended family members—who, where do they live, closeness to the family, kind of relationship (supportive or disruptive)
  D Living arrangements—kind of home, distance from the hospital, people living with them
  E Family life—cultural background, activities done together and separately, discipline used in the home, usual routines, vacation patterns, modes of communication
  F Financial—income, insurance, travel distances, car problems and expenses, motel expenses, babysitting expenses, avenues of help
  G Community—relationship of the family to the larger community, their view of the community, reaction of community to them
  H Religion—church activities, depth of faith, relationship with minister, restrictions of their faith, support which their religion provides them, guilt problems
  I Previous health experiences—any other serious illness, any previous hospitalization, their view of this experience, any previous experiences, or knowledge of someone with leukemia (tumors, cancer)
II Information about the child
  A Parents' description of the child—how do they view him, what does he mean to them, how does he fit into the family constellation
  B Favorite name
  C Brief developmental history
  D Past health history—diseases, susceptibility to disease, previous experience with hospitalization and how he reacted to the situation; allergies (medication, tape, food, merthiolate, zylocaine, etc.)
  E Rest and sleep patterns
  F Elimination patterns
  G Nutrition patterns and needs
  H Play and activity patterns and routines
  I Independence/dependence patterns
  J Temperament
  K Interpersonal and communicative patterns—relationships with peers and siblings and parents
  L Intellectual level—school attainment and problems
  M Senses

III Information related to this illness
  A Events leading up to the illness
  B Preparation of the child for the hospitalization
  C Child and parents understanding about the illness
  D Expectations of the child and parents regarding the hospitalization and the illness
  E Expected visiting patterns of parents
  F Responsibility for care of the siblings during the hospitalization
IV Physical assessment of the child, including the following systems
  A Skin
  B Respiratory
  C Cardiovascular
  D Nutritional
  E Central nervous system
  F Gastrointestinal
  G Genitourinary
  H Developmental level

In the experience of the authors, the nursing history outlined above is the cornerstone for providing truly family-centered nursing care. The information should be written in the patient's chart, available to all members of the team. These data help the nurse to understand the areas of greatest stress and vulnerability for the individual child and family, to know the individual and the community resources available to the family during the crises they will face, to begin to recognize how the family may cope with the stresses, to plan for the teaching approach and needs, and to help other members of the health care team know and understand the family.

Because assessment of the child and family continues throughout the course of the child's illness until months after his death, nurses must become skilled in assessing changing grief reactions and coping patterns of these families. Some of these behaviors seen in parents may puzzle and frustrate nurses unless they understand the importance of the coping pattern for the individual parent.

Coping behavior has been described as "all of the mechanisms utilized by an individual to meet a significant threat to his psychological stability and to enable him to function effectively (Friedman, 1963, p. 616). Since a fatal illness in a child poses a serious threat to his parents, one can expect to find some extreme coping mechanisms (Lowenberg, 1970, p. 270). Coping behaviors may be aimed at helping the parents face the reality at hand; however, a great many are aimed at eliminating or avoiding the reality (Lowenberg, 1970, p. 271). As long as they do not seriously impair reality testing, the avoidance coping behavior must be considered an important protective measure for the individual, which helps him to remain fairly comfortable and to continue facing daily activities in a situation where the stress cannot be realistically alleviated (Lowenberg, 1970, p. 272; Friedman, 1967, pp. 498-499). The coping style used during this crisis will be based on the individual's personality and life style and will usually be similar to mechanisms used during a previous crisis. For example, one mother used denial regarding her child's terminal illness even when the girl was in the final stages of her disease. Her husband described her use of denial also during a previous crisis when her mother was suddenly found dead. Mrs. J. insisted that her mother be taken to the hospital and refused to believe that she was dead for days after the burial.

Some of the common coping behaviors observed by the authors and others include: prolonged use of denial, isolation of affect, intellectualization and identification with the medical personnel, motor activity, religion, search for meaning, withdrawal, aggressive behavior and regression (Friedman, 1963, pp. 616-618; Chodoff, 1964, pp. 745-746; Bozeman, 1955, pp. 4-6).

Examples of some of the coping behaviors may help the reader in identifying them in families. Denial was manifested by the mother mentioned in the previous paragraph during her child's terminal admission when she requested, during a nursing interview, that her child have an IQ test so she could plan for placement in school. Isolation of affect, where there is no emotional response to the diagnosis was seen in the father of a child who was just diagnosed with a tumor. He calmly announced that he had to return to work, rather than seeing the child's doctor. His pronouncement of his child's diagnosis as cancer was said with no signs of emotion or grief. Intellectualization and identification with the doctor was seen in a father whose only daughter had leukemia. He asked many medically oriented questions, read any related medical information he could find, and described the child's disease in medical terms. He insisted on helping to regulate his daughter's intravenous (by counting drops); one day he commented, "I like to help with the IV; I'm almost like a doctor."

Religion, as a coping mechanism, was used by the parents of a child with leukemia who joined a religious sect which was headed by a woman who claimed to have been cured of leukemia after thirty years. They prayed, annointed with oil, and all family members wore a mustard seed around their neck. When this child was in remission, they thought him cured.

A few families will withdraw from all social contacts and may withdraw from medical and nursing personnel as well. One mother quit her job, failed to have relatives and friends to the house, refused to go anywhere, and would not tell the school the diagnosis. Aggressive behavior may be seen as the parents strive to protect their child during hospitalizations. This is manifested by telling nursing personnel how to do procedures, by refusing to allow certain personnel to care for their child, or by becoming angry over slight changes in routines. One family kept a log of nursing activities and checked on them constantly. Regression is seen in a difficulty in making decisions, dependency, and inability to carry on activities of daily living for themselves or other family members. This protects the parent from having any expectations made of him.

PHASES

In any setting, it is important for the nurses involved with these families to anticipate the crises the families will face during the course of the disease, common reactions they exhibit, and appropriate nursing intervention at each period: diagnosis, remission, acute exacerbation, terminal phase, postdeath.

Diagnosis

It is obvious that the time of diagnosis of a terminal illness in a child is a time of great stress for his parents, siblings, and other immediate family members. The diagnosis may be sudden and very unexpected, as with a child who goes to see his pediatrician for a lingering cold, malaise, and irritability, symptoms that are not uncommon in children. Or, the diagnosis may come during a hospitalization for an acute infection or hemorrhage. This family may have had a few days to begin understanding that their child is gravely ill. Often, the child is suddenly transferred to a large medical center, far from his home. The image of the center is usually one of a place for people with serious diseases or people who are dying. This creates even more tension, anxiety, and fear for all.

Some of the reactions commonly seen in the families at the time of diagnosis include: shock and disbelief, denial, guilt and personal responsibility, anger and hostility and depression (Hamovitch, 1964, p. 116; Friedman, 1967, pp. 500-501; Ross, 1969, pp. 142-149). It is important that the nurses working with the families accept each family's unique way of manifesting these reactions in a nonjudgmental manner. Some families will still be in a state of shock and disbelief even at the time of dismissal. One family displayed this reaction by walking aimlessly around the wards in a daze, staring out the window, questioning and answering inappropriately, and by demonstrating an inability to care for their own needs.

Denial may be manifested by doctor shopping, refusing to talk about the illness, or not accepting the reality of the child's physical condition. An exaggerated use of denial was seen in the father of an adolescent girl, his favorite daughter, who was diagnosed with an inoperable brain tumor; he removed her from the hospital and took her on a vacation.

Guilt is usually felt by all parents at some time during the child's illness, particularly at the time of diagnosis. Mothers feel guilty for not taking the child to the doctor sooner or for being angry with the child's irritability and "laziness," which can be symptoms of the disease. Fathers develop guilt for not spending more time with the child or picking up the symptoms earlier. A few parents may feel guilty for some personal "misdeed" such as being negligent about church attendance or a promiscuous sexual relationship. Some couples will create guilt by projecting blame on each other.

Anger and hostility can be vented against anybody or anything. Some parents will be angry with the doctor for telling them such bad news. Others, particularly mothers, will focus on the nursing staff and find fault with the care given their child. Sometimes the anger is vented on each other, siblings, other relatives, or the community. Fathers may express their anger by drinking, promiscuous activity, fighting, or cursing. This behavior is usually exhibited outside the hospital setting when he goes to escape the agonizing reality.

Almost all parents will become depressed at one time or another. Depression may be manifested by withdrawal, an inability to communicate, feelings of hopelessness, and a lack of interest in anything. One family expressed their feelings of hopelessness by stating, "What's the use of treating our child, she'll only die anyway."

One of the most important roles for the nurse at this time is that of listening. The more the parents are able to verbalize and express their reactions of shock, denial, guilt, anger, depression, concerns, questions, fears, and anxieties, the sooner they are able to cope. Often nurses are so concerned about what to say to the parents of a newly diagnosed child, that they shy away from the room, or talk constantly about trivial matters. Tolerating the silences and learning to listen comfortably at these times is an art that must be developed through practice and discipline.

Through the art of listening, understanding, and displaying a nonjudgmental acceptance of them, the nurses' can display empathic concern and interest thus establishing a trusting rapport. Openness, honesty, and thorough information about the hospital, the disease, planned therapy, and tests help to cement the rapport with families.

The parents and the child need a thorough orientation to the hospital and the pediatric unit, including the physical set up, routines such as medical rounds, nap times, and meals; hospital policies; and reasons for various procedures. They should also meet the various medical and nursing personnel who will be working with their child and understand a little about the organizational patterns (medical and nursing teams, shift patterns, etc.).

Usually the doctors will tell the families a great deal about the disease and planned therapy at the time of diagnosis. Studies have shown that parents do not remember very much of this information because of feelings of shock and disbelief (Friedman, 1963, p. 613). In addition they may not understand the terminology used and are too shy or overwhelmed to ask questions. Ideally, the nurse working with the family should be present at these discussions in order to know exactly what they were told. This information will frequently need to be restated and reinforced.

Many questions will be asked about prognosis. Some parents will compare the answers given them by various medical personnel until they hear a prognosis that is not so profound. Answers about the prognosis need to be answered in close collaboration with what the doctors have told the family. In discussing prognosis, the families need to know that there is hope. Feelings of hopelessness regarding the disease on the part of the nursing staff can easily be transmitted to the family and can seriously impair their ability to cope with the diagnosis. One mother was told by a nurses' aide, "I would not have the child treated with chemotherapy because it won't do any good, and it will only put her through unnecessary misery." They need information regarding the drugs and treatment available for therapy, the expected remissions and what they will mean to their child, and the abundant research being done around the world.

After the immediate impact of hearing the diagnosis, the parents will begin asking questions about their sick child. They must reorient their thinking from that of having a healthy child to that of having a child with a terminal illness. The immediate response to this reality is to massively overprotect the child and to want to give him everything. One thirteen-year-old girl, at the time of diagnosis, was bombarded by literally hundreds of gifts from her parents' friends and acquaintances. She asked, "Why would people I don't even know do this? Then I must be going to die." It is important during this period to help parents discuss this change in focus and to see how important it is to treat their child as much like a normal child as possible. He should not be given "special" privileges or vacations; he should be punished when he needs it, although the mode of punishment may need to change from swatting to deprivation of some sort; he should not be kept from school and activities, within the limitations that the disease allows. The parents will need constant encouragement to do this and to see how important this is to their child's feelings of well-being. This problem is particularly difficult during the child's hospitalization, for out of his feelings of insecurity, he will begin to manipulate his parents and the nursing staff. Setting limits on this behavior, at this time, creates many feelings of guilt and anxiety. However, if his behavior is not stopped, the family will have a very difficult adjustment on returning home.

The parents also need guidance regarding what to tell the child about his illness. There are many theories and philosophies regarding whether to tell the child about his diagnosis or not. Research and experience is beginning to show that children as young as four or five eventually know that they have a terminal illness (Waechter, 1971, p. 1172; Morissey, 1965, p. 334; Easson, 1970, pp. 15-16). However, the decision of what the child is told will depend on the philosophy of the entire medical team and on his parents' philosophy and views. This is why it is so important to know the family and their usual patterns of communication. If a family has always been honest with their children, they will tend to be more comfortable at this time in being open. One such family said, "Rita (age seven) will be less frightened and cooperate more if she knows the truth. If we don't tell her, she'll be afraid and think everyone is against her." Many families, however, seem to protect their children from all kinds of feelings and information. These families are very uncomfortable about any mention of telling the child the name of his disease. Some parents will refuse to tell the child anything, yet will talk in front of him about the disease and prognosis or about other children who have died. It is as if they are denying their child's capability of understanding the conversation. It is important that the child does not become isolated and alienated from his parents at a time when he needs them so much. All families should be prepared for the questions that the child may ask; this is usually during remission when he is feeling better. One twelve-year-old child who was not told her diagnosis was found by her mother reading a school textbook on leukemia. She immediately asked, "Do I have leukemia?"

Soon after diagnosis another reaction seen in both the child and parents is severe separation anxiety (Bozeman, 1955, p. 5). Temporary separation appears to remind them of the final separation, death. The authors feel that unlimited visiting hours are very important at this time to ensure their feeling of security. In addition, rooming-in appears very beneficial for the young child especially during the first few days as he adjusts to the hospital routines, personnel, and separation. Rooming-in may also be important for older children during acute and serious crises. In the experience of the authors, however, allowing parents to stay day and night for extended periods of time with older children creates many problems. Regression, aggression, whining, crying, manipulation, and poor cooperation have been seen in these children. When the parents discontinued staying all day and night, the problems disappeared rapidly. As one ten-year-old girl said, "My mom never sleeps in my room at home, even when I'm real sick. Something terrible must be wrong."

Parents will also need help to realize siblings are affected by this illness. Often they are isolated during the time of the illness and are not encouraged to verbalize feelings, fears, and questions. This only adds to their anxiety. They will grieve over the sibling's absence, that of their parents, and will feel the tensions and anxieties of all concerned. The parents will need to return home frequently to see them and communicate with them the reason for their sibling's hospitalization, his current condition, and probable date for returning home. Some hospitals allow the siblings to visit, which is very helpful to them.

It is important at some point during the first week after the diagnosis to help the parents recognize how they can and must help each other. It is very easy for them to move apart and keep their feelings and fears to themselves. The mother soon becomes very involved in the needs of the sick child and expresses her feelings to medical personnel and extended family and friends. If she becomes preoccupied in meeting her own needs and that of her child, she may leave her husband out of these activities. The father returns to work and frequently only visits at night when the child is most irritable and tired. He easily becomes discouraged by the child's inability to relate to him and by his difficulty in defining his role as father to a sick child. In addition, fathers in our society are not encouraged to show their feelings and emotions. To deal with his feelings of inadequacy, he may visit less frequently and withdraw from his family. One father had two jobs, became involved in Little League, Scouts, and a civic organization, leaving only 2 hours per week for his family. Thus, the parents need help to become aware of their need for each other. Communication with each other and sharing the care of the sick child are vital.

Remissions

At the time of the child's remission, he can usually return to most of his usual patterns of living such as school, play, and most recreational activities. Some differences between him and the other children may include: taking medications, frequent out-patient visits, loss of hair, gain or loss of weight and appetite.

Because of the child's return to relatively normal activities, many parents will vacillate between denial and acceptance in their reaction to the diagnosis. Denial may be manifested by their hope that the remission is a cure. Even when acceptance is reached, it is more of an intellectual acceptance than an emotional one. Emotional acceptance comes as they work through anticipatory grief, in later stages of the disease, or during grief work after his actual death (Bozeman, 1955, p. 7).

Almost all families spend this time searching for more information about the disease (Bozeman, 1955, p. 6; Friedman, 1967, p. 501). They find medical texts (frequently old and outdated) and articles in popular magazines or newspapers convincing them the "cure" mentioned in the article is possible for their child. They may receive solicitations in the mail for "sure cures" available at high prices in distant sites across the country. Advice will also come from neighbors and relatives. It is important to advise the families that they will find such information and ask that they bring all articles, letters, or other questions to the nurses and doctors so the information can be discussed and clarified.

Since a child is the creation of one's own being, accepting the fact that he is less than perfect creates many feelings of guilt and inadequacy. It becomes intolerable to accept the child's illness without some meaning or cause. Some families will search through antecedent events to find such a cause (Friedman, 1963, p. 620). Two mothers discovered that both of their children had received gamma globulin injections several months before the diagnosis of cancer was made. They felt sure that this was the causal factor (Galiardi, 1969, p. 94). Other families will turn to religion for an answer and support. Religion is a way of life for some families, whereas others use it only at a time of crisis.

Almost all families live with daily fear and anxiety. They have a great fear of the unknown—what might happen in the future, coupled with a fear of assuming the total responsibility for the child when he is discharged from the hospital. They become overconcerned with the slightest symptoms such as a cold, fever, or pain. They agonize over decisions as whether he should go on a camping trip or on a planned vacation.

As a result of their feelings of inadequacy and fear, they may continue to seriously overprotect the child and make him the focus of all family activities and life. The child responds to this overprotection and concern in his parents by becoming insecure, irritable, manipulative, or withdrawn. He may respond by feeling guilty for ruining family plans or causing his parents such concern.

The siblings may react to the solicitious and overprotective attitude of their parents toward the sick child by becoming resentful, jealous, and angry. These attitudes in turn create feelings of guilt and anxiety, especially after the child has died.

It is understandable that the parents also become frustrated, confused, and sometimes angry at the sick child, adding to their feelings of guilt. In addition, marital problems may begin manifesting themselves as their energies begin to focus more and more on the sick child. Not wanting to upset each other, some couples may begin keeping their feelings to themselves. They may begin to drift apart and become irritable with each other. This process, however, is a gradual and subtle one. Parents may not be cognizant of what is happening; they may need help to face this reality.

One cannot underestimate the amount of support and help the family needs as they try to return to normal patterns of relating to the child and routines of the entire family. Obviously one of the most important nursing roles during this period is to continue to assist them in verbalizing their fears and concerns. Certainly the process of establishing trust continues. The families feel more secure when they know the same health team continues to be vitally interested in them and their child in an individualized manner.

The parents will still have many questions about the child's disease. Help may be needed to formulate, write down, and ask questions of their doctors. Often, they become so nervous about what he will say regarding the child that they forget to ask even the most pressing questions. In addition to understanding the child's disease, it is important that the parents become aware of the drug therapy being used and the various side effects. They will need to become proficient in evaluating their child's reactions to various drugs and their disease status. Assessments such as appetite changes, petecchiae, skin and mouth lesions, bleeding gums, unusual fatigue, bone pain, headache, limp, fever, or backache must be recorded and reported to the doctors. Teaching these aspects is an ongoing process during the course of the disease.

The parents will also need guidance in preparing the child for planned procedures, painful therapies, or anticipated hospitalizations. It is important that all children be told honestly and openly about these planned activities, although the timing will depend upon the child's age and personality. The younger child need only be told shortly before coming to the hospital. The older child will ask questions much sooner, probably at the previous clinic visit. The parents, then, need to know the anticipated therapy so they can adequately prepare him. The unprepared child soon loses trust in his health care personnel as well as his parents. In addition, the siblings will also need explanations for the repeated clinic visits and hospitalizations and for the reactions of the sick child such as fatigue or irritability.

The parents will soon become aware of the reactions of the wider community in regard to their child's illness. They will receive many inquiring phone calls and questions. They will also be faced with anxieties from school personnel regarding the child's needs. Comments may be made to the child by his playmates. They will certainly require help to deal with these varied reactions. One child dismissed from the hospital was met at the car by a playmate who said, "You have leukemia, you should be dead." The well-prepared and informed child replied calmly with a smile, "Do I *look* dead?"

Exacerbation

During the course of his illness, the child will be admitted to the hospital for acute episodes such as overwhelming infection; serious relapse with complications such as bleeding, pneumonia, central nervous system involvement; or experimentation with research drugs. These admissions create a great deal of fear and anxiety and are times of deep stress. The parents are no longer able to use as much denial. At this time there is often a change from intellectual to emotional acceptance of the disease and prognosis. Hope changes from a dream for a cure to a desire for one more remission, one more return home, one more vacation together, one more holiday or birthday to enjoy with their child (Friedman, 1963, p. 621).

It is vitally important during these crises that the same health team care for the child. The parents need to continue to build and sustain their trust in the care he is getting. The staff should display knowledge, competency, and genuine interest as they give care to the child.

The parents will have many questions regarding their child's condition, therapy, and prognosis. It is important that they obtain consistent answers from all members of the team. They will constantly compare what they are told; if the answers differ drastically, they begin to lose trust, become angry, and get confused. It is better to tell the family if one does not know the answer to their question and refer them to the proper person, than to give an incomplete or inaccurate one. Families may need help to make an appointment with the doctor so they can talk with him.

Many of the questions at this time relate to the child's immediate condition: temperature, medications, intravenous, blood counts. The nursing staff can answer many of these questions and explain procedures as they care for the child. At times, parents need assistance in recognizing signs of hope and encouragement, even though small.

Another important nursing function is that of helping parents identify their roles with their acutely ill child. Many will want to stay with their child as much as possible and help in his care in some way. Some will want to do everything possible; others will want to observe, report, and call for help when needed. Individual family assessment regarding their ability and desire to care for their sick child is vital. Care plans should be made to help them accordingly.

The authors have observed two problems facing the staff in their care of the child and family. First, the overzealous family may be abandoned and isolated by the staff. Nursing visits may be made only when necessary. This family needs to know the staff will not abandon them or their child. Secondly, competition between the nursing staff and the mother can develop (Bozeman, 1955, p. 9). Some nurses develop an overprotective and possessive attitude toward a dying child. This nurse can leave the mother out completely and create feelings of anger, inadequacy, and guilt in her.

One of the most frustrating parental experiences at this time involves the behavior of their sick child. Frequently the child becomes depressed, withdrawn, angry, whiney, or extremely irritable due to prolonged pain, repeated injections, procedures, and long hospitalizations. Some of their feelings are vented onto the parents creating guilt and frustration. Nurses can help the parents deal with this problem if they indicate the reasons for the child's behavior. It should be stressed that these reactions are commonly seen in hospitalized children. Parents may then realize the behavior is not directed personally to them.

If the hospitalization is prolonged, the parents, especially the mother, will need to become aware of the needs of their children at home. Frequently they will refuse to leave the hospital for extended periods of time; the siblings suffer as a result. One twelve-year-old brother, who was staying with friends, did not want to go home because, "You'll only leave me again."

With increased hospitalizations, as the disease progresses, the parents begin to face the final reality of the prognosis—the proximity of the final separation. It is usually at this time that the process of anticipatory mourning begins. This grief process involves a gradual detachment of emotional investment from the child and prepares them for the final loss (Friedman, 1963, p. 621; Friedman, 1967, p. 503; Chodoff, 1964, pp. 747–748). The reactions seen in parents at this time include all of those described by Lindemann: somatic distress, preoccupation with thoughts of the child, guilt, hostility, and a loss of patterns of conduct (1944, p. 141).

Listening once again becomes an important part of nursing intervention. Some parents will talk incessantly about the child; his birth, childhood, vacations taken together, important occasions such as school entrance. One mother brought a picture album to help her review her daughter's life with the nurse. Feelings of guilt also need to be expressed. Often the guilt is evoked by minor incidents. One mother who was awake all night with her child expressed guilt for not answering his last call before he lapsed into a coma.

The hostility may be manifested in complaints about the nursing and medical care given the child. It may be focused on medications that are not given exactly on time or a light that is not answered immediately. One particular member of the nursing staff may become the target of one family's anger. Such complaints need to be investigated carefully. The problem may be real or may be a projection of the family's grief. Much tension can be alleviated by helping the families to focus on the underlying causes of their anger and to express their feelings more directly.

Bargaining can be seen with many parents as they begin to compare their child's disease with that of another child who may be progressing. They may beg for the use of the other child's drug protocol or ask for a return to a drug which was used successfully earlier.

Many parents will complete their grief process and reach an accepting stage before the child actually dies. For some parents this may happen during one of his many acute exacerbations. Thereafter, the relationship with the child may be greatly altered. These parents may begin decreasing their visiting hours or become busy with other children when they do visit. The stage of acceptance in parents is very difficult for many nurses to understand or tolerate. The authors have seen instances when an individual nurse or an entire staff become angry with a parent who decreases visiting hours or does not stay in the room with his child. It is very important that we recognize the reason for such behavior. The nursing staff must begin to give the child the support he will no longer receive from his parents, and at the same time, accept their response to the child's terminal state. It should be kept in mind that parents can experience only so much grief, depending upon their previous personality, experiences, and coping mechanisms. As one mother said after her child recovered from a very serious infection in which she almost died, "Now we have to go through this again."

Terminal

At the terminal stage of an illness such as leukemia, the child has usually spent several weeks or months acutely ill with frequent, if not constant, hospitalizations. As we have mentioned, his parents have usually begun to face the certainty of his death. They now begin to ask more specific questions about the terminal process. Questions may be very direct or may come in a very indirect and disguised form. Nurses should anticipate such questions and assist parents to discuss their concerns. Many parents are worried that they will not be present when the child dies. Most of them are terrified that they will be alone in the room when death occurs. They also want to know what the moment of death will be like. Although it is difficult to answer such questions about the death itself, it is very important to be available to listen to their questions and concerns, giving them answers when possible.

If the child remains conscious during this terminal phase, the nurses should help the parents anticipate the possibility that he may ask about his death. One child who asked if he was dying wanted to know if he could take enough bandaides to heaven for Jane and Ted (who died months previously). A simple affirmative answer made him feel very secure and satisfied. Another child asked his parents, "What's gonna happen when I go to heaven?" His parents told him that there would be no more pain, and he responded, "I'm ready."

Most parents experience deep feelings of ambivalence and guilt about their child's death: they have seen him suffer for a long time, have completed much of their grief work, and are anxious for the dying process to be completed. In our culture, these feelings and thoughts are very contrary to the "good parent ideal" and create many guilt feelings. If parents realize that these feelings are shared by other parents of terminally ill children, it lessens the impact.

The parents may need guidance and assistance to prepare the siblings for the death and to help them express grief and concern. The father and mother need to support each other as they face this difficult task. It is ideal if the parents can be open and honest with their children and can share their feelings of grief with them. If there are teen-agers in the family, they may want to be present at the bedside of their sister or brother to help them grieve and prepare for his death. In addition, grandparents often need more help with grief than the parents who have already worked through their feelings.

It is important to the family to continue to provide expert physical care to their child. They should never feel their child has been abandoned. The focus of care may change from curative to comfort measures such as skin care, turning, mouth care, linen change, and pain medications. This kind of care, given with a loving and concerned attitude, is a great relief to the family. Many families may want to continue to participate in all the child's care; however, much support and help from the staff are needed. The danger comes when the child is moved to a private room, for the sake of the family and other patients. Fewer nursing visits and less personal attention may occur. It is also true that the nursing staff may become preoccupied in giving the best physical care, but may appear afraid of getting emotionally involved.

The physical needs of the family should be part of the nursing care plan. They often spend all day at the hospital under the most primitive of conditions—no privacy, no bath facilities, no bed. It is the task of the entire nursing staff to see that they have time away from the child's bedside, spend time together, eat regular meals, and get some sleep. Parents often develop remarkable stamina at this time, only to suddenly collapse with fatigue. Constipation, diarrhea, vomiting, menstrual irregularities, and headaches are common. Many parents feel guilt in mentioning their own complaints, fearing that care will be taken away from their child.

It is very helpful to the families, if, at the time of the child's death, a nurse is present with whom they feel close. Of course, this cannot be planned; however, a call schedule can be worked out whereby one of the nurses who has worked closely with the family is called into the hospital when death appears imminent. As one mother stated, "I wanted so much for Nancy (a favorite nurse) to be present when Theresa died. I felt that I wouldn't feel foolish doing whatever I might do if she was the one there."

It is supportive to the parents if the staff remains calm but concerned at the time of the child's death. If the staff displays anxiety or fear, the family will become confused and lost. Some families will want to remain in the room with their dead child, while others will want to leave immediately. In either case, they should be allowed to express their grief in their own individual way. Some families will want to touch, fondle, and hold their child; and this should be their privilege. One of the staff members who can accept this kind of grieving should be present. One mother stated, "The nurse gave me so much support and let me hold Jim. I was then able to accept that he was really dead."

A private room should be made available to the family in which to cry, talk, and make decisions. Some families desire a minister, while other families want to be alone. The use of religion as a support, as mentioned earlier, is very individual. It is very important not to impose a minister or religious cliches such as "It's God's will" on the family unless they bring it up; imposing religion on a family at this time may be detrimental to their grief process.

A few families have completed many funeral arrangements during the final stages of the illness, whereas others have been unable to consider any type of prearrangement. Some families prefer someone else such as a distant relative or family minister make the beginning arrangements. Frequently, it is the nursing staff who makes the initial contacts with funeral directors. Many hospitals, however, have a mortician on call who initates the first steps.

The authors have noted that leaving the hospital unit can be a very difficult step for some parents. It is the final separation between them and their child. This makes them face the deep loss they have just experienced. Leave taking should not be rushed or hurried; on the other hand, some families will require help in making the move to leave. Accompanying them to the door or car is an assurance of continued support at this very painful time.

It is most appropriate here to mention the needs of the staff caring for the dying child. Unless the staff has worked through their own philosophy and feelings about death and dying, it will be difficult for them to give personal and individual care to the child and his family. In the educational process, it is unfortunate that most health professionals (nurses, doctors, ministers, social workers) are not prepared to deal with their own feelings regarding death. For too long, we have upheld the false assumption that "professionals" should not experience grief or reveal their feelings. However, the staff will go through a grief process with each dying child. It is not unusual for individual staff members to use denial for a time; to experience anger toward the child, family, God, or others; to feel depressed; and finally, in the ambivalence of accepting the child's prognosis, wish that he would soon die so he would not have to suffer any longer. These feelings can cause psychological as well as physical withdrawal on the part of the staff. In addition, unresolved feelings can affect later experiences. Ward conferences should be held solely for the purposes of openly discussing and sharing together the grief reactions.

Staff assignments should be made with these reactions in mind. Although it is important for the child and family to have continuity of nursing care, this care must be shared. On a given day, it may be impossible for Jimmy's favorite nurse to care for him, as she may be too overcome with grief. Given a rest or change of assignment, she will be able to face him the next day or week. Conversely, there may be members of the staff who are unable to give care to the dying child. Their talent could be used elsewhere, rather than forcing something so painful on them. In time, with the support of the group, they may be able to make this step. Staff members should be given time between assignments of terminally ill children.

Postdeath

After sharing such an intimate experience as death of their child with the nursing staff, the family will need some continued contact to sustain and help them in the difficult weeks to come. They will be faced with the entire grief reaction again, in order to reach full acceptance of the reality.

Most families are grateful for visits to the funeral home made by their child's nurses. It helps to cement the feeling that "they really cared." One family told the nurse at the funeral home, "I thought everybody would forget us after we left." Some nurses may not feel comfortable in making such a visit, or it may not be possible because of distance or other time factors. This will largely be an individual matter.

Following the funeral, however, phone calls and home visits can be made. This can be a very important time for helping parents to work through their grief and to realize that their other children will experience a grief process. Our society has developed the attitude that children "don't comprehend," that they have no real feelings about the death of someone they love. Even very young children grieve the loss of a loved one and need help in verbalizing and expressing their feelings. Some children will experience tremendous guilt because of anger or jealousy felt toward the deceased sibling. Other children may feel anger toward parents, God, doctors, or the hospital for taking away their beloved sibling. Some may develop somatic complaints or exhibit behavior problems. One child was hospitalized for seizures 2 weeks after the death of her sister. These "seizures" stopped only after she was able to discuss her fears of death with her mother who reassured the child of her love. The children also need help in developing an understanding of the meaning of death. The approach will depend upon the age of the child and the individual family's religious and philosophical beliefs.

At some point, usually several months to a year after the death, some parents will have a need to return to the hospital. It appears to be a subtle way of saying, "My grief and pain is resolved enough now for me to return and face more realistically what I have experienced." It is also a message of "thank you." These visits should be expected and encouraged as they are helpful to both parents and staff. It enables the staff to realize they have adequately fulfilled their job.